Gerontology: A Clinical Approach

Gerontology: A Clinical Approach

Edited by Riley Carter

AMERICAN
MEDICAL PUBLISHERS
www.americanmedicalpublishers.com

American Medical Publishers,
41 Flatbush Avenue,
1st Floor, New York,
NY 11217, USA

Visit us on the World Wide Web at:
www.americanmedicalpublishers.com

ISBN: 978-1-63927-006-4

Cataloging-in-Publication Data

Gerontology : a clinical approach / edited by Riley Carter.
p. cm.
Includes bibliographical references and index.
ISBN 978-1-63927-006-4
1. Gerontology. 2. Older people--Diseases--Treatment. 3. Geriatrics. I. Carter, Riley.
RC953.5 .G47 2022
615.547--dc23

Table of Contents

Preface

Every book is a source of knowledge and this one is no exception. The idea that led to the conceptualization of this book was the fact that the world is advancing rapidly; which makes it crucial to document the progress in every field. I am aware that a lot of data is already available, yet, there is a lot more to learn. Hence, I accepted the responsibility of editing this book and contributing my knowledge to the community.

Gerontology deals with the scientific study of old age, the process of ageing, and the particular problems of old people. It focuses on the biological, psychological, cognitive, cultural and social aspects of ageing. Some of its subfields are biogerontology, social gerontology, environmental gerontology and jurisprudential gerontology. Biogerontology is associated with the biological aging process and its evolutionary origins. Social gerontology is a specialization in the study and working with older adults. Environmental gerontology deals with the interaction between aging persons and their social and physical environments. Jurisprudential gerontology is concerned with the relationship between laws and the aging process. This book traces the progress of this field and highlights some of its key concepts and applications. It will help the readers in keeping pace with the rapid changes in gerontology. Some of the diverse topics covered in this book address the varied branches that fall under this category.

While editing this book, I had multiple visions for it. Then I finally narrowed down to make every chapter a sole standing text explaining a particular topic, so that they can be used independently. However, the umbrella subject sinews them into a common theme. This makes the book a unique platform of knowledge.

I would like to give the major credit of this book to the experts from every corner of the world, who took the time to share their expertise with us. Also, I owe the completion of this book to the never-ending support of my family, who supported me throughout the project.

Editor

1

Interactions between Identity and Emotional Expression in Face Processing across the Lifespan: Evidence from Redundancy Gains

Alla Yankouskaya,[1,2] Pia Rotshtein,[1] and Glyn W. Humphreys[2]

[1] *School of Psychology, University of Birmingham, Birmingham B15 2TT, UK*
[2] *Department of Experimental Psychology, University of Oxford, Oxford OX1 3UD, UK*

Correspondence should be addressed to Alla Yankouskaya; alla.yankouskaya@psy.ox.ac.uk

Academic Editor: Arshad Jahangir

We tested how aging affects the integration of visual information from faces. Three groups of participants aged 20–30, 40–50, and 60–70 performed a divided attention task in which they had to detect the presence of a target facial identity or a target facial expression. Three target stimuli were used: (1) with the target identity but not the target expression, (2) with the target expression but not the target identity, and (3) with both the target identity and target expression (the redundant target condition). On nontarget trials the faces contained neither the target identity nor expression. All groups were faster in responding to a face containing both the target identity and emotion compared to faces containing either single target. Furthermore the redundancy gains for combined targets exceeded performance limits predicted by the independent processing of facial identity and emotion. These results are held across the age range. The results suggest that there is interactive processing of facial identity and emotion which is independent of the effects of cognitive aging. Older participants demonstrated reliably larger size of the redundancy gains compared to the young group that reflect a greater experience with faces. Alternative explanations are discussed.

1. Introduction

How does the ability to process information from faces change as we age? Prior work indicates that there are effects of aging on a number of aspects of face processing. For example, there is an age-related decline in recognition memory for faces [1–6], an effect that grows as the retention interval lengthens [7, 8] and memory load increases [9, 10].

In other cases though the effects of aging impact perceptual rather than memory processes [11–15]. For example, Obermeyer et al. [14] examined the effect of age on early perceptual stages of face processing by applying horizontal and vertical filtering to face images in a face recognition task. The results indicated a detrimental effect of age on the processing of horizontal information. Daniel and Bentin [12] examined the ability of people aged 70 to 90 years old to apply global, configural, and featural processing strategies to faces and found age-related perceptual changes specifically in integrating face features into global structures.

A number of studies have demonstrated that difficulties in face recognition with age might also reflect declines in high-level perceptual processes. For example, older adults have an impaired ability to (i) transform perceptual information into familiar templates that may explain poor recognition of faces when seen in other than the front view [13], (ii) engage in joint attention by following gaze cues [16], and (iii) ignore task-irrelevant information in faces [17].

There is also evidence that older people can experience difficulties in processing nonidentity related aspects of faces such as their emotional expressions [18–20]. For example, it has been demonstrated that older adults are less accurate in recognizing negative facial emotions, in particular, anger and sadness [19, 21], and they are less accurate in discriminating between some emotions (e.g., surprise and fear) [22], when compared with younger observers. The age-related decline in the processing of emotional expression has been linked to a variety of factors, for example, the tendency to establish a positive emotional preference in tasks as we age [23] and different perceptual demands for emotional processing relative to the coding of face identity, which may depend on cognitive abilities differentially affected by aging [24].

Given the wealth of studies suggesting age-related declines in both face recognition and the processing of emotional expression in faces in older individuals, it is surprising that no studies have attempted to investigate how aging affected the processing of combined information about facial identity and emotional expression, despite facial identities and expressions covarying in everyday life.

Interestingly there is evidence that the ability to integrate information from two signals is spared as we age [25–28] and older participants can even benefit more than younger adults when information from two sources is combined. For example, Laurienti et al. [27] examined the speed of older and young individuals to discriminate the presence of simple visual (a red or blue circle), auditory (the word red or blue), and combined visual-auditory stimuli. RTs were faster to targets with combined attributes and this "redundant target effect" was greater for older adults than for younger adults (see also [25, 26, 29]). These studies suggest that, although the processing of some properties of stimuli may decline in older individuals, there is a benefit when redundant signals are present to define targets. The enhancement in performance from redundant targets has been linked to the greater ability of older participants to exploit redundant information to help compensate for sensory deficits with single stimuli [27]. For example, if aging is associated with increased levels of "noise" in perceptual processing, then the presence of a redundant target may be beneficial if the additional signal information reduces the effects of the noise [29]. Hugenschmidt et al. [30] applied capacity analysis [31–34] to the data in Laurienti et al. [27]. This analysis compares reaction time (RT) distributions expressed through a hazard function [31] to estimate of how much "work" a system does and how much processing is influenced by stimulus manipulations in a task. The analysis indicated that older adults increased their capacity processing 2.5 times as much when redundant signals were present compared with single signals, while younger adults only increased their capacity up to 1.5 times. The mechanisms underlying such effects, however, remain poorly understood. The present study aims to address this last point by studying the dynamics of redundancy effects in face processing across the lifespan focusing on the relations between the processing of facial identity and emotion.

1.1. Processing Facial Identity and Emotion. A controversial issue in studies of face processing is whether facial identity and emotion are processed independently or in a more interactive manner. The influential model of face recognition proposed by Bruce and Young [35] suggests separate-parallel routes for processing identity and emotional expression. The main support for the model came from neuropsychological studies showing double dissociations of patients with impaired recognition of face identity but not emotion [36–39] or vice versa [36, 40]. Studies with healthy participants also provide some support for the parallel route hypothesis [41, 42].

On the other hand, there are a growing number of studies suggesting that the processing of identity and emotional expression in faces is not entirely independent [43–53]. For example, there is evidence that facial expressions have an influence on the perception of familiarity [45, 54] and that the presence of covarying expression improves the recognition of facial identity in patients [55].

Previously we have examined this issue about independent versus integrative processing of facial identity and emotion using a divided attention task where participants had to detect target identities or emotions in faces. The identity and emotion targets could either appear alone (e.g., the target identity might be paired with a neutral emotion) or appear together (the target identity also expressed the target emotion). Young adults showed a strong facilitation effect for faces containing both the target identity and emotion (a redundant target display) [56]. Moreover, tests were carried out to explore the underlying basis of the redundancy effect. In particular, we used the so-called Miller inequality test [57] to assess whether the gains when redundant targets were present were greater than the gains produced when performance with the two single targets was summed. Based on there being independent processing of facial identity and emotion, we would not predict that performance can be better than the summed responses to each target feature alone. The data violated this prediction, with the redundancy gains being greater than predicted from independent processing of each feature. Also by varying the features present on nontarget trials we also tested (and rejected) accounts of performance based on partial information from each feature (identity and emotion) influencing decision-making independently. We concluded that facial identity and emotion were processed in an integrated manner.

The present study is concerned with how the coding of facial identities and emotions is affected by age and, in addition to this, whether older participants, like younger individuals, process facial identity and emotional expression in an integral manner. To test this, we examined the detection of face identity and emotion targets in three groups of participants aged between 20 and 30, 40 and 50, and 60 and 70 years, with target faces carrying either the critical identity, the emotion, or both the identity and the emotion. We evaluated whether responses to redundant target faces were faster than responses to either single target and what is the magnitude of the redundancy effect in the different age groups examined.

1.2. Analyzing Redundancy Gains in Information Processing. There is considerable evidence that, when a visual display contains two targets that require the same response, reaction times (RTs) are faster than when only one target appears [57–60]. There are different explanations that account for this redundant target effect (RTE), with the most relevant being the independent race model [61] and the coactivation model [57]. The independent race model assumes separate and parallel channels for processing distinct types of information (e.g., facial identity and emotional expression) with the response to each trial determined by the fastest process to be completed. In a test using elementary visual targets, Miller [57] demonstrated that predictions made by the independent race model [61] were violated. The critical contrast for the two models compared the probability of responses being made within particular time bins on redundant targets trials relative to sum of the probabilities for responses in the same bins when either single target was present. The independent race model holds that at no point in the cumulative distribution functions for performance should a response to redundant targets exceed the sum of the probabilities for responses to either single target [57]. In contrast, if there is coactivation of a common representation of both features, responses to the redundant targets can be made from this common representation before processing is complete for either single target. The coactivation model put forward by Miller [57] closely resembles the capacity model of Townsend and Nozawa [62] which defines processing in terms of workload capacity [62]. The concept of capacity reflects the efficiency with which the cognitive system performs a task. In terms of this model, full parallel processing of stimuli (as maintained by the independent race model) is associated with unlimited capacity ($C(t) = 1$). Processing with limited capacity ($C(t) < 1$) is associated with decreasing performance (e.g., slowing in RT) when the workload increases. On the other hand super capacity ($C(t) > 1$)) is associated with integrated processing of features and this always violates the predictions made by the independent race model [31].

These models provide a formal framework within which we can explore the relations between the processing of facial identity and emotion in older adults. Here we tested whether redundancy gains in processing facial identity and emotion occur in older as well as young participants and whether the effects are linked to violations of the independent race model and to super capacity ($C(t) > 1$)) in information processing. These tests enable us to elucidate the mechanisms underlying face processing across the age range.

2. Method

2.1. Participants. Three groups of twelve healthy participants were recruited: (1) young (aged 20–30 y, 10 female), (2) middle-aged (aged 40–50 y, 8 female), and (3) elderly (60–70 y, 8 female). The young participants were University of Birmingham undergraduate students (second- and third-year students of Engineering Department); the middle-aged group was recruited from staff at the Queen Elizabeth Hospital in Birmingham (receptionists, statisticians, and nurses) and staff of University of Birmingham (receptionists and demonstrators); the older group consisted of individuals recruited to the School of Psychology's panel for older participants. There were no big variations between elderly and middle-aged participants in terms of educational level and positions held before their retirement. The majority of the older adults were office workers (secretary, administrator, public coordinator, receptionist, assistant in Post Office customer service, a clerical worker in Estate and Letting agent, rent officer, assistant of manager in a library, and a registrar at a job centre); two participants previously worked as school teachers. None of the volunteers had health-related issues or physical and mental disabilities. There was also a consistency across all participants in their experience of performing a face recognition task in an experimental situation; none of the participants has been previously recruited for a face recognition experiment.

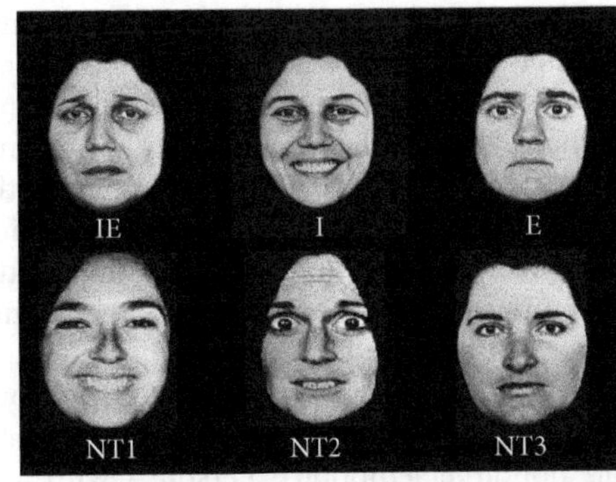

FIGURE 1: An example of the stimuli. IE: a face containing both the target identity and the target emotional expression; I: a face containing the target identity but not the expression; E: a face containing target emotional expression; NT1-NT3 faces containing neither the target identity nor the target emotion. In this study we used faces from the NimStim database, but, because of publication restriction on faces from that database, we present here other faces (taken from Ekman and Friesen [63]) as examples only.

All participants had normal or corrected-to-normal vision and this experiment was carried out in accordance with the ethical guidelines of the British Psychological Society. Each participant gave informed consent at the start.

2.2. Stimuli and Apparatus. A set of 6 photographs was employed (Figure 1).

All the face images were sourced from the NimStim Face Stimuli Set [64]. The recognition of facial expression in all the photographs was rated as 80% and higher [64]. The set consisted of white male faces (original images are not presented here due to restricted permission to publish images from the database).

The photographs were cropped around the hairline to eliminate the possibility of target judgments being based on hairstyle. Any visible background was coloured black. The faces were approximately 10 × 13 cm when displayed on a 17-inch monitor. The presentation of stimuli was controlled using Cogent 2000 and Cogent Graphics developed by the Cogent 2000 team at the FIL and the ICN (http://www.vislab.ucl.ac.uk/cogent_2000.php). The stimuli were presented on the monitor at the viewing distance of 0.8 m. The angular width subtended by the stimulus was approximately 10°.

2.3. Design and Procedure. A "go/no-go" task was employed. Half of the trials used stimuli containing at least one target attribute (target identity, target emotional expression, or both targets; "go" trials). On the other half of the trials, the stimuli did not convey any target attribute ("no-go" trials).

Participants were asked to respond as quickly and accurately as possible when the target identity and/or the emotional expression were displayed by pressing a button "target present" on the keyboard (the right arrow). To minimize bias found for processing positive emotions in older participants (e.g., [65]), the emotion target was a sad expression. The targets were Person 1 expressing a sad emotion (redundant targets), Person 1 with a happy expression (target identity and nontarget expression), and Person 2 with a sad expression (target expression and nontarget identity). The nontargets were a face of Person 3 with an angry expression (nontarget identity and nontarget emotion), Person 4 with a neutral expression (nontarget identity and nontarget emotion), and Person 5 with surprised expression (nontarget identity and nontarget emotional expression) (see examples of stimuli in Figure 1).

Prior to the main task participants completed an initial practice block of 18 trials during which they were given feedback on their accuracy and RT after each trial. After a short break participants performed four blocks of 60 trials with short breaks between the blocks. Each trial started with the presentation of a fixation cross at the centre of the screen for 500 ms. Images were presented successively in random order with random interstimulus intervals from 500 ms to 2 sec. On "go" trials the image was displayed until a response was made. On "no-go" trials the stimulus was displayed 2000 ms.

The procedure for the experiment was kept as consistent as possible across all participants (using the same testing room and computer, performing experiments in morning hours, etc.).

2.4. Analysis of Data. Four analyses were conducted in this study. The first looked at whether the three groups of participants differed in accuracy and RT performance across the different conditions. RTs for correct responses only were used in further analyses.

The second analysis determined whether participants were faster for redundant targets compare to single target trials. Mean RTs across the two single targets (e.g., emotion only or identity only) was subtracted from the mean RT for redundant targets for each participant. A positive value following this subtraction represents a redundancy gain. It has been shown that, when some observers favour one dimension over another, there is an overestimation of the mean RT redundancy gain relative to the fastest single dimension condition for each observer [66, 67]. In contrast, the fixed favored dimension test involves comparing the two single target conditions for each observer against each other. When the two conditions differ, the faster mean RT is retained as the conservative estimate of the single target mean RT; when the two conditions do not differ, the overall mean from both single target conditions is used.

The next analysis assessed whether the independent race model inequality was violated [57]. To test the Miller [57] inequality, empirical CDFs were estimated for every participant and every target condition. All calculations followed the algorithm for testing the independent race model inequality [68]. First, the 100 RTs generated by each participant for all target trials were sorted in ascending order to estimate 19 percentiles (5th through the 95th at 5% intervals). Subsequently these numbers were averaged across participants to produce the composite CDF for redundant targets and each single target condition. To produce the sum of CDFs for the target identity (I) and emotion (E) trials, RTs for the two types of trial were pooled together and 19 quintiles were estimated based on only the fastest 100 of the 200 trials. All calculations were conducted using a modified Matlab script for computing the independent race model test [68]. The nineteen percentiles points and CDFs were calculated for each participant and then averaged. Paired two-tailed t-tests were used to assess the reliability of the difference between redundant targets and the sum of target identity and target emotion responses at each percentile point. Graphic representations of the distributions were constructed using group RT distributions obtained by averaging individual RT distributions [68]. When the CDFs are plotted, the independent race model requires that the CDFs of the redundant targets fall below and to the right of the summed CDFs. Finally we examined whether the groups of young, middle-aged, and older participants were different in the magnitude of any redundancy gains.

The fourth analysis examined capacity processing. Here we used a method of computing the capacity coefficient proposed by Townsend and Eidels [31]:

$$C_{\mathrm{OR}}(t) = \frac{-\log\left[S_{\mathrm{IE}}(t)\right]}{-\log\left[S_{\mathrm{I}}(t) * S_{\mathrm{E}}(t)\right]}, \tag{1}$$

where the survival function of the redundant targets condition is in the numerator and the product of the survival functions of the two single target conditions is in the denominator.

For this assessment, for each condition, we calculated the empirical CDFs using 10 ms time bins. After this the empirical survivor function was computed for each condition at each time bin, which is simply the complement of the cumulative distribution (the proportion of trials that was slower than the specified RT). All computations were performed using Matlab codes [31]. After averaging the CDFs for the redundant targets and either single face property (identity and emotion), the data were converted into survivor functions in order to create integrative hazard functions. Subsequently the capacity coefficients for each group of participants and each face set were generated by creating a ratio of the averaged hazard functions at each time bin [30]. Confidence intervals were defined for each group-capacity coefficient using the bootstrapping technique [31].

3. Results

3.1. Accuracy Performance. Performance accuracy across the three groups of participants is displayed in Table 1.

It is important to note that accuracy was very high across all groups, over 99% accuracy on "go" trials (target(s) present) and 96% on "no-go" trials (target absent). Group comparisons for accuracy performance were made using a 3 (groups) × 6 (conditions) repeated measures analysis of variance

Table 1: The mean percentage of errors for redundant targets (IE), the identity target (I), the emotional expression target (E), and the 3 nontarget faces (NTs) for groups of young, middle-aged, and older participants.

Group of participants	Stimuli					
	IE	I	E	NT1	NT2	NT3
Young	0.2	0.3	0.3	0.6	0.5	0.5
Middle-aged	0.1	0.2	0.4	0.3	1.3	1.6
Older	0	0.4	0.6	0.3	3.4	2.2
Total	0.3	0.9	1.3	1.2	5.2	4.3

(ANOVA). There was a main effect of stimulus ($F(5,165) = 11.3$, $P < 0.001$, $P\mu^2 = 0.025$), in which participants made more errors on "no-go" than on "go" trials (Table 1); a main effect of group ($F(2,33) = 4.0$, $P < 0.05$, $P\mu^2 = 0.02$), in which the older the participants were, the more errors they made; and an interaction of stimuli $*$ group ($F(10,165) = 3.3$, $P = 0.001$, $P\mu^2 = 0.017$). Adjustment for multiple comparisons (Bonferroni) revealed that the interaction was mostly driven by the responses to the "no-go" trials with the young participants being more accurate in responding to nontarget stimuli (see Table 1) as compared to the older participants ($P < 0.05$). There were no reliable differences in the accuracy of performance between young and middle-aged participants or between middle-aged and older groups (all $P > 0.05$).

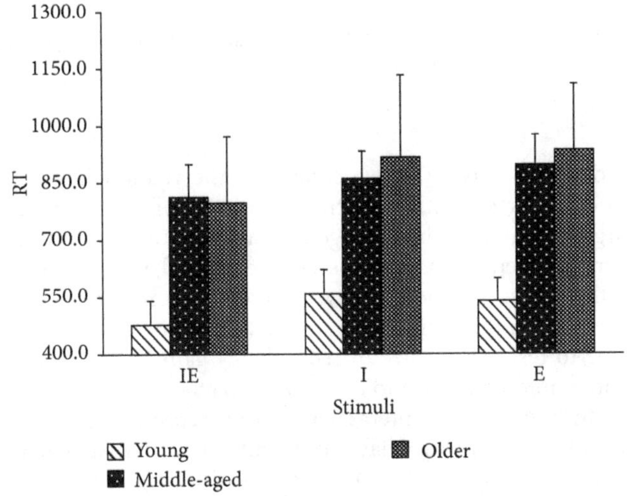

Figure 2: Mean RTs (SD) for images containing both targets (IE), the identity target (I), and the emotional expression target (E), for groups of young, middle-aged, and older participants.

3.2. RT Performance. Mean RTs and standard deviation for correct responses to stimuli containing targets for three groups of participants are displayed in Figure 2.

There was no evidence for accuracy/RT tradeoffs (see Supplementary Material 1 Available online at http://dx.doi.org/10.1155/2014/136073). Group comparisons for RT performance were carried out using a 3 (conditions containing targets) × 3 (groups) ANOVA. As expected, age group had a reliable effect on response times ($F(2,33) = 33.13$, $P < 0.001$, $P\mu^2 = 0.066$), with younger participants being faster than both the middle-aged and older groups on all conditions (all $t(22) > 5.5$, $Ps < 0.001$, $ds > 0.52$), though the middle-aged and the older groups showed no reliable RT differences ($Ps > 0.05$). Target type also had an effect on RT ($F(2,64) = 32.8$, $P < 0.001$, $P\mu^2 = 0.06$), such that RTs on redundant target (IE) trials were faster than both of the single target conditions (IE versus I: $t(35) = 9.3$, $P < 0.001$, $d = 0.96$; IE versus E: $t(35) = 10.8$, $P < 0.001$, $d = 0.97$). This effect was reliable in all three groups: (IE versus I + E: young, middle-aged, and elderly).

More interestingly we also observed an interaction between age group and stimuli ($F(4,64) = 5.4$, $P = 0.001$, $P\mu^2 = 0.021$). Inspection of Figure 2 suggests that the redundancy effect increased with age.

To ensure that our results were not caused by general age-related slowing, which might produce spurious interactions between age group and the experimental conditions [69], we also examined the effects after we converted each individual's RTs to log-transformed scores. Using the log transformation here instead of commonly used z-score transformation [69] was driven by our data which showed correlations for all conditions across the three participant groups (see Supplementary Material 2) and high individual variability in responses to the same stimuli (Supplementary Material 3) that might bias against using z-score transformations. Salthouse [70] suggested that an interaction of Task × Age that remains statistically significant after log transformation of raw RTs is the result of age effects beyond more general influences of task complexity and general slowing, because a logarithmic transformation represents equal ratios as equal intervals. The new transformed scores were then used in a mixed design ANOVA with targets (IE, I, and E) as within-subject factor and age group (young, middle-aged, and older) as a between-subject factor. This analysis revealed a very similar result to the analysis of the nontransformed data; there was a main effect of group ($F(2,32) = 43.8$, $P < 0.001$, $P\mu^2 = 0.068$) and of stimulus ($F(2,64) = 43.7$, $P < 0.001$, $P\mu^2 = 0.05$) and an interaction of stimuli$*$group ($F(4,64) = 5.6$, $P = 0.001$, $P\mu^2 = 0.021$). There were no other effects ($F < 1.0$). Similar to the ANOVA on the nontransformed data, patterns for the three stimuli were obtained after the examination of main effects using independent sample t-tests.

3.3. Redundancy Gains. All three groups showed faster responses for displays containing both targets compared to displays containing either single target (Figure 1). To better

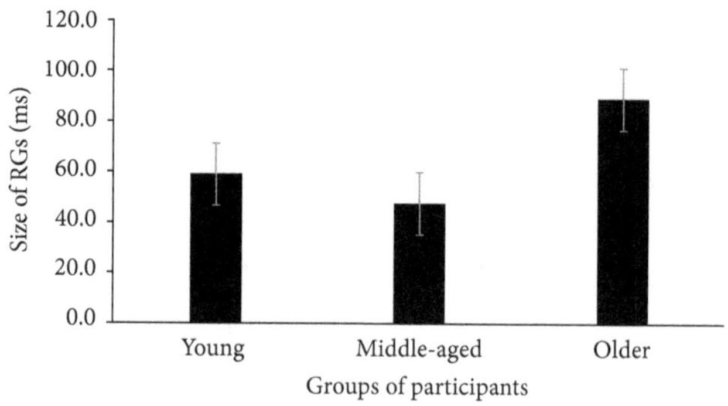

FIGURE 3: The size of the redundancy gains for groups of young, middle-aged, and older participants.

TABLE 2: Overall capacity coefficients for young, middle-aged, and older people.

Capacity coefficient	Groups		
	Young	Middle-aged	Older
	1.12	1.24	2.24

understand this effect we computed the redundancy gain for each participant, by subtracting the RT of the redundant target from each single target, separately. The redundancy gain was then estimated conservatively based on the smallest of the two subtractions. These data were entered into a one-way ANOVA performed on nontransformed data which were used to test for the size of redundancy gains (RGs) among young, middle-aged, and older participants.

In line with the interaction that we reported above, the size of the RGs was reliably different across the participant groups ($F(2,33) = 5.1$, $P = 0.012$, $P\mu^2 = 0.24$). The redundancy gain was larger for the older participants as compared to the middle-aged group ($t(22) = 2.8$, $P < 0.05$, $d = 0.75$) (Figure 3). The differences between the younger and the older groups, and between the younger and the middle-aged groups, were not reliable (all $Ps > 0.05$).

The same analysis using log-transformed data revealed quite similar results for the main effect of group ($F(2,33) = 5.35$, $P = 0.01$, $P\mu^2 = 0.27$). However, post hoc (Bonferroni) comparisons showed that, in contrast to the nontransformed data, the size of the redundancy gain in both younger and older participants was reliably greater than in the middle-aged group ($t(22) = 3.0$, $P = 0.048$, $d = 0.52$, and $t(22) = 2.7$, $P < 0.05$, $d = 0.74$, resp.). Similar to nontransformed data no difference in the size of the redundancy gain was found for comparisons between young and older participants ($t(22) = 0.4$).

3.4. Testing the Independence versus Coactivation. To test whether redundancy gains are determined by statistical sampling of independent channels or coactive processing of identity and emotional expression, we carried out the Miller test [57] for each RT quantile point in the three groups using paired-sample t-tests (comparing mean RTs for the redundant targets to the sum of the identity target and the emotion targets, at each quantile point in each group of participants). As mentioned in the data analysis section, Miller's inequality [57] predicts that, for the independent race model [61] model, the probability of a response in the redundant target condition should never exceed that for the sum of two single targets [57]. Previous studies have reported violations of the Miller inequality [57] for early percentile points (e.g., percentiles 10–25; [26, 58]). In cases where violations of the inequality are observed at multiple percentile points, an appropriate correction for multiple comparisons is needed in order to control Type 1 errors. However, the widely used Bonferroni test for multiple comparisons demands that all the tests be independent of each other [71]. This demand is not fulfilled in our data where correlations between percentiles bins are high (from 0.84 to 0.93). In order to conduct the Miller test [57], but to control Type 1 errors, our strategy was to perform the test at two percentiles (10% and 15%) using paired t-tests but with a strict significance level adopted (1% instead of 5%).

The CDFs for each participant group are displayed in Figure 4. The CDFs for redundant targets fell to the left of the sum of the single target CDFs for the redundant target faces, which indicates violation of the Miller [57] inequality. These violations were statistically significant at the 10th and 15th quantiles ($Ps < 0.01$) in all groups of participants.

To visualize the results above, we plotted the CDFs for each quantile point predicted by the race model (I + E) from the CDFs of corresponding quantiles for redundant targets (IE) (see Figure 5).

The data presented in Figure 5 demonstrate that the time window over which the older group benefitted from redundant targets was larger than that in the young and the middle-aged groups (the part of the curves that are above the horizontal solid line): for the young group the time window for the violation ran across 50 ms (440–390 ms), for the middle-age participants it was 75 ms (840–765 ms), and for the older group it was 201 ms (900–699 ms). Also, the magnitude of the enhancement from redundant targets was reliably greater for the older group ($F(2,33) = 8.92$, $P < 0.05$, $P\mu^2 = 0.053$) than for the young group ($t(22) = 4.2$, $P < 0.05$, $d = 0.54$) and the middle-aged group (t $(22) = 2.8$, $P = 0.045$, $d = 0.21$). The young and middle-aged groups did not differ.

3.5. Testing Capacity Processing. The capacity coefficients at each time bin across participant groups are presented in Figure 6, and the overall capacity coefficients (averaged across time bins) are displayed in Table 2.

Figure 6 and Table 2 demonstrate different magnitudes of capacity processing in the three groups of participants. The overall workload capacity in the older group was significantly greater in the redundant target condition ($F(1,33) = 8.9$, $P < 0.001$, $P\mu^2 = 0.49$) when compared to the young participants ($t(11) = 5.18$, $P < 0.001$, $d = 0.41$) and the middle-aged group $t(11) = 4.6$, $P < 0.001$, $d = 0.62$). The difference between the younger and middle-aged groups was not reliable ($t(11) = 0.8$).

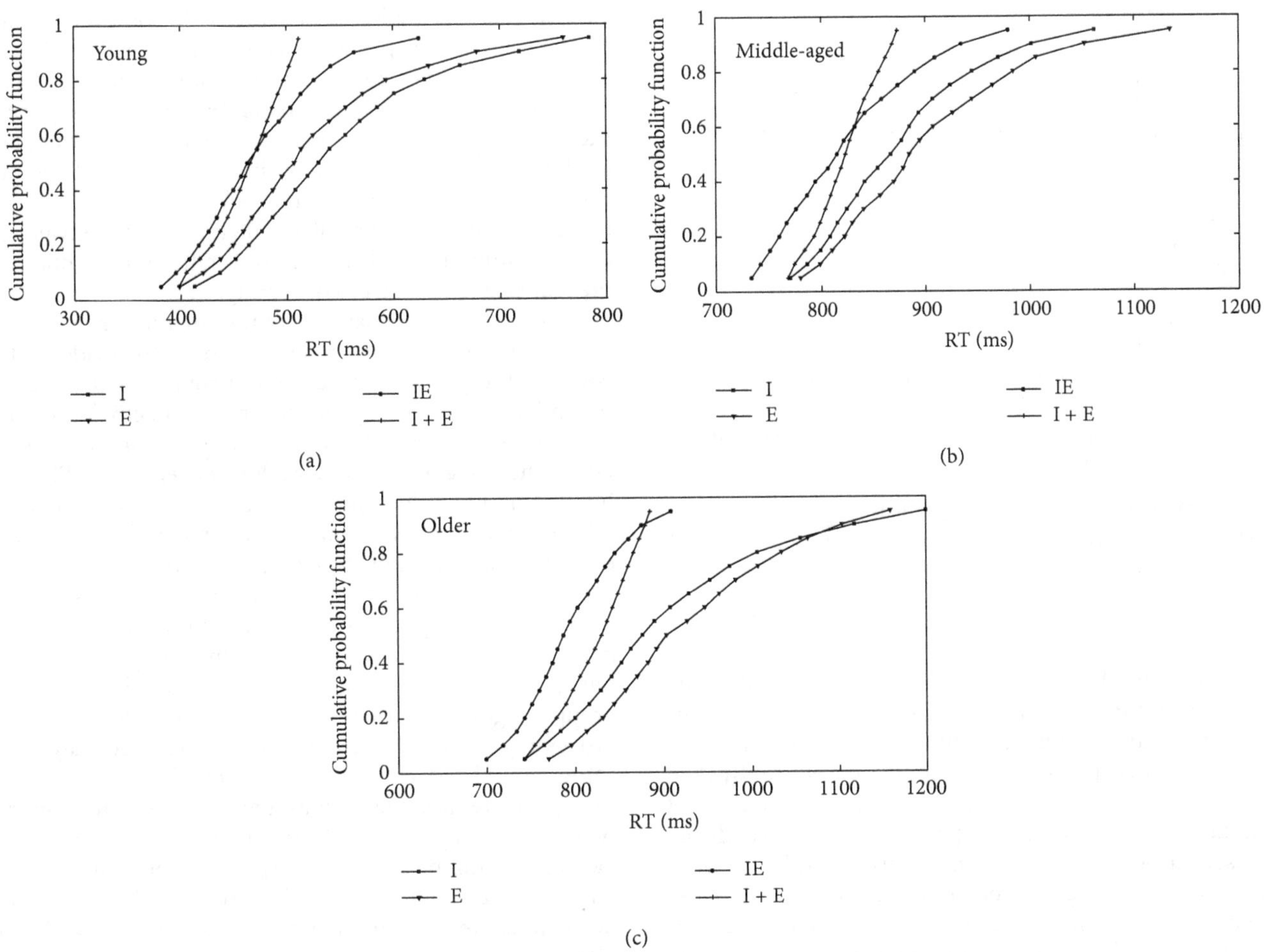

Figure 4: CDFs for redundant targets (IE), the sum of the distributions for emotional expression and identity targets (I + E), and single targets (E) and (I) in groups of young (a), middle-aged (b), and older (c) participants.

4. Discussion

The present study examined the effect of aging on the processing of redundant information in faces. Three findings are striking. First, participants from all three age groups benefitted from combining facial identity and emotional expressions in target faces, but this effect was more pronounced in the older group which showed greater redundancy gains in processing both the identity and emotional expression targets. Second, the results of the Miller test [57] provide clear evidence that enhanced responses to redundant face stimuli are determined by coactive processing of the two facial dimensions (note that Yankouskaya et al. [56] provided evidence against redundancy gains reflecting crosstalk after partial processing of facial identity and emotion.). The coactive processing was present at all ages but had more marked effects on the performance of the older participants. Third, the capacity analysis indicates that older people were able to increase their processing up to 2.4 times with redundant targets, while younger and middle-aged adults increased their capacity only 1.2 times. Most notably, the effects of age here remained even when the data were log transformed, when effects of overall processing speed should be reduced [6, 72, 73].

These findings are consistent with the results of previous studies with elementary visual stimuli showing faster responding for two targets as compared to either single target in elderly participants [25–27, 74] and super capacity in the processing of multisensory stimuli [30]. The new findings here are as follows: (1) the redundant target effect in older people occurs with complex ecological stimuli such as human faces; (2) facial identity and emotional expression are processed interactively, and this effect is preserved across lifespan; (3) the dynamics of the redundancy effect across lifespan have a nonlinear trend.

The results raise the question as to why older adults show improvements in processing of redundant information in faces, despite suffering age-related perceptual and cognitive declines, and what is the origin of this improvement? One possibility is that older people combine information from faces in a more efficient way compared to young adults due to life experience with faces. Indeed, there is evidence that accumulated life and interpersonal experience increases older adults' ability to identify other people's faces and emotions

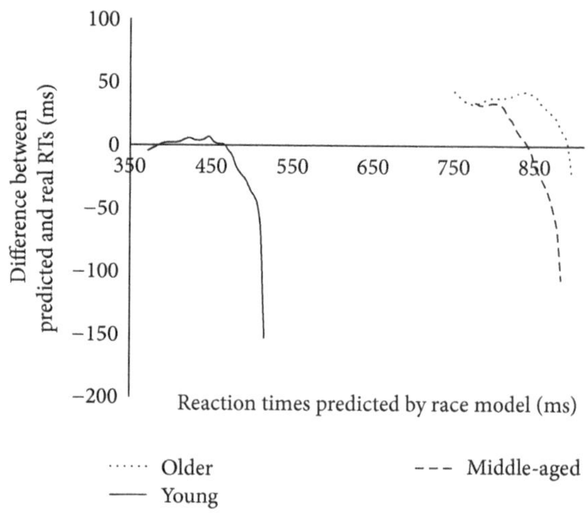

Figure 5: Differences between RTs predicted by the race model (solid horizontal line) and the observed RTs for young, middle-aged, and older groups.

[75, 76]. As a result, this would predict an improved ability to combine information in faces and greater redundancy gains compared to younger adults. On the other hand, older subjects may process facial features less efficiently than younger adults, and the gains produced from redundant target faces are greater for individual features which are processed slower. This explanation is supported by previous studies demonstrating that older people showed increases in scanning behavior when looking at faces and were subsequently less efficient in recognition performance due to disrupted feature processing. There is also the possibility that greater redundancy gains in the older group may reflect a decline in ignoring irrelevant information accompanied either single target. For example, Allen et al. [77] emphasized that older participants have difficulties with ignoring irrelevant information rather than any difficulty associated with activating or selecting targets. If age increases the "internal noise" in information processing [77], then we can think that redundant targets contain no internal noise, while the single target stimuli contain "noise" along the other dimension (the "noise" of the emotional expression for identity targets and of identity information for expression targets). The failure to ignore stimuli along the nontarget dimension when only one facial feature is present would then lead to noise entering any computations on single target trials but also large(r) reductions in noise when both identity and emotion targets are present.

It has to be noted that although all the above explanations may account for the greater redundancy gains in the older group, it is less clear why the older group shows a greater integrative effect and higher workload capacity than younger adults, in the formal analyses presented here. The most pronounced evidence for enhanced integrative processing in elderly participants comes from studies using multisensory signals [25, 27, 74]. For example, similar to our results, Laurienti et al. [27] reported a greater peak and a broader temporal window of audio-visual integration. The authors suggest that the multisensory signals become much more efficient for older participants because these individuals experience declines in each of the unisensory modalities. Furthermore, an additional possibility that may account for the multisensory enhancement was linked to a better ability in the elderly to exploit the redundant nature of the cues. Bucur et al. [25, 26] proposed that older people do exhibit age-related deficits when they divide their attention between two different stimulus modalities; however, this is not sufficient to prevent coactivation from occurring.

Although the mechanisms of the enhanced responses for redundant information remain unknown, the evidence that, compared to younger adults, older people can better exploit redundant cues may explain the greater coactivation in processing both the identity and emotional expression targets. Given the evidence that older adults experience difficulty in integrating individual facial features into a whole representation, capturing covariations in redundant faces may be an efficient compensation strategy to minimize declines in the processing of facial identity and emotional expression. This assumption is supported by results of the capacity analysis here. The finding that the older group was generally slower but greater in processing capacity compared to the young group suggests that there is a qualitative difference in face processing across the groups. This difference may reflect some age-related changes in perceptual mechanisms. We can speculate here that combining target information from two sources may produce "a distinct feature" that makes the face containing both the identity and emotional expressing targets more salient. Responding to the "distinct feature" determines greater redundancy gains as compared with target information in either single target face, because this would require less cognitive resources. The challenge for further research is to examine whether reducing cognitive load by efficient integration information is a function of normal aging.

The data here show that the size of the redundancy gains in the middle-aged group was smaller compared to both the younger and older adults. This indicates nonlinear changes in face processing as people age. As compared to younger adults, middle-aged people experience some declines in face processing that results in smaller size of redundancy gains. Indeed, there is evidence that peak recognition performance for faces occurs around 30–34 years, reflecting the continued development of face processing skills into middle-aged people (Germine, Duchaine, and Nakayama, 2010). Smaller redundancy gains in the middle-aged group as compared to older participants suggest less efficient combining information and indicate that qualitative changes in perceptual mechanisms link to more advanced age. On the other hand, our results on the Miller [57] test of the independent race model, along with the capacity analysis, demonstrate gradual increases in coactivation and capacity processing across the groups. Although the finding needs further investigation, this may indicate that the integration of facial identity and emotional expression information is a function of normal aging.

A number of studies have reported faster RTs and higher accuracy for older participants when recognizing positive as

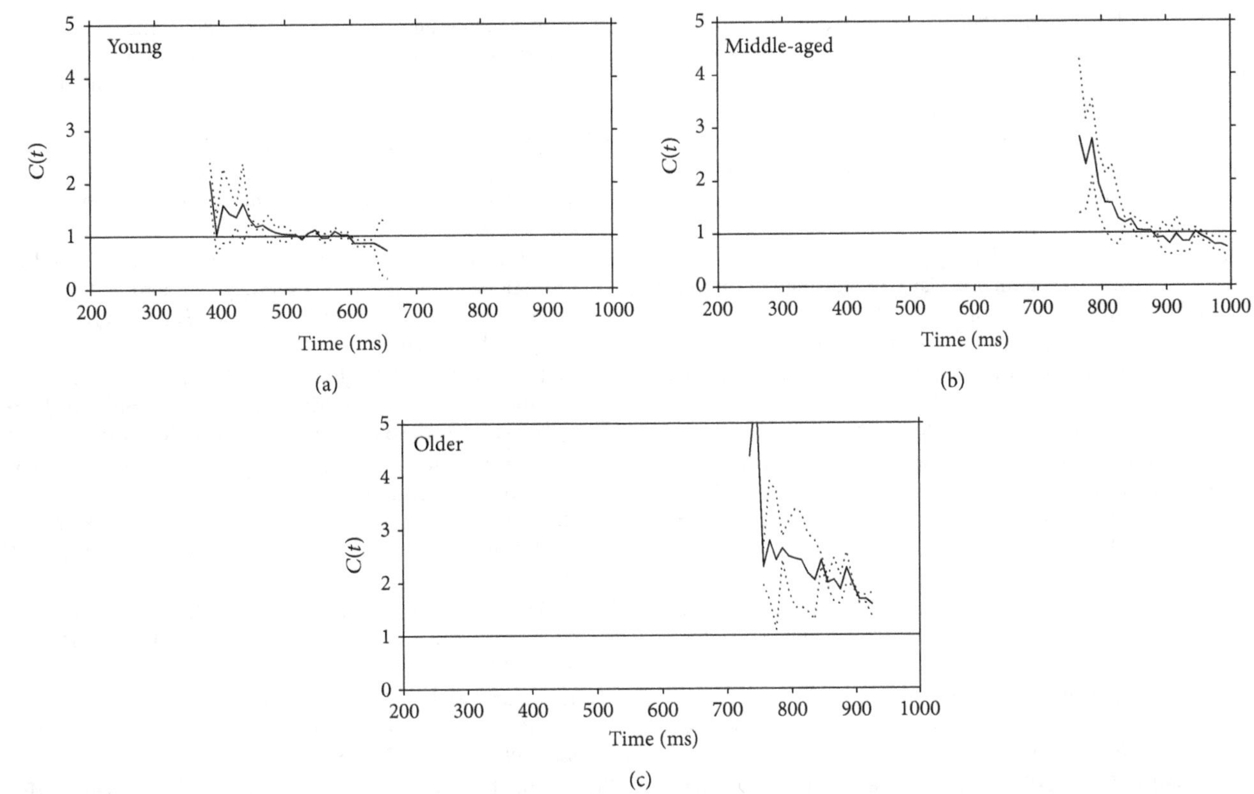

FIGURE 6: Capacity coefficients for the three groups of participants: top row young adult and middle row middle-aged people. The horizontal line at $C(t) = 1$ indicates the reference value for unlimited capacity. The capacity coefficients are depicted in solid line; the confident interval for capacity coefficient is depicted in dash line.

compared to negative emotional expressions [78–80]. In the present study, the identity target only (Person 1) was shown with a happy emotional expression (nontarget emotion), while both the redundant target (Person 1 expressing sadness) and the emotional expression target only (Person 2 expressing sadness) contained a negative emotional expression. The "positive expression bias" predicts that the older group would show better performance for the identity target as compared to the emotional expression target, and there should also be a reduced redundant target effect. However, there were no reliable differences between RTs for the identity and emotional expression targets and an increased redundancy effect, contradicting the "positive emotion" bias account of performance. We did, however, find that the size of redundancy gain in middle-age participants was smaller as compared to both the young and the older groups when the log-transformed data were considered. Although the difference between RTs predicted by the race model and the observed RTs gradually increased with age (Figure 5), this finding needs further investigation to examine which factors may reduce redundancy gains in middle age.

5. Conclusions

The present study provides strong evidence that facial identity and emotional expression are processed interactively and this interaction remains intact with age, with, if anything, older people demonstrating a greater benefit when identity and emotion combine in a redundant manner. This effect does not reflect general age-related slowing but may result from increased distribution of attention to both identity and expression properties of faces in older participants.

Acknowledgments

This work was supported by grants from the BBSRC, ERC, and ESRC to the second author and a studentship to the first author subsidized by the Hilary Green Research Fund.

References

[1] J. C. Bartlett and A. Fulton, "Familiarity and recognition of faces in old age," *Memory & Cognition*, vol. 19, no. 3, pp. 229–238, 1991.

[2] I. Boutet and J. Faubert, "Recognition of faces and complex objects in younger and older adults," *Memory & Cognition*, vol. 34, no. 4, pp. 854–864, 2006.

[3] A. Fulton and J. C. Bartlett, "Young and old faces in young and old heads: the factor of age in face recognition," *Psychology and Aging*, vol. 6, no. 4, pp. 623–630, 1991.

[4] L. A. Lott, G. Haegerstrom-Portnoy, M. E. Schneck, and J. A. Brabyn, "Face recognition in the elderly," *Optometry and Vision Science*, vol. 82, no. 10, pp. 874–881, 2005.

[5] M. Naveh-Benjamin, J. Guez, and S. Shulman, "Older adults' associative deficit in episodic memory: assessing the role of decline in attentional resources," *Psychonomic Bulletin and Review*, vol. 11, no. 6, pp. 1067–1073, 2004.

[6] D. Norton, R. McBain, and Y. Chen, "Reduced ability to detect facial configuration in middle-aged and elderly individuals: associations with spatiotemporal visual processing," *Journals of Gerontology B*, vol. 64, no. 3, pp. 328–334, 2009.

[7] A. C. Lamont, S. Stewart-Williams, and J. Podd, "Face recognition and aging: effects of target age and memory load," *Memory & Cognition*, vol. 33, no. 6, pp. 1017–1024, 2005.

[8] J. M. Logan and D. A. Balota, "Expanded vs. equal interval spaced retrieval practice: exploring different schedules of spacing and retention interval in younger and older adults," *Neuropsychology, Development, and Cognition B*, vol. 15, no. 3, pp. 257–280, 2008.

[9] D. Kidder, D. Park, C. Hertzog, and R. Morrell, "Prospective memory and aging: the effects of working memory and prospective memory task load," *Aging, Neuropsychology, and Cognition*, vol. 4, no. 2, pp. 93–112, 1997.

[10] M. M. Metzger, "Stimulus load and age effects in facial recognition: a comparison of children and adults," *North American Journal of Psychology*, vol. 4, no. 1, pp. 51–52, 2002.

[11] J. C. Bartlett and J. E. Leslie, "Aging and memory for faces versus single views of faces," *Memory & Cognition*, vol. 14, no. 5, pp. 371–381, 1986.

[12] S. Daniel and S. Bentin, "Age-related changes in processing faces from detection to identification: ERP evidence," *Neurobiology of Aging*, vol. 33, no. 1, pp. 206.el–206.e28, 2012.

[13] C. Habak, F. Wilkinson, and H. R. Wilson, "Aging disrupts the neural transformations that link facial identity across views," *Vision Research*, vol. 48, no. 1, pp. 9–15, 2008.

[14] S. Obermeyer, T. Kolling, A. Schaich, and M. Knopf, "Differences between old and young adults' ability to recognize human faces underlie processing of horizontal information," *Frontiers in Aging Neuroscience*, vol. 4, article 3, 2012.

[15] H. R. Wilson, M. Mei, C. Habak, and F. Wilkinson, "Visual bandwidths for face orientation increase during healthy aging," *Vision Research*, vol. 51, no. 1, pp. 160–164, 2011.

[16] G. Slessor, L. H. Phillips, and R. Bull, "Age-related declines in basic social perception: evidence from tasks assessing eye-gaze processing," *Psychology and Aging*, vol. 23, no. 4, pp. 812–822, 2008.

[17] T. W. Schmitz, F. H. Cheng, and E. de Rosa, "Failing to ignore: paradoxical neural effects of perceptual load on early attentional selection in normal aging," *The Journal of Neuroscience*, vol. 344, no. 30, pp. 14750–14758, 2010.

[18] A. Mill, J. Allik, A. Realo, and R. Valk, "Age-related differences in emotion recognition ability: A Cross-Sectional Study," *Emotion*, vol. 9, no. 5, pp. 619–630, 2009.

[19] T. Ruffman, J. D. Henry, V. Livingstone, and L. H. Phillips, "A meta-analytic review of emotion recognition and aging: implications for neuropsychological models of aging," *Neuroscience and Biobehavioral Reviews*, vol. 32, no. 4, pp. 863–681, 2008.

[20] A. Suzuki, T. Hoshino, K. Shigemasu, and M. Kawamura, "Decline or improvement?: age-related differences in facial expression recognition," *Biological Psychology*, vol. 74, no. 1, pp. 75–84, 2007.

[21] N. A. Murphy and D. M. Isaacowitz, "Preferences for emotional information in older and younger adults: a meta-analysis of memory and attention tasks," *Psychology and Aging*, vol. 23, no. 2, pp. 263–286, 2008.

[22] C. McAlpine, K. A. Kendall, and N. N. Singh, "Recognition of facial expressions of emotion by persons with mental retardation," *American Journal on Mental Retardation*, vol. 96, no. 1, pp. 29–36, 1991.

[23] L. L. Carstensen, M. Pasupathi, U. Mayr, and J. R. Nesselroade, "Emotional experience in everyday life across the adult life span," *Journal of Personality and Social Psychology*, vol. 79, no. 4, pp. 644–655, 2000.

[24] D. P. Smith, C. H. Hillman, and A. R. Duley, "Influences of age on emotional reactivity during picture processing," *The Journals of Gerontology B*, vol. 60, no. 1, pp. P49–P56, 2005.

[25] B. Bucur, P. A. Allen, R. E. Sanders, E. Ruthruff, and M. D. Murphy, "Redundancy gain and coactivation in bimodal detection: evidence for the preservation of coactive processing in older adults," *Journals of Gerontology*, vol. 60, no. 5, pp. P279–P282, 2005.

[26] B. Bucur, D. J. Madden, and P. A. Allen, "Age-related differences in the processing of redundant visual dimensions," *Psychology and Aging*, vol. 20, no. 3, pp. 435–446, 2005.

[27] P. J. Laurienti, J. H. Burdette, J. A. Maldjian, and M. T. Wallace, "Enhanced multisensory integration in older adults," *Neurobiology of Aging*, vol. 27, no. 8, pp. 1155–1163, 2006.

[28] E. Linnet and M. E. Roser, "Age-related differences in interhemispheric visuomotor integration measured by the redundant target effect," *Psychology and Aging*, vol. 27, no. 2, pp. 399–409, 2012.

[29] P. A. Allen, D. J. Madden, K. E. Groth, and L. C. Crozier, "Impact of age, redundancy, and perceptual noise on visual search," *Journals of Gerontology*, vol. 47, no. 2, pp. P69–P74, 1992.

[30] C. E. Hugenschmidt, S. Hayasaka, A. M. Peiffer, and P. J. Laurienti, "Applying capacity analyses to psychophysical evaluation of multisensory interactions," *An International Journal on Information Fusion*, vol. 11, no. 1, pp. 12–20, 2010.

[31] J. T. Townsend and A. Eidels, "Workload capacity spaces: a unified methodology for response time measures of efficiency as workload is varied," *Psychonomic Bulletin & Review*, vol. 18, no. 4, pp. 659–681, 2011.

[32] J. T. Townsend and M. J. Wenger, "A theory of interactive parallel processing: new capacity measures and predictions for a response time inequality series," *Psychological Review*, vol. 111, no. 4, pp. 1003–1035, 2004.

[33] M. J. Wenger and B. S. Gibson, "Using hazard functions to assess changes in processing capacity in an attentional cuing paradigm," *Journal of Experimental Psychology*, vol. 30, no. 4, pp. 708–719, 2004.

[34] M. J. Wenger and J. T. Townsend, "Spatial frequencies in short-term memory for faces: a test of three frequency-dependent hypotheses," *Memory & Cognition*, vol. 28, no. 1, pp. 125–142, 2000.

[35] V. Bruce and A. Young, "Understanding face recognition," *British Journal of Psychology*, vol. 77, part 3, pp. 305–327, 1986.

[36] R. Bruyer, C. Laterre, X. Seron et al., "A case of prosopagnosia with some preserved covert remembrance of familiar faces," *Brain and Cognition*, vol. 2, no. 3, pp. 257–284, 1983.

[37] R. Campbell, T. Landis, and M. Regard, "Face recognition and lipreading. A neurological dissociation," *Brain*, vol. 109, no. 3, pp. 509–521, 1986.

[38] R. D. Jones and D. Tranel, "Severe developmental prosopagnosia in a child with superior intellect," *Journal of Clinical and Experimental Neuropsychology*, vol. 23, no. 3, pp. 265–273, 2001.

[39] J. A. Nunn, P. Postma, and R. Pearson, "Developmental prosopagnosia: Should it be taken at face value?" *Neurocase*, vol. 7, no. 1, pp. 15–27, 2001.

[40] G. W. Humphreys, N. Donnelly, and M. J. Riddoch, "Expression is computed separately from facial identity, and it is computed separately for moving and static faces: neuropsychological evidence," *Neuropsychologia*, vol. 31, no. 2, pp. 173–181, 1993.

[41] N. L. Etcoff, "Selective attention to facial identity and facial emotion," *Neuropsychologia*, vol. 22, no. 3, pp. 281–295, 1984.

[42] A. W. Young, K. H. McWeeny, D. C. Hay, and A. W. Ellis, "Matching familiar and unfamiliar faces on identity and expression," *Psychological Research*, vol. 48, no. 2, pp. 63–68, 1986.

[43] L. Aguado, A. Garcia-Gutierrez, and I. Serrano-Pedraza, "Symmetrical interaction of sex and expression in face classification tasks," *Attenion, Perception & Psychophysics*, vol. 71, no. 1, pp. 9–25, 2009.

[44] A. P. Atkinson, J. Tipples, D. M. Burt, and A. W. Young, "Asymmetric interference between sex and emotion in face perception," *Perception & Psychophysics*, vol. 67, no. 7, pp. 1199–1213, 2005.

[45] J. Y. Baudouin, D. Gilibert, S. Sansone, and G. Tiberghien, "When the smile is a cue to familiarity," *Memory*, vol. 8, no. 5, pp. 285–292, 2000.

[46] J. Y. Baudouin, F. Martin, G. Tiberghien, I. Verlut, and N. Franck, "Selective attention to facial emotion and identity in schizophrenia," *Neuropsychologia*, vol. 40, no. 5, pp. 503–511, 2002.

[47] K. M. Curby, K. J. Johnson, and A. Tyson, "Face to face with emotion: holistic face processing is modulated by emotional state," *Cognition and Emotion*, vol. 26, no. 1, pp. 93–102, 2012.

[48] A. D'Argembeau, M. van der Linden, A. M. Etienne, and C. Comblain, "Identity and expression memory for happy and angry faces in social anxiety," *Acta Psychologica*, vol. 114, no. 1, pp. 1–15, 2003.

[49] T. Ganel and Y. Goshen-Gottstein, "Effects of familiarity on the perceptual integrality of the identity and expression of faces: the parallel-route hypothesis revisited," *Journal of Experimental Psychology*, vol. 30, no. 3, pp. 583–597, 2004.

[50] J. M. Kaufmann and S. R. Schweinberger, "Expression influences the recognition of familiar faces," *Perception*, vol. 33, no. 4, pp. 399–408, 2004.

[51] Y. Levy and S. Bentin, "Interactive processes in matching identity and expressions of unfamiliar faces: evidence for mutual facilitation effects," *Perception*, vol. 37, no. 6, pp. 915–930, 2008.

[52] S. R. Schweinberger, A. M. Burton, and S. W. Kelly, "Asymmetric dependencies in perceiving identity and emotion: experiments with morphed faces," *Perception & Psychophysics*, vol. 61, no. 6, pp. 1102–1115, 1999.

[53] S. R. Schweinberger and G. R. Soukup, " Asymmetric relationships among perceptions of facial identity, emotion, and facial speech," *Journal of Experimental Psychology*, vol. 24, no. 6, pp. 1748–1765, 1998.

[54] T. Garcia-Marques, D. M. Mackie, H. M. Claypool, and L. Garcia-Marques, "Positivity can cue familiarity," *Personality and Social Psychology Bulletin*, vol. 30, no. 5, pp. 585–593, 2004.

[55] B. de Gelder, I. Frissen, J. Barton, and N. Hadjikhani, "A modulatory role for facial expressions in prosopagnosia," *Proceedings of the National Academy of Sciences of the United States of America*, vol. 100, no. 22, pp. 13105–13110, 2003.

[56] A. Yankouskaya, D. A. Booth, and G. Humphreys, "Interactions between facial emotion and identity in face processing: evidence based on redundancy gains," *Attention, Perception & Psychophysics*, vol. 74, no. 8, pp. 1692–1711, 2012.

[57] J. Miller, "Divided attention: evidence for coactivation with redundant signals," *Cognitive Psychology*, vol. 14, no. 2, pp. 247–279, 1982.

[58] J. Miller, R. Ulrich, and Y. Lamarre, "Locus of the redundant-signals effect in bimodal divided attention: a neurophysiological analysis," *Perception & Psychophysics*, vol. 63, no. 3, pp. 555–562, 2001.

[59] J. T. Mordkoff and J. Miller, "Redundancy gains and coactivation with two different targets: the problem of target preferences and the effects of display frequency," *Perception & Psychophysics*, vol. 53, no. 5, pp. 527–535, 1993.

[60] M. J. Wenger and J. T. Townsend, "On the costs and benefits of faces and words: process characteristics of feature search in highly meaningful stimuli," *Journal of Experimental Psychology. Human Perception and Performance*, vol. 32, no. 3, pp. 755–779, 2006.

[61] D. H. Raab, "Statistical facilitation of simple reaction times," *Transaction of the New York Academy Sciences*, vol. 24, pp. 574–590, 1962.

[62] J. T. Townsend and G. Nozawa, "Spatio-temporal properties of elementary perception: an investigation of parallel, serial and coactive theories," *Journal of Mathematical Psychology*, vol. 39, pp. 321–360, 1995.

[63] P. Ekman and W. V. Friesen, *Facial Action Coding System: A Technique for the Measurement of Facial Movement*, Consulting Psychologists Press, Palo Alto, Calif, USA, 1978.

[64] N. Tottenham, A. Borsheid, K. Ellertsen, D. J. Marcus, and C. A. Nelson, "Categorization of facial expressions in children and adults: establishing a larger stimulus set," in *Proceedings of the Cognitive Neuroscience Society Annual Meeting*, San Francisco, Calif, USA, 2002.

[65] L. L. Carstensen, "The influence of a sense of time on human development," *Science*, vol. 312, no. 5782, pp. 1913–1915, 2006.

[66] I. Biederman and S. F. Checkosky, "Processing redundant information," *Journal of Experimental Psychology*, vol. 83, no. 3, pp. 486–490, 1970.

[67] J. T. Mordkoff and S. Yantis, "An interactive race model of divided attention," *Journal of Experimental Psychology*, vol. 17, no. 2, pp. 520–538, 1991.

[68] R. Ulrich, J. Miller, and H. Schröter, "Testing the race model inequality: an algorithm and computer programs," *Behavior Research Methods*, vol. 39, no. 2, pp. 291–302, 2007.

[69] M. E. Faust, D. A. Balota, D. H. Spieler, and F. R. Ferraro, "Individual differences in information-processing rate and amount: implications for group differences in response latency," *Psychological Bulletin*, vol. 125, no. 6, pp. 777–799, 1999.

[70] T. A. Salthouse, "Resource-reduction interpretations of cognitive aging," *Developmental Review*, vol. 8, pp. 238–272, 1988.

[71] Y. Benjamini, "Simultaneous and selective inference: current successes and future challenges," *Biometrical Journal*, vol. 52, no. 6, pp. 708–721, 2010.

[72] D. J. Plude and W. J. Hoyer, "Age and the selectivity of visual information processing," *Psychology and Aging*, vol. 1, no. 1, pp. 4–10, 1986.

[73] B. L. Somberg and T. A. Salthouse, "Divided attention abilities in young and old adults," *Journal of Experimental Psychology*, vol. 8, no. 5, pp. 651–663, 1982.

[74] A. Diederich, H. Colonius, and A. Schomburg, "Assessing age-related multisensory enhancement with the time-window-of-integration model," *Neuropsychologia*, vol. 46, no. 10, pp. 2556–2562, 2008.

[75] F. Blanchard-Fields, "Everyday problem solving and emotion: an adult developmental perspective," *Current Directions in Psychological Science*, vol. 16, pp. 26–31, 2007.

[76] L. L. Carstensen, D. Isaacowitz, and S. T. Charles, "Taking time seriously: a theory of socioemotional selectivity," *American Psychologist*, vol. 54, pp. 165–181, 1999.

[77] P. A. Allen, T. A. Weber, and D. J. Madden, "Adult age differences in attention: filtering or selection?" *Journal of Gerontology*, vol. 49, no. 5, pp. P213–P222, 1994.

[78] A. J. Calder, J. Keane, T. Manly et al., "Facial expression recognition across the adult life span," *Neuropsychologia*, vol. 41, no. 2, pp. 195–202, 2003.

[79] C. Kiffel, S. Campanella, and R. Bruyer, "Categorical perception of faces and facial expressions: the age factor," *Experimental Aging Research*, vol. 31, no. 2, pp. 119–147, 2005.

[80] V. Orgeta and L. H. Phillips, "Effects of age and emotional intensity on the recognition of facial emotion," *Experimental Aging Research*, vol. 34, no. 1, pp. 63–79, 2008.

2

Action-Oriented Study Circles Facilitate Efforts in Nursing Homes to "Go from Feeding to Serving": Conceptual Perspectives on Knowledge Translation and Workplace Learning

Albert Westergren

The PRO-CARE Group, School of Health and Society, Kristianstad University, 291 88 Kristianstad, Sweden

Correspondence should be addressed to Albert Westergren, albert.westergren@hkr.se

Academic Editor: Julie Locher

Background. Action-oriented study circles (AOSC) have been found to improve nutrition in 24 nursing homes in Sweden. Little, however, is known about the conceptual use of knowledge (changes in staffs' knowledge and behaviours). *Methods.* Qualitative and quantitative methods, structured questionnaires for evaluating participants' (working in nursing homes) experiences from study circles ($n = 592$, 71 AOSC) and for comparisons between AOSC participants ($n = 74$) and nonparticipants ($n = 115$). Finally, a focus group interview was conducted with AOSC participants (in total $n = 12$). Statistical, conventional, and directed content analyses were used. *Results.* Participants experienced a statistically significant increase in their knowledge about eating and nutrition, when retrospectively comparing before participating and after, as well as in comparison to non-participants, and they felt that the management was engaged in and took care of ideas regarding food and mealtimes to a significantly greater extent than non-participants. The use of AOSC was successful judging from how staff members had changed their attitudes and behaviours toward feeding residents. *Conclusions.* AOSC facilitates professional development, better system performance, and, as shown in previous studies, better patient outcome. Based on a collaborative learning perspective, AOSC manages to integrate evidence, context, and facilitation in the efforts to achieve knowledge translation in a learning organisation. This study has implications also for other care settings implementing AOSC.

1. Background

Promoting nutritional health equity among at risk older populations in nursing homes is of importance. Effective interventions that reduce the risk of undernutrition can help to ensure that people stay healthier in old age. Findings from a couple of studies indicate inequity between the nutritional care provided to patients in hospitals and elderly people in nursing homes. Two surveys conducted in 2007 indicate that patients in hospitals and at risk of undernutrition are more likely to get oral supplements (43–54%) [1] than elderly persons at risk of undernutrition in nursing homes (14–19%) [2]. It is plausible that appropriate nutritional care for older people in nursing homes requires educational interventions.

This study is a part of a larger project that has shown, in a before–during–after controlled trial, that by implementing action oriented study circles (AOSC) for the staff in nursing homes, knowledge translation (KT) regarding eating and nutrition was achieved in terms of instrumental outcomes (had a positive impact both on provider behaviour and on patient outcomes) [2, 3]. The means by which this was achieved is believed to be inconsistent and complex, and what occurred can be described as a "black box phenomenon" [4]. It is presumed that evidence, context, and facilitation influenced the KT in the previous studies [2, 3], but this remains to be explored. This study puts action-oriented study circles (AOSC), a pedagogical method for work based collaborative learning, and KT into a theoretical context. It also looks into the "black box" of KT and reveals some of its content.

Knowledge Translation. It is a challenge to achieve improvements in nutritional care in an environment that is complex and evolving, and there is a tendency to measure the success of projects only in terms of instrumental outcomes of KT (better system performance (care) and measurable change in patient outcomes (health)). However, besides instrumental outcomes, also conceptual outcomes are of interest when it comes to improving nutritional care. The conceptual outcomes describe changes in understanding, knowledge and attitudes [5]. It is suggested that research translation should be used as an intermediate outcome, while patient outcomes and provider behaviour are endpoint outcomes [6, 7].

KT can be defined as "the exchange, synthesis, and ethically-sound application of knowledge—within a complex system of interactions among researchers and users—to accelerate the capture of the benefits of research ... through improved health, more effective services and products, and a strengthened health care system" (Canadian Institutes of Health Research, cited in [8] page 1). KT is a processual phenomenon that is dynamic and interactive [9]. The purpose of KT is to decrease the gap between what is known from research and knowledge synthesis, and the implementation of this knowledge by key stakeholders, in order to improve care delivery, efficiencies of the health care system and health outcomes [5]. Graham and Tetroe [10] highlight the importance of improving our knowledge about KT. For instance, more research is needed that focuses on developing theory-based KT interventions and on testing their effectiveness.

The Organisational Influence and the PARiHS Framework. In this study, the success of the implementation of change is believed to be linked to the nursing home organisation. Thus, in order to succeed, the type of organisation and decentralised decision making, in relation to the teams, are regarded as important [11]. A framework for successful implementation that incorporates organisational factors (such as facilitation and context) is the PARiHS framework (Promoting Action on Research Implementation in Health Sciences), developed since 1998 [12, 13]. The framework can be used to theory-based KT, and to better understand the "black box" of implementation. According to Kitson and colleagues [12], a "successful implementation" (SI) of new ideas (evidence, guidelines, etc.) is a function (f) of the interrelations between three key elements—evidence (E), context (C), and facilitation (F): SI = f (E, C, and F).

The dimension *Evidence* includes research, clinical experience, patient experience, and routine data. Thus, it is important to not only consider evidence within the "evidence-based medicine" framework. Instead, in the PARiHS framework, also other sources of knowledge are considered, including research evidence, clinical experience, professional craft knowledge, patient preferences and experiences, and local information [12]. Graham et al. [5] conceptualise, in relation to KT, that "knowledge" can be empirically derived (research based) but also encompass other forms of knowing, such as experiential knowledge. Both local and external knowledge creation or research can be integrated in the knowledge to action process [5]. For instance, local research can be carried out in order to determine the magnitude of the problem and the care gap [5]. The *Context* in a care setting is made up of several factors, factors that are interdependent [12, 14]. Among others such as leadership, culture (prevailing beliefs, values of relationships, teamwork, power, and reward systems), feedback processes (information sharing), and organisational slack (human resources, space, time) are part of the context [14]. *Facilitation* includes purpose, role, skills, and attributes. The subelement "Purpose" (in the *Facilitation* dimension) can be technical or holistic. "Technical" means introducing a discrete method, while "holistic" means sustaining and enabling personal development and system transformation [12]. Facilitation refers to the process of "enabling (making easier) the implementation of evidence into practice" and "facilitation is achieved by an individual carrying out a specific role (a facilitator), which aims to help others" ([13] page 579). The facilitator has an appointed role, internal or external to the organisation, in which the change is being implemented. Facilitators are said to have a key role in helping teams and individuals understand what and how they need to change practice. The role of facilitator is more about helping and enabling than persuading or telling [13]. In the two previously mentioned studies [2, 3], the intervention with study circles was theory based in the PARiHS framework.

The success of the implementation of change is believed to be linked to the professionals' needs and motivation and to the fact that people change their behaviour on the basis of experienced problems in practice [11]. Thus, in order to achieve improved nutritional care, a pedagogical method is needed to increase professional competence, to better serve the care recipients, to meet external expectations (including pressure from colleagues), and to inspire to change by learning through social interaction. Action-oriented study circles might have these qualities.

Action Oriented Study Circles . By adding "action oriented" to "study circles," I want to emphasise that it is not only "studies" that are expected but also "action" (knowledge to act). Action-oriented study circles (AOSC) is a pedagogical method that might increase the likelihood of achieving KT, as it emphasises work-based learning in the local social context. Often, different theoretical perspectives must be considered in order to develop a good KT [11], and using AOSC makes it possible to integrate pedagogical, social, and organisational theoretical perspectives. Furthermore, the study circle methodology can be linked to the PARiHS framework in that the facilitation aspect is very much connected to enabling self directive learning and cooperative learning approaches [12]. Facilitative learning approaches that are student centred and problem based emphasise critical reflection and focus on experimental learning, and by achieving local consensus they have the potential to enhance changes in practice culture, as well as evidence-based improvements.

The "birth year" for the study circle is regarded to be 1902. It started in the temperance movement, and its instigator was Oscar "with the beard" Olsson. It has since then been the core method used by the Workers' Educational Association (ABF) in Sweden [15]. The idea of the study circle can be connected to Vygotsky's ideas about cultural mediation and internalisation, namely, that by interacting in a group, individuals come to share the knowledge of a culture. In this way, knowledge becomes internalised, one "knows how" [16]. Also Piaget's thoughts on "cooperative relations" are applicable to the ideas behind study circles. In cooperative relations, power is evenly distributed between participants so that a symmetrical relationship emerges. In cooperative relations, authentic forms of intellectual exchange become possible; each partner has the freedom to project his or her own thoughts, consider the positions of others, and defend his or her own point of view. According to Piaget, the knowledge that emerges is open, flexible, and regulated by the logic of argument rather than determined by an external authority [17]. Study circles also have similarities with problem-based learning (PBL), and pedagogical research has shown that learning is enhanced when the student is active [18, 19].

The fundamental concepts of the study circle are voluntary, informal, and participant-centred learning in which flexibility of format and structure is important [20]. If pedagogical models are divided into the persuasion model, the information model and the discussion model, the study circle belongs to the discussion model. The discussion model means that the participants engage in conversations, identify and analyse problems, and take actions [21]. In addition, the study circle places great emphasis on the broader environmental and social context in which individuals work and where the interventions for change are expected to occur. By using a discussion model for learning, one assumes that knowledge acquisition is a collaborative process and that individual understanding is rooted in social interaction. Because of its simple, flexible structure, and its capacity to address contextual factors, the study circle could serve as a model for educational interventions in care and service. The overall aim of study circles is to identify key problems and to learn how to master them [22]. Several positive experiences have been described by participants in study circle activities arranged within the popular education framework in Sweden (folkbildning), such as personal development, increased self-esteem, changed ways of thinking, increased courage, learning how to study, increased social and cultural competence, and improved cooperation and solidarity [15].

Study circles are becoming increasingly popular in Sweden in care and service. The Swedish Institute for Health Sciences (Vårdalinstitutet) [23], for instance, has several manuals for study circles for different areas such as dementia, ethics, culture, eating and nutrition, palliative care, pain, stroke, and elderly health. However, study circle interventions in care and service have been explored only in a few studies [2, 3, 22, 24–28], and some of these have focused on nutrition in nursing homes and instrumental outcomes of KT [2, 3, 28]. It was shown that study circle interventions with focus on nutrition in nursing homes can improve the care (more residents with risk of undernutrition get the right treatment) [2, 3] and the care recipients' outcome (decreased number of residents with undernutrition) [2, 3, 28] in a short- [2, 28] and long-term perspective [3]. Wallin [7] states that "if we want to understand what strategies are working in changing practice to be more evidence-based, then we must test these strategies" (page 579). Thus, research has shown that study circle interventions improve instrumental outcomes, and now we need to show what impact they have on staff knowledge and attitudes, that is, conceptual outcomes. Furthermore, Wallin [7] highlights that there is a need for examining the PARiHS framework through intervention studies. Thus, when exploring the process of KT with focus on nutrition using the AOSC methodology, it should be done in relation to a theoretical framework.

This study reports on the use of AOSC as an intervention to promote the conceptual use of new knowledge concerning eating and nutrition in nursing homes in Sweden, using the Promoting Action on Research Implementation in Health Sciences (PARiHS) framework as the explanatory theoretical model.

Aim. The aims were to explore nursing home staffs' views of participating in action-oriented study circles focused on eating and nutrition, to compare participants with non-participants, and to describe goals set by study circle participants.

2. Methods

In this study, both quantitative methods (structured questionnaires, comparisons between groups and over time) and qualitative methods (knowledge-to-action goals and focus group interviews) were used. The quantitative data focused on the content of the AOSC, the participants and non-participants self-evaluation of their knowledge about eating and nutrition, and on how they thought the management acted upon ideas regarding food and mealtimes. The qualitative methods were used to explore nursing home staffs' views of participating in AOSC and to capture the knowledge-to-action goals set by the study circle participants.

2.1. Description of the Project as a Whole. The project as a whole is built up by one all-embracing "knowledge-to-action process" [5] as well as by smaller action processes within each study circle. The knowledge-to-action process described in this study is based on Graham et al. [5]. First of all, the problems with nutrition were identified by a large survey of nutritional status and nutritional care in 2005, capturing the care gap [29]. Following this, a study circle manual, with reference to relevant literature, was developed [30]. Thus, based on the manual, as well as on the findings from the survey in 2005, the identified knowledge was adapted to the local context by the participants in AOSC. In addition, each study circle had the possibility to further adapt the knowledge to their particular setting. Barriers to using the knowledge were continuously assessed by regular evaluations and through dialogues with the front-line staff. Within each study circle, interventions were selected, tailored, and implemented to promote the use of knowledge (i.e., implement the change). The instrumental use of

TABLE 1: Number of study circles and participants every six months.

Period	Number of study circles	Number of participants
Spring 2006	6	49
Autumn 2006	11	92
Spring 2007	14	111
Autumn 2007	7	63
Spring 2008	12	109
Autumn 2008	21	168
Total	71	592

knowledge was monitored in 2007, by repeating the survey of nutritional status and nutritional care, and comparing findings with baseline data from 2005 [2]. The conceptual use of knowledge was monitored every six months (during the two years in which the study circles were going on). To evaluate whether sustained instrumental knowledge use was achieved, a final survey (with the same methodology as in 2005 and 2007) was conducted in 2009 [3].

2.2. This Study. The focus of this study was the conceptual use of knowledge. In order to evaluate the process of change and the important ingredients in that process, both qualitative and quantitative methods were used, that is, focus group interviews and questionnaires. Wallin [7] states that qualitative research is particularly helpful in uncovering why something happens and in identifying the active ingredients of an intervention. Further, Titler [31] advocates using "natural experiments," in the study of KT, as it makes it possible to capture "real world" initiatives that otherwise are not feasible to investigate or would be too costly [31].

2.3. Sample. The study involved 24 nursing homes (with one to nine units in each nursing home) and three home care areas. The number of participants from each nursing home or home care area was in median 24 (range 6–74 participants).

This study describes the results from three to some extent overlapping samples:

(A) Participants ($n = 592$) in all study circles (71 study circles, about 8 participants/AOSC) continuously evaluated their experiences (structured questionnaires) (during spring 2006 till autumn 2008) (Table 1). The target group for the study circles was front-line staff working in the nursing homes (long-term care facilities) as well as staff working in the kitchens (Table 2).

(B) AOSC participants ($n = 74$) and AOSC non-participants ($n = 115$), staff working in nursing homes attending an education day (spring 2007) with focus on eating and nutrition. Thus, the non-participants were those that no yet had been involved in AOSC but were attending the education day.

(C) At the end of the project period (December 2008), a focus group interview was carried out with project leaders ($n = 2$), study circle leaders ($n = 5$), both leader and participant ($n = 1$), and participants ($n = 4$) (in total $n = 12$). The managers contacted the previous AOSC participants and asked if they would like to participate in the focus group.

TABLE 2: Characteristics of participants and their evaluation of the study circles.

	$n = 592$
Age, mean (SD)	45.2 (10.0)
Gender, men/women, %	4/96
Profession, %	
Auxiliary nurses or nursing assistants	80
Cook, kitchen helpers	12
Registered nurses	3
Team head, students, dietician	3
Home care, auxiliary nurses	2
Number of years in current workplace, %	
Less than one year	2
One to five years	14
Six to ten years	18
Eleven to fifteen years	6
Sixteen to twenty years	16
More than twenty years	44
Content–interesting, %	
Very interesting	42
Interesting	56
Neither nor	2
Fairly/totally uninteresting	0
Content–relevant, %	
Very relevant	33
Relevant	61
Somewhat relevant	6
Not very/not at all relevant	0
Level of difficulty, %	
Very difficult	0
Difficult	1
Neither difficult nor easy	46
Easy	46
Very easy	7

2.4. Intervention: Action Oriented Study Circles. Inspired by Kitson and colleagues' [12] ideas about the three key elements (evidence, context and facilitation) for a successful implementation of evidence and knowledge into practice, the AOSC intervention is here described.

2.4.1. Evidence. A manual for the study circles was developed by Elisabet Rothenberg and the author of this paper (AW) [30]. Six themes were discussed: (1) the importance of food for the care recipient, (2) difficulties with eating, (3) routines, tools and responsibility, (4) food as medicine, (5) food hygiene and (6) when the mealtime becomes a question of life and death. In the manual, references were made to chapters in two books from the National Food Administration [32, 33], as well as to scientifically based texts online written by researchers in the field. Besides this, the staff also had access to results from the survey of nutritional status and care done in 2005 [29].

The pedagogical method included the identification of specific nutritionally related problems that the participants decided to discuss and a brainstorming session about ways to solve the problem in their own context, at their own unit. A structured plan of action was developed in order to achieve the necessary changes, bridging the gap between knowledge and care. The participants were encouraged to use the power of the group to achieve the changes. More than one study circle could be held at each unit.

2.4.2. Facilitation. The facilitation that was provided can mainly be considered "holistic," that is, sustained and enabled personal development and system transformation [12]. External facilitation was provided by the project leaders for the study circle intervention and the management. The project leaders coordinated the circles and evaluated them regularly (every six months). They also ordered and distributed the material and had discussions with politicians and managers. The project leaders were not involved in the study circles but could be invited to the groups for discussions. The intervention was supported by the management. Thus, managers ensured that the staff got time to prioritise the study circles. Internal facilitation was provided by the study circle leaders, who acted as facilitators for the participants.

The role of the study circle leader was to administer the circles, facilitate discussions, and ensure that the participants focused on the issues. The study circle leader did not need to be an expert in the focused field. As Strombeck ([20] page 10) states, "the function of the leader is to help promote a positive environment in which participants are encouraged to analyze, discuss and critically examine what they have read." The study circle leaders were provided training in their forthcoming role. Before the first six months of study circles the leaders were given half a day of training, and after the six-month evaluation, it was decided that the new leaders should be given a full day of training. In addition, it was decided after six months that the management should work towards recruiting homogenous groups (persons from the same nursing home and ward) instead of having the groups be heterogeneous (persons from different nursing homes and wards), and that instead of having six meetings that last for one and a half-hour each, there should be three meetings that last for three hours each. Thus, most (about 65) of the AOSC had three meetings that lasted for three hours each.

Based on the study circle manual and related references, the individuals made decisions about the value, usefulness, and appropriateness of the particular knowledge to their settings and circumstances. The topic area, the particular knowledge to implement, was agreed upon (local consensus) in each study circle and arose from the awareness that there was a need to improve the older persons' experiences from mealtimes and outcomes relating to nutrition. Each of the study circle teams was required to define the problem, work on how to create a potential for change, and then hopefully improve the older persons' experiences and outcomes. Thus, they tailored or customised the knowledge to their particular context. What knowledge to implement could vary from circle to circle, and it was not at all stressed that they should focus on screening for undernutrition and on what measures to take for those who were at risk for undernutrition, that is, the outcomes measured in the previously mentioned two studies [2, 3] of which this study is a part.

2.5. Data Collection. Structured questionnaires after each study circle, focusing on content, level of difficulty [23], and knowledge were used (sample a). The participants retrospectively rated their knowledge, thus, they rated their knowledge before the intervention and after in the same questionnaire. Besides this, qualitative data regarding goals for quality improvements set within each study circle (n = 71) were collected.

In addition, a questionnaire was given to participants attending an education day (sample b). They filled in the questionnaire before the education began. Both staff that previously had been AOSC participants (n = 74) and staff that no yet had been involved in AOSC (n = 115) answered the questionnaire that focused on knowledge development and perception of management engagement.

Within the focus group (sample c), experiences from participating or leading study circles were discussed. The interview took three hours. Each participant gave written consent to participate and agreed to have the interview tape-recorded. The interview was transcribed verbatim and analysed using conventional and directed content analysis [34–36].

2.6. Analysis

2.6.1. Quantitative analysis. Parametric and non-parametric statistics were used depending on the level of data and based on unpaired comparisons between two groups. The following tests were applied: T-test, Chi-square test, Wilcoxon signed ranks test, and Mann Whitney U test. The level of statistical significance was set at P-value < 0.05. Analyses were performed using PASW Statistics 18.0.

2.6.2. Qualitative analysis. Conventional (latent and manifest) and directed content analysis was chosen as the method of analysis for the focus group interviews in order to clarify deeper or latent meanings in the text [34, 36]. Both manifest and latent content analysis include an interpretation of the text material, although both vary with regard to interpretation depth and abstraction level [35].

The text was read several times in order to gain an overall understanding. On the basis of the first readings, distinguished patterns emerged from the texts. These patterns made up the first results: "the naive understanding". These first thoughts and reflections on the text contents were

Table 3: Study circle participants' ($n = 592$) retrospective self-evaluation of their knowledge development.

	Study circles		
	Before, %	After, %	P-value
Knowledge, %			
I have sufficient/great knowledge	72	96	<0.0005[(1)]
I feel insecure whether my knowledge is sufficient or not	25	3	
I do not have sufficient knowledge	3	1	

[(1)] Wilcoxon signed ranks test.

recorded in the margins and were used continuously during the remaining stages of the analysis. Step-by-step, the material was analysed with the aim of the study in mind. "Meaning units" were then identified, that is, assertions from the contents of the text. Meaning units with similar content were organised into different areas (categories) with the study aim in focus. The meaning units were condensed (the sentences were shortened while preserving the core) [34]. Subcategories were created for sorting out the analysed material. At the last stage, the subcategories were linked together into two main categories that in turn were linked to a core category. Afterwards, the concepts from the PARiHS framework [12] were deduced to the qualitative findings (directed content analysis) [36]. Categories at different levels were ordered in relation to *Evidence*, *Context*, *Facilitation* and *Successful Implementation*.

2.7. Ethics. The ethics for conducting scientific work were followed. This study was approved in each municipality. The respondents were asked for informed consent. Both verbal and written information were given and respondents were guaranteed confidentiality (no personal identification numbers or names were collected). Within the focus group, each participant gave written consent to participate and agreed to have the interview tape recorded. As the study was part of an overall quality development project, no formal approval by an ethical committee was required, according to the Swedish Act concerning the Ethical Review of Research Involving Humans [37].

3. Results

3.1. All Study Circles. During three years (2006–2008), 592 persons from 24 nursing homes participated in the study circles, according to the filled-in and returned questionnaires. There were 71 study circles in total with an average of eight persons per circle (Table 1).

566 women (96%) and 26 men (4%) participated, with a mean age of 45 years (min 20, max 66, q1–q3 39–51 years). The most common profession participating in study circles was auxiliary nurses or nursing assistants (80%). Most participants had been working in their current line of work for more than 20 years (Table 2).

The most common combination of staff in each circle was one person working in the kitchen, who usually also was the circle leader, and seven auxiliary nurses or nursing assistants. The staff members attending each study circle usually came from the same unit, except during the first six months of study circles (six study circles).

3.1.1. Evidence and Knowledge. Of those attending the study circles, 98% regarded the content as interesting/very interesting, 94% thought that it was relevant/very relevant and 92% considered that the difficulty level was easy/neither difficult or easy (Table 2).

When participants retrospectively rated their knowledge about food and nutrition before and after having participated in the study circle, there was a significant improvement. Before the study circle, 72% stated that they had sufficient or great knowledge and afterwards 96% stated the same thing (Table 3).

3.1.2. Action Orientation Goals for Quality Improvement. The action orientation of the study circles included the identification of specific nutritionally related problems that the participants decided to discuss and brainstorm in order to find ways to solve the problem in their own context, at their own unit. A structured plan of action was developed by the participants in order to achieve the necessary changes. Thus, each study circle worked with setting goals to work towards within each group's workplace. These goals could be grouped into environment, food, hygiene, routines, shortening overnight fast, the ability to choose, and cooperation (Table 4).

3.2. Comparisons between Those Participating and Those Not

3.2.1. Facilitation and Knowledge. In total 189 structured questionnaires were returned during the education day and it is unclear how many did not answer them. There were no differences in age, gender, or in number of years in current workplace between AOSC participants and non-participants. However, there was a significant difference in professions, with more cook/kitchen helpers and less registered nurses among the AOSC participants (Table 5).

More among those who had participated than among those who had not participated in the study circles agreed totally/partly that the management was engaged in and took care of ideas regarding food and mealtimes (80% and 66%, P-value = 0.009). In addition, more of those who had participated in study circles than among those who had not felt that they had great or sufficient knowledge about the field (69% versus 63%, P-value = 0.044) (Table 5).

Table 4: Knowledge-to-action goals set within study circles focusing on eating and nutrition.

Goal category	Example of focus
Mealtime environment	Create a homelike environment Bake at the unit, fragrance impressions from food, tease the appetite Create a calm atmosphere in the dining room
Food	Offer alternatives to oral supplements Spices on the table Individually adapted food and consistencies
Hygiene	Be careful with hand hygiene Keep cold food cold and warm food warm (check temperature) Improve mouth care
Routines	Ask newly admitted about food habits Control weight for those moving in and continually Inform substitute staff about goals and routines
Shorten the overnight fast	Offer evening coffee/tea/sandwich Postpone evening meal Have night staff offer sandwich and milk
The ability to choose	Have the residents serve themselves food Have the residents choose between different dishes Offer the residents assistance to go to the dining room
Cooperation	Improve cooperation between kitchen, registered nurses and other professions

3.3. Focus Group Interview. The analysis of the focus group interview with project leaders ($n = 2$, one man and one woman), circle leaders ($n = 5$, all women of whom two worked in kitchen), and participants ($n = 4$, all women) in the study circles resulted in one core category: "nutritional knowledge translation expressed as *going from feeding to serving*." This was the most concluding description of what was achieved. This core category captures an awareness that includes both the meaning of the mealtime environment, being together, and staff that is service minded, lays the table and presents the food in an appealing way. It also captures the two categories that it was built up from (Table 5).

(i) Socioculturally Mediated knowledge spread.

(ii) Facilitation of knowledge spread and sustainability

3.3.1. Socio-Cultural Mediated Knowledge Spread. The main impression from this category was that the socio-culturally mediated knowledge spread contributed to a shared vision among the staff. This category was built up from three subcategories (Table 6).

(i) Together and from the same place we are stronger.

(ii) Getting together broadens one's perspective and improves the work atmosphere.

(iii) Through discussions, the gap between knowledge and practice can be bridged.

The participants expressed both that one person achieves less change than many and that one study circle achieves less change than many. "One swallow does not make a summer" can here be used as a metaphor (developed by the researcher) to illustrate that one single person who attends a training was described as having difficulties in achieving changes in the workplace. Staff members say that attending a training day as the only representative from their workplace made it difficult to gain interest and understanding for what they had learned and what they wanted to change. It became clear that the staff experienced the study circle as the superior method, since it meant that several persons from the same setting came together and discussed and set goals that were adapted to their own workplace, their own context. In addition, many participants expressed a preference for homogenous groups rather than heterogeneous groups. Study circles with participants from different workplaces made it difficult for participants to mutually agree on the same goals, and more difficult to communicate the goals to their own workplace. Furthermore, "rings on the water" can be used as a metaphor to say that the more study circles that had taken place at the same workplace, the greater was the possibility of achieving positive changes. To summarise, "together and from the same place we are stronger."

Broadening one's perspective signifies that the participants in the study circles experienced a greater understanding for each other and each other's work tasks, saw new dimensions of their work, and communicated more with each other. The understanding between the staff improved, especially between those working in the ward and those working in the kitchen. The work atmosphere improved.

The participants felt that the gap between knowledge and practice could be bridged through the discussions in the study circles. The ward culture and personal engagement were thought to have improved as a consequence of the knowledge-focused discussions between colleagues. The staff

TABLE 5: Comparisons between staff members who had participated in study circles ($n = 74$) and those not ($n = 115$).

	Study circles		
	Non-participants, $n = 115$	Participants, $n = 74$	P-value
Age, mean (SD)	45.7 (9.7)	47.5 (10.0)	0.241⁽¹⁾
Gender, men/women %	3/97	6/94	0.286⁽²⁾
Profession, %			<0.0005⁽²⁾
Auxiliary nurses or nursing assistants	75	86	
Cook, kitchen helpers	0	11	
Registered nurses	20	3	
Home care, auxiliary nurses	5	0	
Number of years in current workplace, %			0.677⁽³⁾
Less than one year	3	0	
One to five years	13	8	
Six to ten years	15	16	
Eleven to fifteen years	12	16	
Sixteen to twenty years	10	11	
More than twenty years	47	49	
Knowledge, %			0.044⁽³⁾
I have sufficient/great knowledge	63	69	
I feel insecure whether my knowledge is sufficient or not	33	31	
I do not have sufficient knowledge	4	0	
The management is engaged in and takes into account ideas regarding food and mealtimes, %			0.009⁽³⁾
Completely/partly agree	66	80	
Can't decide	23	10	
Completely/partly disagree	11	10	

(1) t-test.
(2) Chi-square test.
(3) Mann Whitney U test.

felt that they had gained a deeper knowledge about food and mealtimes, knowledge that was based on evidence and the groups' experiences, and not only on the individuals' own experiences. They also said that they had changed their attitudes regarding the food, from being negative to being more positive. The food and mealtime was regarded more and more important. In addition, they described how incorrect routines or a negative ward culture could be improved through relearning.

3.3.2. Facilitation of Knowledge Spread and Sustainability. The category "facilitation of knowledge spread and sustainability" was built up from three subcategories (Table 6):

(i) action-oriented goals

(ii) facilitation by anchoring and feedback

(iii) facilitation of sustainability

It was seen as valuable to set and evaluate goals within the study circles. At wards where there had been many study circles, it became, in the end, difficult to set new goals. Participants also described different ways of making the staff more aware of the goals, for instance, to write down all goals in a document that was framed and hung in a place where everyone could see it. Staff members also talked about how they informed new staff and substitutes about the goals. Many improvements were also described as being an effect of the set goals, improvements that for instance meant a calmer and more homelike mealtime environment, and better measuring and followup of weight, and so forth.

Facilitation by anchoring and feedback of results was seen as important. A lot of information and persuasion were required in order to make the management understand the importance of the study circles. When management got feedback of the results from each six-month evaluation, their motivation to support and back up the intervention increased.

Table 6: Inductive results structured into core category, categories, subcategories, and quotations (different quotations are separated by a slash). The PARiHS (Promoting Action on Research Implementation in Health Sciences) framework deduced to the inductive results.

Core category	Categories	Subcategories	Quotations	PARiHS framework
Nutritional knowledge translation expressed as "going from feeding to serving"[(a)]	Socioculturally mediated knowledge spread	Together and from the same place we are stronger	After training, when you come back, usually alone, it is hard to get people to listen. It is difficult to adapt the new knowledge to your own workplace. / . . .initially, we had one participant from each unit, then with participants from the same unit, there was an enormous difference. / If you carry out one study circle at a unit, then you might achieve some things, but it is when the second study circle is formed that you can really achieve changes.	Context
		Getting together broadens one's perspective and improves the work atmosphere	People have a greater understanding for one another, are more open, and feel free to ask questions about different things. One broadens one's views, one can actually do things differently, if you don't try–nothing happens.	Context
		Through discussions, the gap between knowledge and practice can be bridged	You get a new perspective, think differently than before./ I would absolutely not want to have missed this time, never in my life, I have learned so much that I can make use of. / We will try to figure out everything that we can do, instead of focusing on things we can't do. / A culture can develop that is not justified.	Evidence
	Facilitation of knowledge spread and sustainability	Action-oriented goals	The study circles have been goal-directed, it is easier to explain to the others together what to do. / These documents stating goals. . .they have led to so many changes at the units. / There is cooperation between all of us: team manager, staff, kitchen, and the actual health care. Everyone works towards the same goal: we have a human being who we want to feel well, and it is our job to do what we can to make it possible.	Evidence
		Facilitation by anchoring and feedback	There has been a lot of persuasion, and a lot of marketing. . .geared towards team managers and the management group. Then there are the politicians as well.	Facilitation
		Facilitation of sustainability	We have put in a lot of work on this and we have to make sure that it continues even though the study circles end. / It is not supposed to end just because the three years have passed, it is a process that is supposed to continue. / Yes, it is easy to fall back into old habits. . .there should perhaps be some sort of follow-up. / Finally, we have made a dent at the shortcomings we have had, and now we will continue forward.	Facilitation

[(a)] "Successful implementation" is deduced using the PARiHS framework. The idea for labelling this core category stemmed from an actual statement in the focus group interview, "we are thinking more in terms of service, it is not a matter of feeding anymore."

Facilitation of sustainability in order to maintain and achieve new improvements in practice was mainly focused on the time after finishing the project. It was clear from the focus group interviews that both the study circle participants and the leaders wanted to maintain and further develop the improvements that were initiated or achieved from the study circles. Suggestions were put forward regarding how the work could be continued, for instance, by discussing food and mealtimes at workplace meetings and to continue with study circles for those who had still not participated in any (Table 6).

3.4. Directed Content Analysis. The deductive/directed content analysis, using the PARiHS framework, of the findings from the conventional/inductive analysis showed that the category "socio-culturally mediated knowledge spread" related to the components context and evidence, while the category "Facilitation of knowledge spread and sustainability" was related to the two categories facilitation and evidence. The core category "nutritional knowledge translation expressed as *going from feeding to serving*" was considered to manifest successful implementation.

4. Discussion

Study circles focusing on eating and nutrition were found to have a positive effect on learning and the workplace context (conceptual use of knowledge). In an earlier study, the study circle intervention was shown to also have positive effects on nutritional care and on care recipients' nutritional status (instrumental knowledge use) [2, 3]. The study circle intervention seems to give quality improvements leading to professional development (learning), better system performance (care), and better patient outcomes (health), by integrating evidence, context, and facilitation in the efforts to achieve KT.

Different methods were used to evaluate the effects of study circles. In some cases, the findings from using one method were confirmed by using another method. For instance, through the focus group interview some results found through the quantitative continuous evaluations were confirmed. This can be considered a methodological strength. It could be seen as a shortcoming that the results are based on the staff's self-reflections, for instance, when it comes to reflecting on one's own knowledge development retrospectively. Anyhow, this result was indirectly confirmed when comparing the results of those who had participated in the intervention and those who had not, and it was confirmed by the focus group interviews. Another example of what could be studied more directly is the improvements related to the working place context, for instance better working routines and work atmosphere. However, staff members are a part of and create the working place context, and their views are important to capture. In addition, some actual improvements in the provided care were described in the previous studies [2, 3]. Even so, it seems worthwhile to conduct more studies directly focusing on the actual interaction between team members and between staff and care recipients during an intervention with study circles.

In the efforts to achieve a successful implementation, it is of utmost importance to consider the context and the power of teamwork. This was evident in several ways in the results, not the least in the category "socio-culturally mediated knowledge spread." Thus, the systematic implementation of study circles creates a favourable context, including workplace climate, that also leads to a more positive view among management and staff of what the circles can achieve for individuals, for the team, and for the care recipients.

Improving teamwork is not easily achieved by traditional methods, and single interventions have limited impact in KT [38, 39]. In this study, using multifaceted interventions, it was found that skills were developed within the study circles, by the teams, and that this in time could develop the overall capacity of the organisation, allowing further improvements. In a study by Zeitz et al. [40], it was found that the complexity behind the so-called "simple care" (providing warm drinks, appetizing food, energy enriched food, and oral supplements) relied on the active management and broader transformation of the system. In order to achieve improvements in such pragmatic issues as giving care recipients good nutrition, organisational aspects had to be tackled, such as teamwork, communication processes, and organisational and individual values and beliefs [40]. When using AOSC as an intervention method, it is important to have homogenous groups and to understand that more study circles in the same workplace can possibly lead to better transformation of the system. AOSC seems to be an optimal pedagogical method that gives priority to the context in order to achieve KT. These conceptual outcomes of KT are most likely generalizable also to other care settings implementing AOSC with focus on nutrition and eating.

The focus on eating and nutrition, and the fact that the staff came together in the study circles, contributed to competence development and led to positive outcomes. Overall, participants experienced a high degree of satisfaction through participating in the study circles. This could be attributed to the format of the study circle, which provided the opportunity for participants to engage in sustained and meaningful discussions about eating and nutrition. It might, however, come as a surprise that the work atmosphere improved through an intervention focusing on improving nutritional care. There could be at least two reasons for this: first of all that the staff came together from the same workplace, and secondly that the focus was on eating and nutrition. In another study, "food" seemed to be a medium through which other themes were discussed, for example respect, teamwork, communication and redesigning systems of care delivery [40]. Thus, the successful conceptual outcome could be due to both the AOSC and the actual focus within these, that is, an integration of context and evidence. This might in turn strengthen the fact that the directed content analysis connected both the PARiHS concept context and evidence to the category "socio-culturally mediated knowledge spread". Also, Gougoulakis [15] states in a thesis that learning in study circles is socio-culturally conditioned—knowledge is created and grows in the meeting and communication with others in study circles. In this perspective, knowledge is not something that is only registered. Instead, it is developed in collaboration, relates to the participants' context, and a propitious learning atmosphere that comes about when participants have an exchange without competition [15].

By attending study circles, individuals felt that they developed their competence. This became apparent in several ways. For instance, when staff retrospectively self-rated their knowledge, before and after attending the study circles, a significant improvement was indicated. In addition, the participants in the SC considered their knowledge more sufficient than what non-participants rated. Thus, in study circles a socio-culturally mediated knowledge spread, including collaborative learning, takes place that can form the basis for KT and quite likely a successful implementation of evidence.

In order to be successful in the KT, staff needed support from project leaders, management, and from trained circle leaders. The intervention needed to be anchored in the management and the management received feedback that in turn made them more eager to support the intervention. Anchoring and feedback (every six months) was provided by the project leaders. Both quantitative and qualitative findings support the need for facilitation. Participants experienced that the management was engaged in and took care of ideas regarding food and mealtimes to a greater extent than what the non-participants experienced. In addition, the need for facilitation was evident in the category "facilitation of knowledge spread and sustainability." In addition, the staff needed facilitation from the circle leaders. A full-day training in the study circle leader role was effective in helping them to get the group to focus on the tasks for the circle, which in turn most likely enhanced learning in the group.

There were no experts involved in the study circles, which might have contributed to the high degree of satisfaction, as the power was evenly distributed between participants and symmetric relationships emerged, corresponding to Piaget's ideas about "cooperative relations" [17]. Participants also found it important that kitchen staff attended the study circles. This contributed to better communication between staff at the unit and staff working in the kitchen. From a project leader perspective, there needed to be a balance between structuring the process of study circles and enabling teams to maintain ownership and control. It might be that if the study circles had a more explicit focus on nutritional screening and management of residents with nutritional risk, the instrumental outcomes would have been even better than found in previous studies [2, 3]. However, this could be at the cost of conceptual outcomes, that is, understanding, knowledge, and attitudes. Correspondingly, not only improvements in knowledge but also in the perception of how work was carried out, in the view of care recipients, working atmosphere and cooperation were described.

The study circle participants and leaders wanted to continue the work, and felt that the work had only just begun—similarly to what was found in a study by Wiechula et al. [39]. Thus, facilitation was emphasised to continue also after the intervention period. also it most likely did continue to some extent, as some positive instrumental outcomes (provision of energy enriched food and/or oral supplements) were seen also one year after the project ended [3]. Thus, facilitation from different levels in the organisation, together with regular evaluations and feedback from project leaders, is likely to contribute to a "learning organisation", and it needs to continue also after the project has been completed. In the concept "a learning organisation" the two PARiHS concepts facilitation and evidence get connected, as it is also evident in the category "facilitation of knowledge spread and sustainability" found in this study.

By making the study circles action oriented, several positive effects are achieved. Besides the findings in this paper, also a few earlier studies have shown positive effects, both in the care provided and for the care recipients [2, 3, 28]. The PARiHS framework can be used to understand the interactions and complexities involved in KT activity. The positive changes achieved can possibly be attributed to the fact that complex interventions were developed in the study circles that fit the local contexts. Melding and implementing evidence involves negotiation and shared understanding [12]. In addition, the need to consider the context in order to achieve quality improvements as emphasised by Kitson and colleagues [12] is supported by the findings from this study.

5. Conclusions

KT in nursing homes is a complex and challenging activity. Through action-oriented study circles, priority is given to the staff's experiences, feelings, values and beliefs, and teamwork when striving towards quality improvements. Knowledge to action is achieved through socio-culturally mediated knowledge spread, including collaborative learning, and through facilitation of knowledge spread and sustainability in a learning organisation.

The study circle seems to be an outstanding pedagogical method for getting staff in care and service from the same unit, in the same context, to focus on a specific knowledge area. By making study circles action oriented, several positive effects can be achieved for the staff's learning, team collaboration, care provision, and most importantly, for the care recipients' health. The findings from this study have implications for other care settings implementing AOSC with focus on eating and nutrition.

Conflict of Interests

The author declares that no Conflict of interests.

Acknowledgments

The author (A. Westergren) is supported by the Swedish Research Council and the Skåne County Council's Research and Development Foundation. The study circle intervention was supported by the "competence ladder," a government investment in competence improvement for staff in social service. The author gives special thanks to the Swedish Institute for Health Sciences (Vårdalinstitutet) for the support in the development of the study circle manual focusing on eating and nutrition. A. Westergren would like to thank the residents and the staff, teachers and students for their cooperation. The study was conducted in cooperation with the Network for Eating and Nutrition in North-East Skåne (NEN-NES, founded in 2003 by the author), research group PRO-CARE (Patient Reported Outcomes—Clinical Assessment Research and Education), and research platform Health in Collaboration at Kristianstad University. Also he gives special thanks to Professor Alison Kitson for the valuable input on earlier papers and to the Swedish house in Kavalla, Greece.

References

[1] A. Westergren, C. Wann-Hansson, E. B. Börgdal et al., "Malnutrition prevalence and precision in nutritional care differed in relation to hospital volume ? A cross-sectional survey," *Nutrition Journal*, vol. 8, no. 1, article 20, 2009.

[2] A. Westergren, C. Axelsson, P. Lilja-Andersson, C. Lindholm, K. Petersson, and K. Ulander, "Study circles improve the precision in nutritional care in special accommodations," *Food and Nutrition Research*, vol. 53, no. 1, pp. 1–8, 2009.

[3] A. Westergren and G. Hedin, "Do study circles and a nutritional care policy improve nutritional care in a short- and long-term perspective in special accommodations?" *Food and Nutrition Research*, vol. 54, no. 1, 2010.

[4] C. A. Estabrooks, L. Wallin, and M. Milner, "Measuring knowledge utilization in health care," *International Journal of Policy Evaluation & Management*, vol. 1, no. 3, pp. 3–36, 2003.

[5] I. D. Graham, J. Logan, M. B. Harrison et al., "Lost in knowledge translation: time for a map?" *The Journal of Continuing Education in the Health Professions*, vol. 26, no. 1, pp. 13–24, 2006.

[6] C. A. Estabrooks, "Prologue: a program of research in knowledge translation," *Nursing Research*, vol. 56, no. 4, supplement, pp. S4–S6, 2007.

[7] L. Wallin, "Knowledge translation and implementation research in nursing," *International Journal of Nursing Studies*, vol. 46, no. 4, pp. 576–587, 2009.

[8] M. Eccles, J. Grimshaw, A. Walker, M. Johnston, and N. Pitts, "Changing the behavior of healthcare professionals: the use of theory in promoting the uptake of research findings," *Journal of Clinical Epidemiology*, vol. 58, no. 2, pp. 107–112, 2005.

[9] I. D. Graham and J. Logan, "Innovations in knowledge transfer and continuity of care," *Canadian Journal of Nursing Research*, vol. 36, no. 2, pp. 89–103, 2004.

[10] I. D. Graham and J. Tetroe, "Whither knowledge translation: an international research agenda," *Nursing Research*, vol. 56, no. 4, supplement, pp. S86–S88, 2007.

[11] R. P. T. M. Grol, M. C. Bosch, M. E. J. L. Hulscher, M. P. Eccles, and M. Wensing, "Planning and studying improvement in patient care: the use of theoretical perspectives," *Milbank Quarterly*, vol. 85, no. 1, pp. 93–138, 2007.

[12] A. L. Kitson, J. Rycroft-Malone, G. Harvey, B. McCormack, K. Seers, and A. Titchen, "Evaluating the successful implementation of evidence into practice using the PARiHS framework: theoretical and practical challenges," *Implementation Science*, vol. 3, no. 1, article 1, 2008.

[13] G. Harvey, A. Loftus-Hills, J. Rycroft-Malone et al., "Getting evidence into practice: the role and function of facilitation," *Journal of Advanced Nursing*, vol. 37, no. 6, pp. 577–588, 2002.

[14] T. J. Schultz and A. L. Kitson, "Measuring the context of care in an Australian acute care hospital: a nurse survey," *Implementation Science*, vol. 5, no. 1, article 60, 2010.

[15] P. Gougoulakis, *The Study Circle: Lifelong Learning-in Swedish*, Stockholm Institute of Education , HLS förl, Stockholm, Sweden, 2001.

[16] H. Daniels, *An Introduction to Vygotsky*, Routledge, London, UK, 1996.

[17] R. DeVries, "Piaget's social theory," *Educational Researcher*, vol. 26, no. 2, pp. 4–17, 1997.

[18] L. O. Dahle, J. Brynhildsen, M. B. Fallsberg, I. Rundquist, and M. Hammar, "Pros and cons of vertical integration between clinical medicine and basic science within a problem-based undergraduate medical curriculum: examples and experiences from Linköping, Sweden," *Medical Teacher*, vol. 24, no. 3, pp. 280–285, 2002.

[19] S. Toohey, *Society for Research into Higher Education: Designing Courses for Higher Education*, Open University Press, Buckingham, UK, 1999.

[20] R. Strombeck, "The Swedish study circle—possibilities for application to health education in the United States," *Health Education Research*, vol. 6, no. 1, pp. 7–17, 1991.

[21] I. Dahn, "Let health education become adult education," *Landstingsvärlden*, vol. 3, pp. 16–17, 1987.

[22] A.-M. Landtblom, C. Lang, and G. Flensner, "The study circle as a tool in multiple sclerosis patient education in Sweden," *Patient Preference and Adherence Patient Preference and Adherence*, vol. 2, pp. 225–232, 2008.

[23] Vårdalinstitutet, The Swedish Institute for Health Sciences, 2010, http://www.vardalinstitutet.net/.

[24] E. Sönnerberg, L. Edgren, and L. Welin, "The Patient role in a changing world. Follow-up of a study circle for diabetes patients," *Vård i Norden*, vol. 4, pp. 38–41, 2001 (Swedish).

[25] A. Sarkadi and U. Rosenqvist, "Study circles at the pharmacy—a new model for diabetes education in groups," *Patient Education and Counseling*, vol. 37, no. 1, pp. 89–96, 1999.

[26] W. Jansson, B. Almberg, M. Grafstrom, and B. Winblad, "The Circle Model—support for relatives of people with dementia," *International Journal of Geriatric Psychiatry*, vol. 13, no. 10, pp. 674–681, 1998.

[27] K. A. Forsberg, T. Björkman, P. O. Sandman, and M. Sandlund, "Physical health—a cluster randomized controlled lifestyle intervention among persons with a psychiatric disability and their staff," *Nordic Journal of Psychiatry*, vol. 62, no. 6, pp. 486–495, 2008.

[28] K. Wikby, A. C. Ek, and L. Christensson, "Implementation of a nutritional programme in elderly people admitted to resident homes," *Scandinavian Journal of Caring Sciences*, vol. 23, no. 3, pp. 421–430, 2009.

[29] A. Westergren, C. Lindholm, C. Axelsson, and K. Ulander, "Prevalence of eating difficulties and malnutrition among persons within hospital care and special accommodations," *Journal of Nutrition, Health and Aging*, vol. 12, no. 1, pp. 39–43, 2008.

[30] Vårdalinstitutet, *Study Plan for Study Circles with Focus on Nutrition and Eating*, 2005.

[31] M. G. Titler, "Methods in translation science.," *Worldviews on Evidence-Based Nursing*, vol. 1, no. 1, pp. 38–48, 2004.

[32] B. Karlström and M. Andersen, *Food and Nutritional Treatment for Elderly People: Problems and Possibilities*, Statens Livsmedelsverk, Uppsala, Sweden, 1998.

[33] U. Nilsson-Balknäs and M. Andersen, *Food and Nutrition for Sick People in Care and Service*, Statens Livsmedelsverk, Uppsala, Sweden, 2003.

[34] B. Berg, *Qualitative Research Methods for Social Sciences*, 2001.

[35] U. H. Graneheim and B. Lundman, "Qualitative content analysis in nursing research: concepts, procedures and measures to achieve trustworthiness," *Nurse Education Today*, vol. 24, no. 2, pp. 105–112, 2004.

[36] H. F. Hsieh and S. E. Shannon, "Three approaches to qualitative content analysis," *Qualitative Health Research*, vol. 15, no. 9, pp. 1277–1288, 2005.

[37] SFS, *The Act Concerning the Ethical Review of Research Involving Humans on the website of the Central Ethical Review Boards*, 2003.

[38] R. Robertson and K. Jochelson, *Interventions that Change Clinician Behaviour: Mapping the Literature*, The National Institute for Health and Clinical Excellence, London, UK, 2006.

[39] R. Wiechula, A. Kitson, D. Marcoionni, T. Page, K. Zeitz, and H. Silverston, "Improving the fundamentals of care for older people in the acute hospital setting: facilitating practice improvement using a Knowledge Translation Toolkit," *International Journal of Evidence-Based Healthcare*, vol. 7, no. 4, pp. 283–295, 2009.

[40] K. Zeitz, A. Kitson, H. Gibb et al., "Working together to improve the care of older people: a new framework for collaboration," *Journal of Advanced Nursing*, vol. 67, no. 1, pp. 43–55, 2011.

3

Which Part of a Short, Global Risk Assessment, the Risk Instrument for Screening in the Community, Predicts Adverse Healthcare Outcomes?

Rónán O'Caoimh,[1,2] Carol FitzGerald,[1] Una Cronin,[1] Anton Svendrovski,[3] Yang Gao,[1] Elizabeth Healy,[4] Elizabeth O'Connell,[5] Gabrielle O'Keeffe,[6] Eileen O'Herlihy,[1] Elizabeth Weathers,[1,7] Nicola Cornally,[1,7] Patricia Leahy-Warren,[7] Francesc Orfila,[8] Constança Paúl,[9] Roger Clarnette,[10] and D. William Molloy[1,2]

[1] *Centre for Gerontology and Rehabilitation, University College Cork, St. Finbarr's Hospital, Douglas Road, Cork, Ireland*
[2] *COLLAGE (Collaboration on Ageing), University College Cork, Cork City and Louth Age Friendly County Initiative, County Louth, Ireland*
[3] *UZIK Consulting Inc., 86 Gerrard Street E, Unit 12D, Toronto, ON, Canada M5B 2J1*
[4] *Centre for Public Health Nursing, Ballincollig and Bishopstown, County Cork, Ireland*
[5] *Centre for Public Health Nursing, Mahon and Ballintemple, Cork, Ireland*
[6] *Health Service Executive, South Lee, St. Finbarr's Hospital, Cork, Ireland*
[7] *School of Nursing & Midwifery, University College Cork, Brookfield Health Sciences Complex, College Road, Cork, Ireland*
[8] *Primary Healthcare University Research Institute, IDIAP Jordi Gol, Barcelona, Spain*
[9] *UNIFAI/ICBAS, Institute of Biomedical Sciences Abel Salazar, University of Porto, 4050-313 Porto, Portugal*
[10] *School of Medicine and Pharmacology, University of Western Australia, 35 Stirling Hwy, Crawley, WA 6009, Australia*

Correspondence should be addressed to Rónán O'Caoimh; rocaoimh@hotmail.com

Academic Editor: F. R. Ferraro

The Risk Instrument for Screening in the Community (RISC) is a short, global risk assessment to identify community-dwelling older adults' one-year risk of institutionalisation, hospitalisation, and death. We investigated the contribution that the three components of the RISC (*concern*, its *severity*, and the ability of the *caregiver network* to manage concern) make to the accuracy of the instrument, across its three domains (mental state, activities of daily living (ADL), and medical state), by comparing their accuracy to other assessment instruments in the prospective Community Assessment of Risk and Treatment Strategies study. RISC scores were available for 782 patients. Across all three domains each subtest more accurately predicted institutionalisation compared to hospitalisation or death. The *caregiver network's* ability to manage ADL more accurately predicted institutionalisation (AUC 0.68) compared to hospitalisation (AUC 0.57, $P = 0.01$) or death (AUC 0.59, $P = 0.046$), comparing favourably with the Barthel Index (AUC 0.67). The *severity* of ADL (AUC 0.63), medical state (AUC 0.62), Clinical Frailty Scale (AUC 0.67), and Charlson Comorbidity Index (AUC 0.66) scores had similar accuracy in predicting mortality. Risk of hospitalisation was difficult to predict. Thus, each component, and particularly the *caregiver network*, had reasonable accuracy in predicting institutionalisation. No subtest or assessment instrument accurately predicted risk of hospitalisation.

1. Introduction

Population ageing [1] is associated with rising numbers of frail and functionally impaired community-dwelling older adults [2]. As time is limited in clinical practice, short risk prediction instruments are useful in identifying frailty [3] and quantifying the potential for adverse healthcare outcomes in this population [4]. Traditionally, healthcare practitioners have used demographic details and a battery of cognitive and functional tests in an attempt to predict risk [5], triage patients and rationalize the provision of limited healthcare resources [4]. Although multiple measures of frailty exist; few have been tested for reliability or validity [6].

More recently, instruments to identify specific adverse outcomes have been developed. These include tools to measure the likelihood of hospitalisation [7], readmission [8], institutionalisation [9], and mortality [10], often within a defined period of time. Few have targeted risk of institutionalisation, an important marker of healthcare utilisation [11]. Institutionalisation in turn is associated with other adverse outcomes such as risk of death [12]. Identifying risk is important as it singles out those who may benefit from more intensive, targeted interventions [4]. Few instruments are available in the community to screen large numbers of patients quickly and in their own environment for risk of functional decline, while simultaneously measuring risk of hospitalisation, institutionalisation, and death.

The Risk Instrument for Screening in the Community (RISC) is a new, short [13, 14], reliable [15], and valid [16] global subjective assessment of risk, designed for use by community healthcare workers. It was developed as part of Irelands' European Innovation Project on Active and Healthy Ageing three-star reference site the COLLaboration on AGEing (COLLAGE) [17]; see the Community Assessment of Risk and Treatment Strategies (CARTS) study at http://www.collage-ireland.eu/. The RISC identifies the presence and severity of concern in three domains (mental state, ADL, and medical state) [14]. Based upon the ability of an individuals' caregiver network to manage the patients' care needs, the one-year risk of three adverse outcomes, hospitalisation, institutionalisation, and death, is scored according to the magnitude and likelihood of an event, from 1 (minimal and rare) to 5 (extreme and certain). Short, often single, question screens similar to this have been used successfully in other studies. These include the "surprise question" [18], an independent predictor of one-year mortality, validated in different patient groupings [19], and the "Yale-Brown" [20] and "down-hearted and blue?" [21] single depression questions. Similarly, a single question "is the patient frail?" correlates with the Clinical Frailty Scale [13].

The contribution that each part of the RISC contributes to the overall predictive validity of the tool is unknown. Given this, we sought to investigate which part of the RISC contributes to the sensitivity and specificity of the instrument and how the components of the RISC compare to a traditional battery of screening instruments and to identify the components of the RISC which predict each of the three adverse healthcare outcomes under consideration.

2. Materials and Methods

2.1. The Risk Instrument for Screening in the Community (RISC). The RISC collects demographic data and scores three domains: mental state, ADL (functional state), and medical state. Each has three components, called steps. The first step identifies whether there is a *concern* about this domain and is scored dichotomously (Yes/No). If there is no concern, the rater moves on to the next domain. If there is concern, the rater assesses the *severity* of the *concern* on a scale from one to three (mild, moderate, or severe). The ability of the *caregiver network* to manage the concern, within each domain, is then scored using a five-point Likert scale from 1 to 5 (1: can manage; 2: carer strain; 3: some gaps; 4: cannot manage; 5: absent/liability). The *caregiver network* includes the formal and informal resources and services that are available to the person. Finally, the *severity* of concern and the ability of the *caregiver network* are taken into account when completing the three global risk scores *of institutionalisation, hospitalisation,* and *death*, within one-year of assessment. These are also scored on a Likert scale from 1 (minimal/rare) to 5 (extremely likely/certain). In order to analyze the data, patients were subsequently divided into minimum (global risk score of 1 or 2) and maximum (global risk score of 3, 4, or 5) risk of each adverse healthcare outcome [14].

2.2. Patients. This study includes a secondary analysis of 803 patients included in the CARTS study. All patients were community-dwelling older adults, aged over 65 years. Only those recently reviewed and under long-term follow-up by their public health nurse (PHN) were included. The baseline characteristics of these patients have been published previously [13]. In summary, the median age of patients was 80 years (interquartile range 10) and 64% were females. Additional demographics and the results of a selection of cognitive and functional assessments were also available. The median Barthel Index (BI) score was 18 (+/−6), abbreviated mental test score (AMTS) [22] was ten (+/− <1), Charlson Comorbidity Index [23] score was one (+/− two), and the Clinical Frailty Scale (CFS) [24] was five (+/− two).

2.3. Data Collection and Sampling. The collection of data in the CARTS study has been described previously [13]. In summary, all PHN sectors in County Cork were invited to participate. Two, Ballincollig and Bishopstown and Mahon and Ballintemple, were the first respondents and were sampled based on the nonprobability method of convenience sampling using a quota method. All PHNs ($n = 15$) from these centres were trained and certified in scoring the RISC [15, 25]. Scoring was based on the PHNs knowledge of the patients. Each PHN only scored patients directly under their care. Demographic data were recorded from PHN records by a clinician blinded to the RISC scores. One year follow-up data on hospitalisation and death were obtained from the hospital in-patient enquiry system of all hospitals in Cork. Follow-up data on institutionalisation were obtained from the Cork Local Placement Forum. Ethical approval for the CARTS study was granted by the Clinical Research Ethics Committee of the Cork Teaching Hospitals and adhered to the tenants of Declaration of Helsinki.

2.4. Statistical Analysis. Data were analysed using SPSS version 20.0. Accuracy of components was determined from the AUC, calculated from receiver operating characteristic (ROC) curves. ROC scores above 0.50 indicated that the component had better predictive power than by chance alone. Nonoverlapping 95% confidence intervals (CI) suggested statistically significant differences between components.

Cronbach's alpha coefficient (α) and the intraclass correlation coefficient (ICC) measured internal consistency.

3. Results

One-year outcomes comparing the RISC to the CFS have been presented previously [16]. In summary, RISC scores were available for 782 with 21 missing as patients were lost to follow-up. At baseline, 88%, 64%, and 79% were scored as minimum risk for institutionalisation, hospitalisation, and death, respectively. At one year, the incidence of the three adverse outcomes were 10.2% for institutionalisation, 17.7% for hospitalisation (at least one), and 15.6% for death. The accuracy of the global risk score to predict the outcomes was higher for risk of institutionalisation (AUC of 0.70) and death (AUC of 0.70) than hospitalisation (AUC of 0.61). Patients scored as maximum risk of institutionalisation had a 31.3% incidence of admission to long-term care compared with 7.1% for patients scored as minimum risk. Those scoring maximum RISC had a 25.4% and 33.5% incidence of hospitalisation and death compared to 13.2% and 10.8% for minimum risk patients, respectively.

Internal consistency between the three domains of the RISC, assessed with Cronbach's alpha, was high ($\alpha = 0.72$) with scores above 0.7 indicating a high degree of reliability. The ICC, using one-way random effect model, was 0.68 (95% CI 0.61–0.70, $P < 0.001$), indicating a relatively high degree of agreement between the three domains of the RISC.

3.1. Components (Steps) of the RISC. Each step was examined to determine how accurately they predicted one-year outcomes. For the first step, assessing whether a *concern* was present or not, the AUC for predicting institutionalisation was 0.62 (95% CI: 0.55–0.69) for the mental state domain compared with 0.60 (95% CI: 0.54–0.66) for ADLs and 0.54 (95% CI: 0.48–0.61) for the medical state. *Concern* (Yes/No) on its own was a poor predictor of both hospitalisation and death, with all AUC values being less than 0.60 (see Table 1). The *severity* (mild, moderate, or severe) of each domain more accurately predicted institutionalisation compared to hospitalisation or death. The *severity* score of each domain was least accurate in predicting hospitalisation. The ability of the *caregiver network*, irrespective of domain assessed, more accurately predicted institutionalisation compared to the other adverse outcomes. The *caregiver networks'* ability to manage concern for ADL was significantly more accurate in predicting one-year risk of institutionalisation (AUC of 0.68, 95% CI: 0.62–0.74) compared to hospitalisation (AUC of 0.57, 95% CI: 0.52–0.63, $P = 0.01$) or death (AUC of 0.59, 95% CI: 0.53–0.65, $P = 0.046$). The *caregiver networks'* ability to manage mental and medical states predicted institutionalisation better than hospitalisation or death.

The AUC values for the global RISC scores, the caregiver components of the RISC, the CFS, the PHNs perception of frailty, and a battery of cognitive and functional instruments routinely collected by PHNs are presented in Table 2 and Figure 1. The global RISC scores most accurately predicted all three adverse outcomes. The *caregiver networks'* ability to manage ADLs (AUC of 0.68) had similar accuracy in identifying one-year risk of institutionalisation as the BI (AUC of 0.67, $P = 0.84$), the AMTS (AUC of 0.66, $P = 0.68$), and the CFS (AUC of 0.63, $P = 0.30$) but was significantly more accurate than the Charlson Comorbidity Index (AUC of 0.55, $P < 0.01$). The BI was significantly more accurate in predicting institutionalisation (AUC of 0.67 95% CI: 0.61–0.73, $P = 0.04$) and death (AUC of 0.65 95% CI: 0.60–0.71, $P \leq 0.05$) than hospitalisation (AUC of 0.58 95% CI: 0.50–0.61). The Charlson Comorbidity Index was a significantly more accurate predictor of death at one year (AUC of 0.66) than hospitalisation (AUC of 0.57), $P = 0.02$. The AMTS was only accurate for predicting institutionalisation (AUC of 0.66).

4. Discussion

This study describes the relationship between the components of the RISC across its three domains (mental state, ADL, and medical state), their accuracy in predicting the incidence of three adverse outcomes (institutionalisation, hospitalisation, and death), and the contribution that the components of the RISC provide in predicting each adverse healthcare outcome within one year of assessment, compared with a battery of assessment instruments, in a sample of community-dwelling older adults.

The results suggest that all components of the RISC were better able to predict institutionalisation than hospitalisation and death. The perceived ability of the *caregiver network* to manage patients' ADL was most accurate in predicting institutionalisation and hospitalisation. This component contributes much to the predictive power of the instrument as a whole. This would be expected, particularly for institutionalisation, as patients' social and caregiver networks play an important role in the mental [26] and physical health [27] of community-dwelling older adults. Indeed, caregiver burden is an established risk factor for all three adverse outcomes evaluated in this study [28].

The overall accuracy of the RISC subtests for predicting hospitalisation, within one year of the assessment, was poor. Only the perceived *severity* of concern of a patients' medical state and the ability of an individuals' *caregiver network* to manage a persons' ADLs had some, albeit weak (AUC < 0.60), ability to predict the one-year rate of hospitalisation. This difficulty in predicting hospitalisation was seen in the validation of the RISC [16] and may reflect the complexity associated with predicting hospital admission in such a frail population (median Clinical Frailty Scale score of 5/9). Several studies and instruments have been developed to predict readmission to hospital, many with poor accuracy [8]. The Hospital Admission Risk Profile, for example, stratifies patients into low, medium, and high risk based on three factors: age, cognitive function, and preadmission ADL function, with an AUC of 0.65 for predicting hospitalisation [29]. In part, this may relate to the fact that short risk prediction instruments fail to incorporate other complex factors influencing hospitalisation including system-specific and patient-specific factors [8]. While the RISC was designed to measure risk within one year, most instruments measure risk of hospitalisation or readmission within a short period such as 30 days [8]. Available studies predicting outcomes over longer periods, up

Table 1: Receiver operating characteristic (ROC) curve area under the curve scores and 95% confidence intervals (CI) for the global risk score and components of the Risk Instrument for Screening in the Community (RISC) scores including mental state, activities of daily living (ADL), and medical state domains, the primary caregiver, and primary cohabitant (who the patient is living with), for predicting one-year risk of institutionalisation, hospitalisation, and death.

Variable		Actual outcomes	
	Institutionalization	Hospitalization	Death
RISC global risk score (CI)	0.70 (0.62–0.76)***	0.61 (0.55–0.66)***	0.70 (0.64–0.75)***
Mental state			
Mental state *concern*	0.62 (0.55–0.69)***	0.52 (0.47–0.58)	0.56 (0.50–0.61)*
Mental state *severity* of concern	0.64 (0.57–0.71)***	0.53 (0.47–0.58)	0.56 (0.51–0.62)*
Mental state *caregiver network*	0.64 (0.57–0.71)***	0.53 (0.47–0.58)	0.56 (0.50–0.61)
ADLs			
ADLs *concern*	0.60 (0.54–0.66)**	0.55 (0.50–0.60)	0.56 (0.50–0.61)*
ADLs *severity* of concern	0.66 (0.60–0.72)***	0.54 (0.49–0.59)*	0.63 (0.58–0.69)***
ADLs *caregiver network*	0.68 (0.62–0.74)***	0.57 (0.52–0.63)**	0.59 (0.53–0.65)**
Medical state			
Medical state *concern*	0.54 (0.48–0.61)	0.52 (0.47–0.58)	0.53 (0.48–0.59)
Medical state *severity* of concern	0.62 (0.55–0.69)***	0.57 (0.52–0.62)*	0.62 (0.56–0.67)***
Medical state *caregiver network*	0.63 (0.56–0.69)***	0.54 (0.49–0.59)	0.56 (0.50–0.61)*

*Statistically significant with P value <0.05.
**Statistically significant with P value <0.01.
***Statistically significant with P value <0.001.

Table 2: Comparison of the accuracy and area under the curve (AUC) scores with 95% confidence intervals (CI), of the Risk Instrument for Screening in the Community (RISC), the caregiver network for each domain and a selection of cognitive and functional tests including the Barthel Index, abbreviated mental test score, Charlson Comorbidity Index, and the Clinical Frailty Score.

Variable	Institutionalization AUC (95% CI)	Hospitalization AUC (95% CI)	Death AUC (95% CI)
RISC global risk score	0.70 (0.62–0.76)***	0.61 (0.55–0.66)***	0.70 (0.64–0.75)***
Mental state *caregiver network*	0.64 (0.57–0.71)***	0.53 (0.47–0.58)	0.56 (0.50–0.61)
ADL *caregiver network*	0.68 (0.62–0.74)***	0.57 (0.52–0.63)**	0.59 (0.53–0.65)**
Medical state *caregiver network*	0.63 (0.56–0.69)***	0.54 (0.49–0.59)	0.56 (0.50–0.61)*
Barthel Index	0.67 (0.61–0.73)***	0.58 (0.50–0.61)*	0.65 (0.60–0.71)***
Abbreviated mental test score	0.66 (0.59–0.73)***	0.51 (0.46–0.56)	0.51 (0.46–0.57)
Charlson Comorbidity Index	0.55 (0.49–0.62)	0.57 (0.52–0.62)**	0.66 (0.60–0.72)***
Clinical Frailty Scale	0.63 (0.57–0.67)***	0.55 (0.50–0.61)*	0.67 (0.61–0.72)***
PHNs perception of frailty	0.56 (0.49–0.62)	0.53 (0.47–0.58)	0.64 (0.59–0.70)***

*Statistically significant with P value <0.05.
**Statistically significant with P value <0.01.
***Statistically significant with P value <0.001.

to one year, have found similar albeit higher accuracy [30]. Given that predictors of short- and long-term adverse healthcare outcomes are likely to be different [31], the accuracy of the RISC in predicting hospitalisation within one year seems reasonable. The accuracy of the RISC for predicting one-year mortality was superior to hospitalisation. This was consistent with other studies [32, 33] including those incorporating multidimensional interdisciplinary CGA, which is a better predictor of one-year mortality than comorbidity or prognostic indices [34]. The reasons for this are complex and unclear. The factors predicting hospitalisation and hospital readmission are more complex than those predicting death and include hospital and healthcare system-level factors which are often location specific and cannot easily be incorporated into short and generalizable risk prediction models [8, 33]. Further, while these outcomes are not mutually exclusive, not all hospitalisations result in death and vice versa.

Comparing the accuracy of the other instruments used in the CARTS study to the components of the RISC suggests that the *caregiver network* component of the RISC (ADLs) had comparable accuracy in identifying risk of institutionalisation as the Clinical Frailty Scale, a marker of frailty. Likewise, both had similar accuracy for one-year mortality. The Charlson Comorbidity Index, a well-validated measure of comorbidity studied across a wide variety of clinical settings, was better able to predict mortality than hospitalisation. This is similar to the Cumulative Illness Rating Scale [35], another measure of comorbidity, which is more accurate at predicting

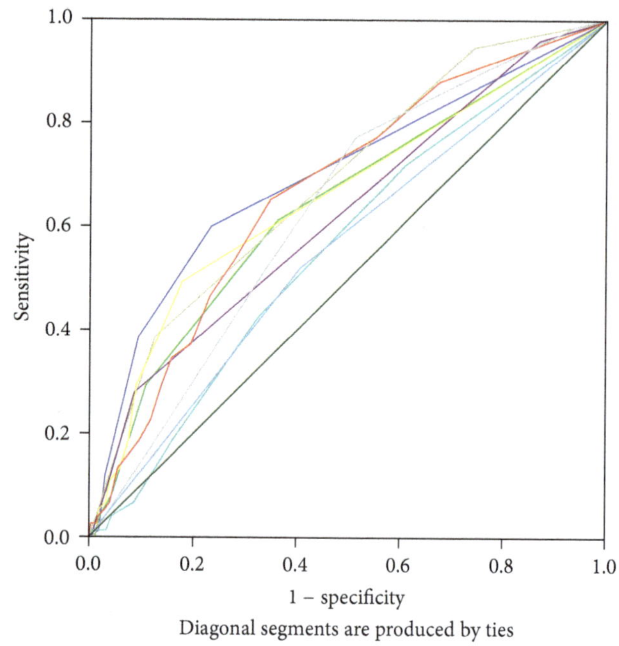

(a) ROC curve predicting actual institutionalization

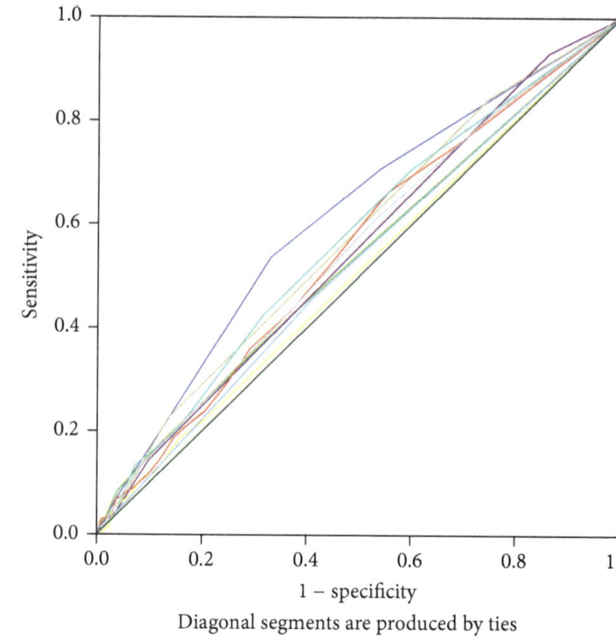

(b) ROC curve predicting actual hospitalization

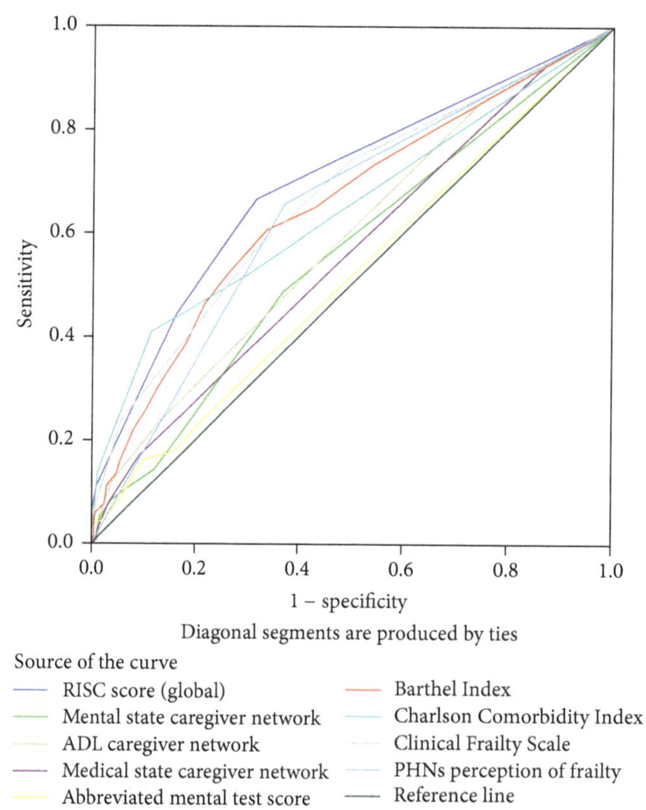

(c) ROC curve Predicting actual death

FIGURE 1: Receiver operating characteristic curves demonstrating the accuracy of the Risk Instrument for Screening in the Community (RISC), mental state, activities of daily living (ADL) and medical state domains, the abbreviated mental test score (AMTS), Barthel Index, Charlson Comorbidity Index, Clinical Frailty Scale, and public health nurses' (PHNs) perception of frailty in identifying one-year risk of (a) institutionalisation, (b) hospital admission (at least one), and (c) death.

institutionalisation than death [24]. The BI, a measure of ADL had similar accuracy to a measure of cognition (AMTS) in predicting institutionalisation. This would be expected given that function is important in determining nursing home placement in patients with [36] and without cognitive impairment [37]. This was mirrored in the greater accuracy of the *caregiver networks'* ability to manage ADL over its ability to manage patients' mental state.

The strengths of this study are the large numbers of community-dwelling older adults included and the comprehensive nature of the PHN records and that the instrument was validated in a sample of urban-suburban community-dwelling older adults in busy health centres. Another strength is that this tool employs a simple Likert scale to score the ability of the caregiver network to manage concerns in three domains. To our knowledge, there is no other instrument that measures the caregiver network in this way. This study does have limitations. Collection of demographic data was based upon a retrospective review of the patients' PHN records. Furthermore, the sample only included patients under active follow-up by their PHN, which may have created selection bias. Likewise, patients were predominantly functionally independent (median BI score of 18), cognitively intact (median AMTS score 10), and without significant comorbidity (median Charlson Comorbidity Index score of one), which may also have contributed to this bias. However, most patients were mildly frail as judged by the CFS (median score of five). Future studies should investigate the use of the RISC in other populations including those not under PHN surveillance and those more or less frail than this current sample. As the RISC is designed to detect outcomes within one year of assessment, the "predictive window" in this study differs from other studies, reducing the ability to directly compare outcomes and predictive validity. Likewise, the performances of many of the RISC subtests were low with AUCs at best between 0.6 and 0.7. This generally indicates low accuracy in correctly identifying outcomes [38]. That said, the objective of this study was to compare a lengthy battery of assessment instruments with a single, short subjective screen for risk. The accuracy of the test compares favourably with the other instruments included in this study and in other published papers.

5. Conclusion

In conclusion, the ability to identify high-risk individuals constitutes the first step in any strategy to target vulnerable, frail patients. The RISC is a short, reliable, and validated risk prediction screen for use in the community to identify risk of adverse healthcare outcomes. The RISC is similar to other short screening instruments like the Clinical Frailty Scale, the application of which, like the RISC, requires judgment and a degree of subjectivity [24]. In this study, the most accurate RISC subtest for institutionalisation was the ADL *caregiver network*. The most accurate subtest for death was ADL *severity*. The measurements of internal consistency suggest that all components of the RISC contribute to the overall predictive validity of the instrument. The RISC performed better than a selection of other assessment instruments, routinely collected by PHNs, in this sample of community-dwelling older adults. Further research is now required to compare the RISC with other validated risk tools, single-question screens, frailty measures, and comprehensive assessment instruments such as the InterRAI [39].

References

[1] B. Rechel, E. Grundy, J.-M. Robine et al., "Ageing in the European Union," *The Lancet*, vol. 381, no. 9874, pp. 1312–1322, 2013.

[2] R. M. Collard, H. Boter, R. A. Schoevers, and R. C. Oude Voshaar, "Prevalence of frailty in community-dwelling older persons: a systematic review," *Journal of the American Geriatrics Society*, vol. 60, no. 8, pp. 1487–1492, 2012.

[3] N. M. de Vries, J. B. Staal, C. D. van Ravensberg, J. S. M. Hobbelen, M. G. M. Olde Rikkerte, and M. W. G. van der Nijhuis-Sanden, "Outcome instruments to measure frailty: a systematic review," *Ageing Research Review*, vol. 10, pp. 104–114, 2011.

[4] J. J. Armstrong, P. Stolee, J. P. Hirdes, and J. W. Poss, "Examining three frailty conceptualizations in their ability to predict negative outcomes for home-care clients," *Age and Ageing*, vol. 39, no. 6, pp. 755–758, 2010.

[5] J. Vermeulen, J. C. Neyens, E. van Rossum, M. D. Spreeuwenberg, and L. P. de Witte, "Predicting ADL disability in community-dwelling elderly people using physical frailty indicators: a systematic review," *BMC Geriatrics*, vol. 11, no. 1, article 33, 2011.

[6] K. Bouillon, M. Kivimaki, M. Hamer et al., "Measures of frailty in population-based studies: an overview," *BMC Geriatrics*, vol. 13, no. 1, article 64, 2013.

[7] J. T. Wagner, L. M. Bachmann, C. Boult et al., "Predicting the risk of hospital admission in older persons—validation of a brief self-administered questionnaire in three European countries," *Journal of the American Geriatrics Society*, vol. 54, no. 8, pp. 1271–1276, 2006.

[8] D. Kansagara, H. Englander, A. Salanitro et al., "Risk prediction models for hospital readmission: a systematic review," *The Journal of the American Medical Association*, vol. 306, no. 15, pp. 1688–1698, 2011.

[9] A. Slade, J. Fear, and A. Tennant, "Identifying patients at risk of nursing home admission: the Leeds Elderly Assessment Dependency Screening tool (LEADS)," *BMC Health Services Research*, vol. 6, article 31, 2006.

[10] Y. Stern, M.-X. Tang, M. S. Albert et al., "Predicting time to nursing home care and death in individuals with Alzheimer disease," *Journal of the American Medical Association*, vol. 277, no. 10, pp. 806–812, 1997.

[11] M. Luppa, T. Luck, S. Weyerer, H.-H. König, E. Brähler, and S. G. Riedel-Heller, "Prediction of institutionalization in the elderly. A systematic review," *Age and Ageing*, vol. 39, no. 1, pp. 31–38, 2009.

[12] F. D. Wolinsky, C. M. Callahan, J. F. Fitzgerald, and R. J. Johnson, "The risk of nursing home placement and subsequent death among older adults," *The Journals of Gerontology*, vol. 47, pp. 173–182, 1992.

[13] R. O'Caoimh, Y. Gao, A. Svendrovski et al., "Screening for markers of frailty and perceived risk of adverse outcomes using the Risk Instrument for Screening in the Community (RISC)," *BMC Geriatrics*, vol. 14, no. 104, 2014.

[14] P. Leahy-Warren, R. O'Caoimh, C. Fitzgerald et al., "Components of the risk instrument for screening in the community

(RISC) that predict public health nurse perception of risk," *Journal of Frailty & Aging*. In press.

[15] R. O'Caoimh, E. Healy, E. O'Connell, Y. Gao, and D. W. Molloy, "The Community Assessment of Risk Tool, (CART): investigation of inter-rater reliability for a new instrument measuring risk of adverse outcomes in community dwelling older adults," *Irish Journal of Medical Science*, vol. 181, supplement 7, p. 227, 2012.

[16] C. FitzGerald, R. O'Caoimh, E. Healy et al., "Risk Instrument for Screening in the Community (RISC): predicting adverse outcomes in older adults," *Irish Journal of Medical Science*, vol. 183, no. 7, pp. S306–S307, 2014.

[17] C. Sweeney, D. W. Molloy, R. O'Caoimh et al., "European innovation partnership on active and healthy ageing: Ireland and the COLLAGE experience," *Irish Journal of Medical Science*, vol. 182, no. S6, pp. 278–279, 2013.

[18] R. D. Penna, "Asking the right question," *Journal of Palliative Medicine*, vol. 4, no. 2, pp. 245–248, 2001.

[19] W.-F. Pang, B. C.-H. Kwan, K.-M. Chow, C.-B. Leung, P. K.-T. Li, and C.-C. Szeto, "Predicting 12-month mortality for peritoneal dialysis patients using the 'surprise' question," *Peritoneal Dialysis International*, vol. 33, no. 1, pp. 60–66, 2013.

[20] S. A. Montgomery and M. Asberg, "A new depression scale designed to be sensitive to change," *British Journal of Psychiatry*, vol. 134, no. 4, pp. 382–389, 1979.

[21] D. W. Molloy, T. I. Standish, S. Dubois, and A. Cunje, "A short screen for depression: the AB Clinician Depression Screen (ABCDS)," *International Psychogeriatrics*, vol. 18, no. 3, pp. 481–492, 2006.

[22] H. M. Hodkinson, "Evaluation of a mental test score for assessment of mental impairment in the elderly," *Age and Ageing*, vol. 1, no. 4, pp. 233–238, 1972.

[23] M. E. Charlson, P. Pompei, K. A. Ales, and C. R. MacKenzie, "A new method of classifying prognostic comorbidity in longitudinal studies: development and validation," *Journal of Chronic Diseases*, vol. 40, no. 5, pp. 373–383, 1987.

[24] K. Rockwood, X. Song, C. MacKnight et al., "A global clinical measure of fitness and frailty in elderly people," *Canadian Medical Association Journal*, vol. 173, no. 5, pp. 489–495, 2005.

[25] R. M. Clarnette, J. P. Ryan, E. O'Herlihy et al., "The community assessment of risk instrument: investigation of inter-rater reliability of an instrument measuring risk of adverse outcomes," *The Journal of Frailty & Aging*. In press.

[26] K. L. Fiori, T. C. Antonucci, and K. S. Cortina, "Social network typologies and mental health among older adults," *Journals of Gerontology, Series B: Psychological Sciences and Social Sciences*, vol. 61, no. 1, pp. P25–P32, 2006.

[27] D. Reeves, C. Blickem, I. Vassilev et al., "The contribution of social networks to the health and self-management of patients with long-term conditions: a longitudinal study," *PLoS ONE*, vol. 9, no. 6, Article ID e98340, 2014.

[28] B. Miller and S. McFall, *Caregiver Burden and Institutionalization, Hospital Use, and Stability of Care*, US Government Printing Office, 1989.

[29] M. A. Sager, M. A. Rudberg, M. Jalaluddin et al., "Hospital Admission Risk Profile (HARP): identifying older patients at risk for functional decline following acute medical illness and hospitalization," *Journal of the American Geriatrics Society*, vol. 44, no. 3, pp. 251–257, 1996.

[30] L. Wang, B. Porter, C. Maynard et al., "Predicting risk of hospitalization or death among patients receiving primary care in the veterans health administration," *Medical Care*, vol. 51, no. 4, pp. 368–373, 2013.

[31] D. J. Kumbhani, B. J. Wells, A. M. Lincoff et al., "Predictive models for short- and long-term adverse outcomes following discharge in a contemporary population with acute coronary syndromes," *American Journal of Cardiovascular Disease*, vol. 3, no. 1, pp. 39–52, 2013.

[32] C. van Walraven, I. A. Dhalla, C. Bell et al., "Derivation and validation of an index to predict early death or unplanned readmission after discharge from hospital to the community," *Canadian Medical Association Journal*, vol. 182, no. 6, pp. 551–557, 2010.

[33] R. O'Caoimh, N. Cornally, E. Weathers et al., "Risk prediction in the community: a systematic review of case-finding instruments that predict adverse healthcare outcomes in community-dwelling older adults," *Maturitas*, 2015.

[34] N. Martínez-Velilla, B. Ibáñez-Beroiz, K. Cambra-Contin, and J. Alonso-Renedo, "Is comprehensive geriatric assessment a better 1-year mortality predictor than comorbidity and prognostic indices in hospitalized older adults?" *Journal of the American Geriatrics Society*, vol. 61, no. 10, pp. 1821–1823, 2013.

[35] Y. Conwell, N. T. Forbes, C. Cox, and E. D. Caine, "Validation of a measure of physical illness burden at autopsy: the cumulative illness rating scale," *Journal of the American Geriatrics Society*, vol. 41, no. 1, pp. 38–41, 1993.

[36] A. Bianchetti, A. Scuratti, O. Zanetti et al., "Predictors of mortality and institutionalization in Alzheimer disease patients 1 year after discharge from an Alzheimer Dementia Unit," *Dementia*, vol. 6, no. 2, pp. 108–112, 1995.

[37] M. Luppa, T. Luck, H. Matschinger, H.-H. König, and S. G. Riedel-Heller, "Predictors of nursing home admission of individuals without a dementia diagnosis before admission-results from the Leipzig Longitudinal Study of the Aged (LEILA 75+)," *BMC Health Services Research*, vol. 10, article 186, 2010.

[38] A. K. Akobeng, "Understanding diagnostic tests 3: receiver operating characteristic curves," *Acta Paediatrica*, vol. 96, no. 5, pp. 644–647, 2007.

[39] L. McDermott-Scales, D. Beaton, F. McMahon et al., "The National Single Assessment Tool (SAT) a pilot study in older persons care-survey results," *Irish Medical Journal*, vol. 106, no. 7, pp. 214–216, 2013.

4

Falls Risk and Simulated Driving Performance in Older Adults

John G. Gaspar,[1] Mark B. Neider,[2] and Arthur F. Kramer[1]

[1] *Department of Psychology and Beckman Institute for Advanced Science and Technology, University of Illinois at Urbana-Champaign, Urbana, IL 61801, USA*
[2] *Department of Psychology, University of Central Florida, Orlando, FL 32816, USA*

Correspondence should be addressed to John G. Gaspar; jgaspar2@illinois.edu

Academic Editor: Karl Rosengren

Declines in executive function and dual-task performance have been related to falls in older adults, and recent research suggests that older adults at risk for falls also show impairments on real-world tasks, such as crossing a street. The present study examined whether falls risk was associated with driving performance in a high-fidelity simulator. Participants were classified as high or low falls risk using the Physiological Profile Assessment and completed a number of challenging simulated driving assessments in which they responded quickly to unexpected events. High falls risk drivers had slower response times (~2.1 seconds) to unexpected events compared to low falls risk drivers (~1.7 seconds). Furthermore, when asked to perform a concurrent cognitive task while driving, high falls risk drivers showed greater costs to secondary task performance than did low falls risk drivers, and low falls risk older adults also outperformed high falls risk older adults on a computer-based measure of dual-task performance. Our results suggest that attentional differences between high and low falls risk older adults extend to simulated driving performance.

1. Introduction

Per mile driven, adults over age 65 are more likely to be involved in motor vehicle collisions than are younger experienced drivers [1], and declines in attention are related to older driver impairment [2, 3]. Attention is also critical to balance and gait, especially for older adults. Walkers must monitor for changes in environment and plan their next step. When a walking or balance task is combined with a cognitively challenging secondary task (e.g., memorizing a list of words), performance decrements are found for both tasks relative to performing each task separately [4]. These dual-task costs suggest that walking competes for shared attentional resources, as predicted by resource models of attention [5–9].

Older adults often have increased difficulty when multitasking, including paradigms that involve balancing or walking [10–12]. For example, older adults show larger dual-task costs on walking while memorizing task than do younger adults [13–16]. Such declines in multitasking ability are theorized to result in an increased risk for falls among older adults. Approximately 30% of community-dwelling older adults experience one or more falls annually [17, 18]. Age-related declines in the ability to multitask are related to an increase in falls risk. For example, performance on a counting while walking task predicts falls in older adults ([19]; see also [20–22]). Similarly, older adults at high risk for falls are less successful than low falls risk adults when crossing the street in a simulated environment while talking on a hands-free cell phone [23].

Differences in multitasking ability that have been associated with falls risk are theorized to result from declines in executive control, the functions which select, schedule, and coordinate task processes. Low falls risk older adults outperform high falls risk adults on tasks theorized to index executive control abilities [24–26]. Further, measures of executive control predict laboratory dual-task performance [27]. This suggests that older adults with poorer executive control are worse at managing complex task demands pertaining to balance or gait and are, therefore, more likely to fall.

Executive control is also important for other real-world tasks, such as driving. Drivers must attend to several areas of the environment and plan and execute responses to avoid collisions. Indeed, poorer performance on executive control tasks is predictive of retrospective crashes in a sample of older male drivers [28], and models of crash risk often comprise multidisciplinary factors, including physical ability, attention, and health [29–31]. Importantly, data also suggest a link between falls risk and driving. A history of falls is associated with older driver crashes [32], and some models of crash risk actually incorporate falls risk among other physical and cognitive measures [33]. Importantly, however, the results linking falls risk and driving performance rely on crash reports and subjectively rated driving performance and do not identify the behaviors related to unsafe driving in high falls risk older adults.

The goal of the present study was to explore the relationship between falls risk and driving in older adults in greater detail using a high-fidelity driving simulator, which allowed us to place drivers in potentially dangerous situations and to collect objective performance measures. We also included a battery of cognitive tasks to examine the relationship between falls risk, cognition, and simulated driving. Given previous findings of heightened crash risk, we predicted that low falls risk drivers would outperform high falls risk drivers on our simulator driving assessments. We further predicted that high falls risk drivers would show the greatest performance decrements in simulated driving performance under high multitasking load (i.e., when responding to unexpected events). Finally, we predicted that low falls risk older adults would outperform high falls risk adults on a desktop computer dual-task paradigm.

2. Methods

2.1. Participants. 36 independent-living older adults were recruited from the Urbana-Champaign community and paid $8 per hour for participating. All participants demonstrated normal or corrected-to-normal visual acuity (20/30 or better using a Snellen chart) and normal color vision (Ishihara Color Vision Test) and scored above 28 (of 30) on the Folstein minimental state exam. All participants had valid drivers' licenses and drove regularly. Mobility and balance were assessed using the Timed Up and Go test (TUAG) [34]. Descriptive data are provided in Table 1.

2.2. Apparatus and Falls Risk Assessment. The Beckman Institute Driving Simulator at the University of Illinois (http://isl.beckman.illinois.edu/) was used to assess simulated driving performance. The simulator consists of a General Motors Saturn automobile surrounded by eight screens. Traffic environments and experimental scenarios were developed using HyperDrive Authoring Suite. Data was recorded at 60 Hz. A PC with a 19-inch screen was used for neuropsychological testing. All tasks were programmed using E-prime (Psychology Software Tools). Viewing distance was approximately 77 cm for all tasks, although participants were free to move their heads.

2.2.1. Falls Risk. Participants completed a falls history questionnaire (i.e., "have you fallen in the last 6 months?" "how many times?"). Only three individuals reported falling in the previous 6 months. Thus, we classified participants as high or low falls risk based on scores from the Physiological Profile Assessment (PPA), as described by Lord and colleagues [35]. The PPA is a composite falls risk score based on measures of edge contrast sensitivity, hand reaction time, proprioception, leg muscle strength, and sway, which have shown to reliably predict falls in community and institutional settings [36, 37]. We set an a priori cutoff score of 0.6 to classify high and low falls risk (i.e., high falls risk ≥ 0.6) [38]. Fifteen participants were classified as high falls risk (mean age = 75.8, age range = 71–80), and 15 participants were classified as low falls risk (mean age = 74.4, age range = 67–80). The high and low falls risk groups were statistically similar in age, driving experience, and current driving habits. PPA scores were significantly correlated with times on the TUAG test ($r = .61$, $P = .001$).

2.3. Cognitive Battery

2.3.1. Computer Dual Task. Participants performed two tasks both separately and simultaneously. For one task, participants determined whether a letter was an A or B and pressed corresponding keys with their right hand. In the second task, participants determined whether a number was a 2 or 3 and pressed a corresponding key with their left hand. On single-task trials (50%), participants performed only one task. On dual-task trials (50%), they performed both tasks. The primary performance measure was reaction time. Participants completed single-task and dual-task practice trials, followed by a block of forty intermixed single- and dual-task test trials.

2.3.2. Functional Field of View (FFOV). Participants searched for a white triangle within a circle among square distracters in a briefly (44 ms) presented display. Targets were presented with equal probability on one of 8 radial spokes at eccentricities of 10°, 20°, and 30° from fixation. The search display was followed by a 100 ms mask consisting of random black and white lines and shapes. Participants then clicked with the mouse on the spoke where the target appeared. The percentage of targets correctly localized was the critical measure of performance. This task is similar to the peripheral localization subtask of the Useful Field of View [3], and we theorized that this measure might be predictive of older drivers' ability to respond to peripheral events. Participants completed 24 practice trials followed by 120 test trials.

2.3.3. Realistic Change Detection. Participants performed a flicker change detection task [37]. Stimuli were 80 pairs of photographs of real driving scenes taken from the driver's perspective. Each pair of images differed in one detail (e.g., a car in one image was removed from the other image). On each trial, participants saw a repeating cycle of 4 images, first image (240 ms), a gray mask screen (80 ms), the modified image (240 ms), and a gray mask screen (80 ms), and pressed a key when they detected the change. The screen froze, and participants clicked on the change location with the mouse.

Reaction time and accuracy were used as performance measures. Participants had 30 seconds to respond and completed 1 practice trial followed by 40 test trials.

2.4. Simulator Driving Assessment

2.4.1. Following Task. Drivers followed a lead vehicle (LV) along a straight, two-lane highway for approximately 15 minutes. Participants were instructed to maintain a 5-second gap from the LV, which traveled at 45 mph. During the practice drive, participants received auditory feedback to help visualize the 5-second gap. At 20 random times during the test drives, the LV's brake lights illuminated and its speed decreased. Drivers were instructed to brake as soon they detected LV slowing. When the driver pressed the brake, the LV accelerated back to 45 mph. Performance measures included response time to LV braking, following distance, and lane keeping.

2.4.2. Hazard Task. Drivers responded to potentially hazardous events as they drove along a straight, two-lane urban road for approximately 15 minutes. Ambient traffic and pedestrians were randomly generated such that there was a constant stream of traffic in the opposite lane, and the sidewalks were crowded with pedestrians. Participants were instructed to maintain a speed of 35 mph. There were a total of 20 randomly spaced potential hazards in each drive. Hazards comprised pedestrians crossing the roadway and cars on the right shoulder beginning to pull out and stopping (Figure 1). Participants were instructed to press the brakes as soon as detecting a hazard. Performance measures included brake response time and lane keeping.

2.4.3. Secondary Task. Participants completed two versions of two separate simulated driving tasks. The order of the task conditions was counterbalanced across participants. In the drive-only condition, participants drove without secondary task distraction. In the drive + 1-Back condition, participants performed cognitively demanding secondary task, a continuous 1-Back task where they heard a letter every 3 seconds and indicated whether the letter was the same as or different from the previous letter via buttons on the steering wheel, while driving. Accuracy was considered the primary measure of secondary task performance.

2.5. Procedure. Participants completed three 1.5-hour sessions. Session 1 consisted of a screening drive for simulator sickness, descriptive measures, and falls risk assessment (6 potential participants showed signs of simulator sickness and were not included in the study). In sessions 2 and 3, participants completed the three computer-based cognitive tasks, followed by practice with the secondary task and two driving assessments in the simulator. The order of the cognitive tasks and driving task conditions was counterbalanced across subjects.

TABLE 1: Demographic and cognitive measures.

Measure	High falls risk (N = 14)	Low falls risk (N = 14)
Age (years)	75.8 (3.3)	74.4 (5.5)
Physiological Profile Assessment score**	1.67 (.64)	.33 (.26)
Timed up and go (seconds)**	13.94 (2.6)	10.18 (2.2)
Activities balance confidence score (of 16)*	14.17 (1.4)	15.43 (.42)
Miles driven per week	55.36 (9.9)	61.42 (7.0)
Years licensed	58.86 (5.3)	57.86 (3.2)
Crashes in last 12 months	3	2
FFOV Accuracy (% Correct)	44.29 (19.9)	47.13 (18.7)
Flicker CD RT (s)	7.40 (1.13)	7.70 (1.28)
Flicker CD Accuracy (% Correct)	53.7 (10.3)	55.39 (8.4)
Computer dual-task cost (ms)*	572.7 (207.2)	354.8 (207.8)
Collisions	8	6

Data expressed as mean (SD).
*$P < .05$; **$P < .001$.
FFOV: functional field of view.
CD: change detection.
RT: response time.
Dual-task cost = dual RT − single RT.

3. Results

3.1. Cognitive Battery. Three participants (2 high falls risk and 1 low falls risk) did not complete the cognitive battery (due to technical issues) and were not included in analyses of the cognitive tasks. Dual-task cost was calculated by subtracting the single-task reaction time from the dual-task reaction time. High falls risk participants had a significantly higher dual-task cost compared to the low falls risk group, $F(1,23) = 6.88$, $P < .05$. Single-task reaction times on the computer dual-task paradigm did not differ between the groups, $F(1,23) = .19$, $P = .67$, indicating that differences were not due to general slowing. Localization accuracy on the FFOV task did not differ between the falls risk groups ($P > .70$), nor did reaction time or accuracy on the change detection task (P's $> .35$; see Table 1).

3.2. Driving Assessment. Analyses were performed separately for each driving task. Driving measures were entered into an ANOVA with falls risk group (high versus low) as a between-subjects factor and task condition (drive-only versus drive + 1-Back) as a within-subjects factor. Two participants (1 high falls risk and 1 low falls risk) who had passed the screening drive showed signs of simulator sickness during the experimental drives, did not complete the study, and were excluded from analyses.

Collisions were infrequent in both driving tasks (Table 1), precluding statistical analysis. Response time (RT) was defined as the time it took a driver to press the brake pedal following the onset of the LV brake lights or the triggering of a hazard event (Figure 2). Only events where the driver avoided a collision were included in the analyses. Low falls

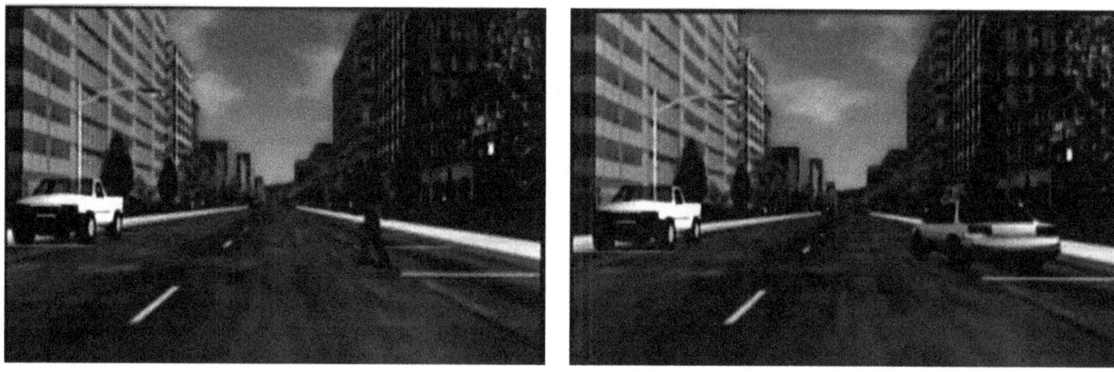

FIGURE 1: Examples of potential hazards in the hazard driving task. In (a), a pedestrian crosses the street in front of the driver. In (b), a parked vehicle starts to pull out in front of the driver.

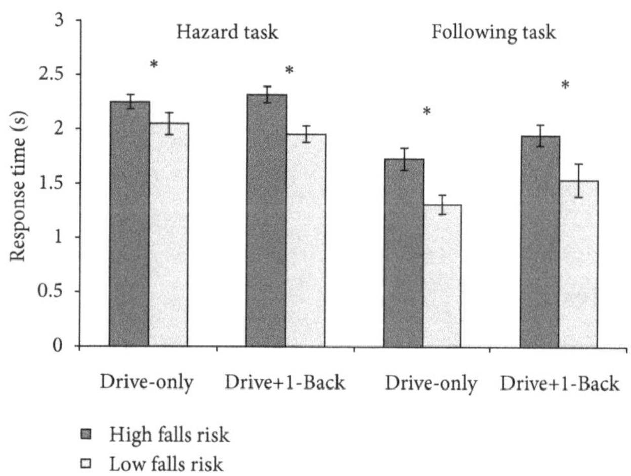

FIGURE 2: Brake response times. Mean brake response time in seconds for the high and low falls risk driver groups in drive-only and drive + 1-Back task conditions in the hazard response and car following paradigms. Error bars represent one standard error of the mean. $^*P < .05$.

risk drivers responded significantly faster than high falls risk drivers to LV braking events, $F(1,26) = 11.28$, $P < .01$. Low falls risk drivers also responded faster than high falls risk drivers to the onset of hazard events, $F(1,26) = 9.32$, $P < .01$. In the following task, performing the auditory 1-Back task slowed responses, $F(1,26) = 5.24$, $P < .05$, though this was not the case for the hazard drive, $F(1,26) = .083$, $P = .78$.

We ran separate analyses using hand reaction time, contrast sensitivity, and the combination of hand reaction time and contrast sensitivity as covariates to investigate the impact of specific components of the PPA [38]. With hand reaction time as a covariate, low falls risk drivers still had significantly faster RTs than did high falls risk drivers (P's $< .05$). When contrast sensitivity was included as a covariate, low falls risk drivers responded faster than did high falls risk drivers in the hazard ($F(1,26) = 4.90$, $P < .05$) but not the following ($F(1,26) = 1.21$, $P > .10$) simulated driving tasks. When both hand reaction time and contrast sensitivity were included as covariates, brake RT differences between groups were no longer significant (P's $> .10$).

High and low falls risk drivers did not differ in average velocity or lane keeping performance (all P's $> .10$). On the following task, headway distance was defined as the average distance between the driver's vehicle and the LV. Drivers increased their headway in the drive + 1-Back condition, $F(1,26) = 4.078$, $P = .05$. However, performing the concurrent secondary task did not differentially impair high falls risk drivers ($P > .40$).

3.2.1. Does Computer Dual-Task Performance Predict Driving Performance? To examine whether performance on the computer dual-task paradigm predicted simulated driving, we computed the correlation between dual-task cost on the computer paradigm and RT in the driving tasks. Participants with a lower computer dual-task cost responded faster to both LV braking events ($r = .42$, $P < .05$) and to hazard events ($r = .45$, $P < .05$). Conversely, single-task performance in the computer dual-task paradigm was not correlated with RT in the simulated driving assessments (P's $> .20$; Figures 3(c) and 3(d)).

3.2.2. Secondary Task Performance. We compared accuracy on the auditory 1-Back task during 1-Back only (during the last half of practice) and 1-Back + driving performances to examine whether there were costs to secondary task performance when driving (Figure 4) [39]. There was a significant cost to 1-Back accuracy in both the following drive ($F(1,26) = 254.5$, $P < .001$) and the hazard drive ($F(1,26) = 173.0$, $P < .001$), though there was no difference between falls risk groups ($P > .15$). To determine if a group difference existed when the driving task was most demanding, we divided 1-Back accuracy into critical segments (i.e., during peripheral hazard or LV braking events) and noncritical segments (i.e., periods between critical events). High falls risk participants were marginally worse than were low falls risk participants during critical periods in both the following ($F(1,26) = 3.27$, $P = .084$) and the hazard drives ($F(1,26) = 3.57$, $P = .071$). There were no differences in 1-Back accuracy between groups

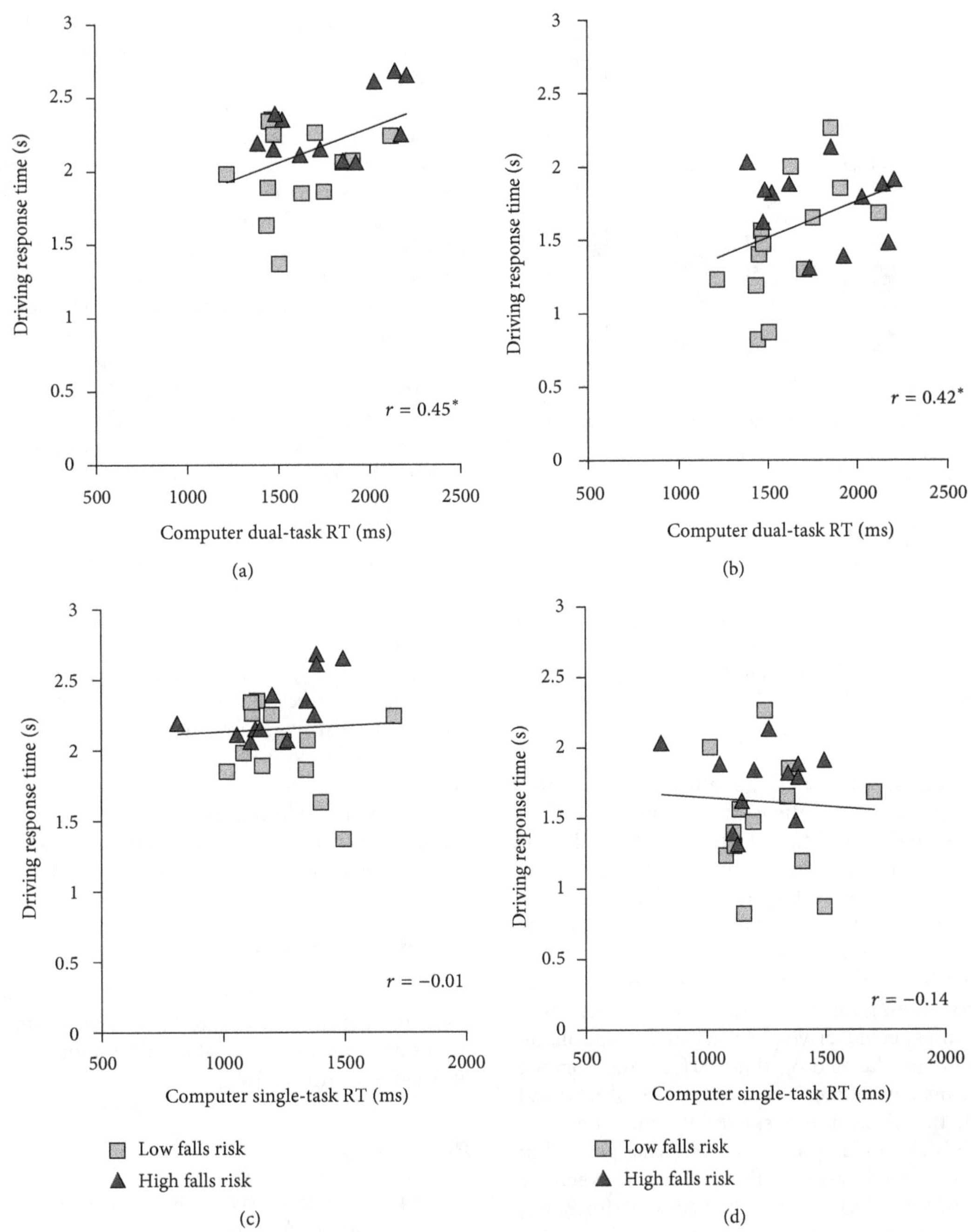

FIGURE 3: Driving response times and dual-task performance. Response time in seconds in the hazard (a) and (c) and following (b) and (d) driving tasks plotted against single-task and dual-task reaction time in milliseconds on the computer dual-task paradigm. $^{*}P < .05$.

in the noncritical segments for either drive (P's $>$ .70; see Figure 3). This indicates that, when responding to critical events, high falls risk drivers showed larger costs to secondary task performance than did low falls risk drivers. Though this may have been a compensatory strategy, it did not eliminate group differences in RT to critical driving events.

4. Discussion

The current study compared the driving performance of high and low falls risk older adults in a high-fidelity driving simulator. Of greatest importance is the finding that high falls risk drivers responded approximately 400 ms slower than did low falls risk drivers to critical events. High falls risk drivers responded slower than did low falls risk drivers to both central lead vehicle braking events and to peripheral hazards. Such slower responses may be a contributing factor to heightened crash rates for high falls risk older adults reported elsewhere [32]. Indeed, the ability to detect hazards has been linked to crash involvement [40].

Our data extend the literature that examines multitasking performance in older adults at high and low risk for falls

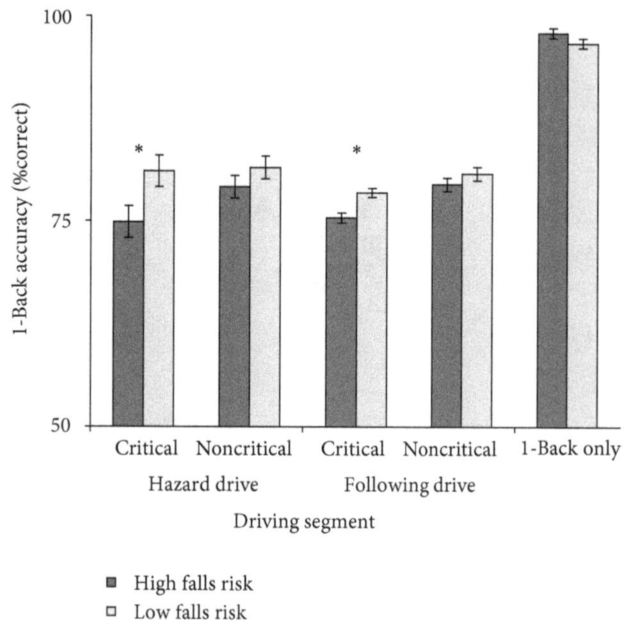

FIGURE 4: 1-Back accuracy. Accuracy on the 1-Back task in critical and noncritical segments of the hazard and following drives and in the single-task (1-Back only) condition. Error bars represent one standard error of the mean. $^*P < .05$.

[19–23]. In our cognitive battery, high falls risk participants had greater dual-task costs on the computer paradigm than did low falls risk older adults, and, importantly, this was not due to differences in general slowing. In much the same way as walking, responding to critical events while driving requires the ability to multitask; drivers must scan the environment and plan and execute evasive responses while controlling the vehicle. In our study, the ability to efficiently allocate attention among different tasks was most critical to responding to unexpected driving events in the simulator. This is supported by the finding that performance on the computer dual-task paradigm predicted driving RTs and further suggests that these multitasking differences between high and low falls risk older adults are somewhat general in nature. Previous research suggests that deficits in executive function likely underlie declines in multitasking performance and mediate the relationship between balance and falls [24, 25, 27], as well as crash risk for older drivers [28]. Changes in executive control likely contribute to the general multitasking differences shown in our cognitive battery and simulator driving assessments.

Our results indicate that contrast sensitivity and response time were the most important components of the PPA relating to simulated driving RT. Previous work has found that contrast sensitivity and response time are important abilities in responding to driving hazards [41]. The present data suggest that these abilities are important to both walking and simulated driving.

We failed to find differences between high and low falls risk drivers on other simulator driving performance measures such as lane keeping. Hazard responses posed the highest multitasking demand in our driving assessments. Previous research has shown that multitasking differences in older adults and differences between high and low falls risk older adults arise primarily at the highest levels of task demand [13, 16, 23]. Thus, in the present study, high and low falls risk drivers performed equally well during relatively low-demand driving intervals, but high falls risk drivers were more impaired in high-demand situations, resulting in slower responses. In the driving + 1-Back condition, dual-task costs were found primarily in 1-Back accuracy. This may reflect a strategy whereby older adults compensated for higher task demands by sacrificing performance on the less safety-critical task [14]. During responses to critical events, high falls risk drivers sacrificed 1-Back accuracy more than did low falls risk drivers, which again suggests high falls risk participants struggled under high multitasking demand.

Future work should explore the contribution of different components of executive control (e.g., switching and inhibition) to deficits in real-world tasks such as walking and driving. Eye tracking techniques could inform as to whether high and low falls risk drivers differ in the way they deploy attention within a driving scene. Research should also explore other driving tasks where older adults are differentially involved in crashes, such as busy intersections [42]. The examination of on-road driving measures is also needed to validate that response time differences in the simulator translate to real-world driving.

In summary, our results demonstrate that high falls risk older drivers respond slower than do low falls risk drivers when responding to potential dangers in a driving simulator. A multidimensional approach that includes falls risk may be useful in more accurately assessing older driver impairment.

Acknowledgments

The authors would like to thank the Illinois Simulator Lab for their support and J. C. and K. L. for subject running. A subset of this data was presented at the Cognitive Aging Conference in Atlanta, in April 2012.

References

[1] L. Evans, *Traffic Safety*, Science Serving Society, Bloomfield Hills, Mich, USA, 2004.

[2] O. J. Clay, V. G. Wadley, J. D. Edwards, D. L. Roth, D. L. Roenker, and K. K. Ball, "Cumulative meta-analysis of the relationship between useful field of view and driving performance in older adults: current and future implications," *Optometry & Vision Science*, vol. 82, no. 8, pp. 724–731, 2005.

[3] L. Hoffman, P. Atchley, J. M. McDowd, and R. Dubinsky, "The role of visual attention in predicting driving impairment in older adults," *Psychology and Aging*, vol. 20, no. 4, pp. 610–622, 2005.

[4] M. Woollacott and A. Shumway-Cook, "Attention and the control of posture and gait: a review of an emerging area of research," *Gait & Posture*, vol. 16, no. 1, pp. 1–14, 2002.

[5] B. Kerr, S. M. Condon, and L. A. McDonald, "Cognitive spatial processing and the regulation of posture," *Journal of Experimental Psychology*, vol. 11, no. 5, pp. 617–622, 1985.

[6] S. Kemper, R. E. Herman, and C. H. T. Lian, "The costs of doing two things at once for young and older adults: talking while walking, finger tapping, and ignoring speech or noise," *Psychology and Aging*, vol. 18, no. 2, pp. 181–192, 2003.

[7] H. E. Pashler, *The Psychology of Attention*, The MIT Press, Cambridge, Mass, USA, 1998.

[8] C. D. Wickens, "Multiple resources and performance prediction," *Theoretical Issues in Ergonomics Science*, vol. 3, no. 2, pp. 159–177, 2002.

[9] A. F. Kramer and D. Madden, "Attention," in *The Handbook of Aging and Cognition*, F. I. M. Craik and T. A. Salthouse, Eds., pp. 189–249, Psychology Press, New York, NY, USA, 3rd edition, 2008.

[10] J. Kray and U. Lindenberger, "Adult age differences in task switching," *Psychology and Aging*, vol. 15, no. 1, pp. 126–147, 2000.

[11] P. S. Tsang and T. L. Shaner, "Age, attention, expertise, and time-sharing performance," *Psychology and Aging*, vol. 13, no. 2, pp. 323–347, 1998.

[12] A. F. Kramer, J. Larish, T. Weber, and L. Bardell, "Training for executive control: task coordination strategies and aging," in *Attention and Performance XVII*, D. Gopher and A. Koriat, Eds., The MIT Press, Cambridge, Mass, USA, 1999.

[13] U. Lindenberger, M. Marsiske, and P. B. Baltes, "Memorizing while walking: increase in dual-task costs from young adulthood to old age," *Psychology and Aging*, vol. 15, no. 3, pp. 417–436, 2000.

[14] K. Z. H. Li, U. Lindenberger, A. M. Freund, and P. B. Baltes, "Walking while memorizing: age-related differences in compensatory behavior," *Psychological Science*, vol. 12, no. 3, pp. 230–237, 2001.

[15] O. Huxhold, S. C. Li, F. Schmiedek, and U. Lindenberger, "Dual-tasking postural control: aging and the effects of cognitive demand in conjunction with focus of attention," *Brain Research Bulletin*, vol. 69, no. 3, pp. 294–305, 2006.

[16] M. B. Neider, J. G. Gaspar, J. S. McCarley, J. A. Crowell, H. Kaczmarski, and A. F. Kramer, "Walking and talking: dual-task effects on street crossing behavior in older adults," *Psychology and Aging*, vol. 26, no. 2, pp. 260–268, 2011.

[17] M. E. Tinetti, M. Speechley, and S. F. Ginter, "Risk factors for falls among elderly persons living in the community," *The New England Journal of Medicine*, vol. 319, no. 26, pp. 1701–1707, 1988.

[18] A. J. Blake, K. Morgan, M. J. Bendall et al., "Falls by elderly people at home: prevalence and associated factors," *Age and Ageing*, vol. 17, no. 6, pp. 365–372, 1988.

[19] O. Beauchet, V. Dubost, G. Allali, R. Gonthier, F. R. Hermann, and R. W. Kressig, "'Faster counting while walking' as a predictor of falls in older adults," *Age and Ageing*, vol. 36, no. 4, pp. 418–423, 2007.

[20] L. Lundin-Olsson, L. Nyberg, and Y. Gustafson, "'Stops walking when talking' as a predictor of falls in elderly people," *The Lancet*, vol. 349, no. 9052, p. 617, 1997.

[21] J. Verghese, H. Buschke, L. Viola et al., "Validity of divided attention tasks in predicting falls in older individuals: a preliminary study," *Journal of the American Geriatrics Society*, vol. 50, no. 9, pp. 1572–1576, 2002.

[22] K. A. Faulkner, M. S. Redfern, J. A. Cauley et al., "Multitasking: association between poorer performance and a history of recurrent falls," *Journal of the American Geriatrics Society*, vol. 55, no. 4, pp. 570–576, 2007.

[23] L. S. Nagamatsu, M. Voss, M. B. Neider et al., "Increased cognitive load leads to impaired mobility decisions in seniors at risk for falls," *Psychology and Aging*, vol. 26, no. 2, pp. 253–259, 2011.

[24] J. M. Hausdorff, G. M. Doniger, S. Springer, G. Yogev, N. Giladi, and E. S. Simon, "A common cognitive profile in elderly fallers and in patients with Parkinson's disease: the prominence of impaired executive function and attention," *Experimental Aging Research*, vol. 32, no. 4, pp. 411–429, 2006.

[25] L. J. Rapport, R. A. Hanks, S. R. Millis, and S. A. Deshpande, "Executive functioning and predictors of falls in the rehabilitation setting," *Archives of Physical Medicine and Rehabilitation*, vol. 79, no. 6, pp. 629–633, 1998.

[26] G. Yogev-Seligmann, J. M. Hausdorff, and N. Giladi, "The role of executive function and attention in gait," *Movement Disorders*, vol. 23, no. 3, pp. 329–342, 2008.

[27] S. Springer, N. Giladi, C. Peretz, G. Yogev, E. S. Simon, and J. M. Hausdorff, "Dual-tasking effects on gait variability: the role of aging, falls, and executive function," *Movement Disorders*, vol. 21, no. 7, pp. 950–957, 2006.

[28] G. Daigneault, P. Joly, and J. Y. Frigon, "Executive functions in the evaluation of accident risk of older drivers," *Journal of Clinical and Experimental Neuropsychology*, vol. 24, no. 2, pp. 221–238, 2002.

[29] J. M. Wood, K. J. Anstey, G. K. Kerr, P. F. Lacherez, and S. Lord, "A multidomain approach for predicting older driver safety under in-traffic road conditions," *Journal of the American Geriatrics Society*, vol. 56, no. 6, pp. 986–993, 2008.

[30] P. A. Hoggarth, C. R. H. Innes, J. C. Dalrymple-Alford, J. E. Severinsen, and R. D. Jones, "Comparison of a linear and a non-linear model for using sensory-motor, cognitive, personality, and demographic data to predict driving ability in healthy older adults," *Accident Analysis and Prevention*, vol. 42, no. 6, pp. 1759–1768, 2010.

[31] C. A. Fischer, G. V. Kondraske, and R. Malcolm Stewart, "Prediction of driving performance using nonlinear causal resource analysis," in *Proceedings of the 2nd Joint Engineering in Medicine and Biology, 24th Annual Conference and the Annual Fall Meeting of the Biomedical Engineering Society EMBS/BMES Conference*, pp. 2473–2474, 2002.

[32] K. L. Margolis, R. P. Kerani, P. McGovern, T. Songer, J. A. Cauley, and K. E. Ensrud, "Risk factors for motor vehicle crashes in older women," *Journals of Gerontology A*, vol. 57, no. 3, pp. M186–M191, 2002.

[33] K. K. Ball, D. L. Roenker, V. G. Wadley et al., "Can high-risk older drivers be identified through performance-based measures in a department of motor vehicles setting?" *Journal of the American Geriatrics Society*, vol. 54, no. 1, pp. 77–84, 2006.

[34] D. Podsiadlo and S. Richardson, "The timed 'Up & Go': a test of basic functional mobility for frail elderly persons," *Journal of the American Geriatrics Society*, vol. 39, no. 2, pp. 142–148, 1991.

[35] S. R. Lord, H. B. Menz, and A. Tiedemann, "A physiological profile approach to falls risk assessment and prevention," *Physical Therapy*, vol. 83, no. 3, pp. 237–252, 2003.

[36] S. R. Lord and J. Dayhew, "Visual risk factors for falls in older people," *Journal of the American Geriatrics Society*, vol. 49, no. 5, pp. 508–515, 2001.

[37] S. R. Lord, R. D. Clark, and I. W. Webster, "Physiological factors associated with falls in an elderly population," *Journal of the American Geriatrics Society*, vol. 39, no. 12, pp. 1194–1200, 1991.

[38] K. Delbaere, J. C. T. Close, J. Heim et al., "A multifactorial approach to understanding fall risk in older people," *Journal of*

the American Geriatrics Society, vol. 58, no. 9, pp. 1679–1685, 2010.

[39] E. Becic, G. S. Dell, K. Bock, S. M. Garnsey, T. Kubose, and A. F. Kramer, "Driving impairs talking," *Psychonomic Bulletin & Review*, vol. 17, no. 1, pp. 15–21, 2010.

[40] M. S. Horswill, K. J. Anstey, C. G. Hatherly, and J. M. Wood, "The crash involvement of older drivers is associated with their hazard perception latencies," *Journal of the International Neuropsychological Society*, vol. 16, no. 5, pp. 939–944, 2010.

[41] M. S. Horswill, S. A. Marrington, C. M. McCullough et al., "The hazard perception ability of older drivers," *Journals of Gerontology B*, vol. 63, no. 4, pp. P212–P218, 2008.

[42] M. R. E. Romoser and D. L. Fisher, "The effect of active versus passive training strategies on improving older drivers' scanning in intersections," *Human Factors*, vol. 51, no. 5, pp. 652–668, 2009.

5

Optimal Approaches for Measuring Tongue-Pressure Functional Reserve

Catriona M. Steele

Toronto Rehabilitation Institute, University Health Network, 550 University Avenue, Toronto, ON, Canada M5G 2A2

Correspondence should be addressed to Catriona M. Steele; catriona.steele@uhn.ca

Academic Editor: Paula Bickford

Tongue-palate pressure is a parameter of considerable interest in the field of dysphagia. Maximum isometric tongue-palate pressures (MIPs) decline in healthy aging and in dysphagia. Functional reserve (FR) is the difference between MIPs and swallowing pressures. Reduced FR is thought to constitute a risk for developing functional swallowing impairments. We compare different approaches for calculating FR and recommend an optimal approach. Tongue-palate pressure data were collected from 78 healthy adults (40 < age 40; 38 > 60) during anterior and posterior MIPs, regular (RESS) and effortful (ESS) saliva swallows, and water swallows (4 repetitions per task). Six different measures of reserve were calculated using maximum anterior MIPs or ESS pressures at the top, and mean or maximum RESS or water swallow pressures at the bottom of the range. Correlations with age and MIPs were explored to confirm suitability for measuring FR. The impact of normalization to maximum MIP range was explored. We conclude that an optimal measure of FR involves the comparison of maximum MIP with mean saliva swallowing pressures. This parameter declines with age, but when normalized to an individual's MIP range, the relationship is no longer evident. This suggests that FR does not necessarily decline in healthy aging.

1. Introduction

The ability to generate tongue-palate pressure has emerged as a measure of considerable clinical and research interest in the field of dysphagia over the past two decades. Key to this interest is that tongue strength, measured during maximum isometric tongue-palate pressure tasks (MIPs), appears to decline in healthy aging [1–6]. This has been argued to resemble sarcopenia, a degenerative loss of skeletal muscle mass and strength seen in aging in the limb musculature. Reduced tongue strength has also been observed in adults with dysphagia [7–10]. These observations have prompted research into exercise-based methods for tongue strengthening in the hope that greater tongue strength and endurance will lead to improved swallowing function [9, 11, 12].

Functional reserve is the term coined to describe the difference in pressures generated in maximum isometric pressure (MIP) tasks compared to swallowing tasks. Robbins and colleagues were the first to point out that swallowing pressures appear to be preserved in healthy older adults, even in the presence of reduced MIPs. Reductions in functional reserve, due to reductions in MIPs, were argued to have important clinical implications and to place a person at greater risk of developing functional swallowing impairments, particularly in the case of decompensation [2, 13].

Functional reserve describes a tongue-palate pressure range that is bounded at the top by a maximum pressure task and at the bottom by a swallowing task. The swallowing task used to define the bottom of the functional reserve range has varied across studies, leading to some confusion regarding the measure. Furthermore, different instruments have been used across studies, without clear demonstration that measures can be generalized across instruments. We are conducting a program of research exploring the relationship between tongue pressure capacity and swallowing behaviors. We are specifically interested in confirming whether or not limited tongue pressure capacity contributes to constrained variability in swallowing behaviors and whether such constraints are seen as a function of healthy aging. We have recently reported that functional reserve, which we defined as the difference between MIPs and regular effort saliva swallow (RESS) pressures, does not necessarily decline with age

[14]. Although overall groupwise trends showed significantly larger functional reserve in individuals aged 20–40 compared to those over the age of 60, we noticed that 18% of our older participant group had excellent functional reserve above the 75th percentile for pooled functional reserve in our sample. Similarly, 13% of our younger group had limited functional reserve, below the 25th% percentile.

Of particular note is the study of Youmans et al. [5], which involved a functional reserve calculation using bolus swallowing pressures at the bottom of the range, with these pressure measures transformed to a percentage value relative to each participant's MIP range, thereby controlling individual differences in strength. These authors found no significant age-group differences using this transformation, although women were found to use a higher percentage of their MIP range when swallowing boluses compared to men. Youmans and colleagues argued that these results challenged the conventional view that functional reserve declines in healthy aging. Similarly, a previous study by Yeates and colleagues [15] measured a parameter that they called "swallow reserve," comparing effortful saliva swallows to regular effort saliva swallows, and failed to find age-related differences in this measure.

These observations led us to question whether functional reserve is indeed a parameter that changes in healthy aging and to explore which elements need to be included in a robust and psychometrically valid measure of functional tongue pressure reserve. We propose that such a parameter should display three characteristics.

(a) A measure of functional reserve should be sensitive to, and positively correlated with, changes in maximum strength measures (MIPs).

(b) A measure of functional reserve should be sensitive to changes that occur across the age span, but in order for these to support a hypothesis that functional reserve declines with age, the trend should be visible in a parameter where swallowing pressures are expressed as a percentage of a person's maximum tongue strength, in order to control for individual variations in strength.

(c) A measure of functional reserve should be one that can be collected easily, without posing a risk of aspiration for the patient.

In this paper, we explore 6 different candidate measures of functional reserve to determine an optimum method for capturing functional reserve in future research and clinical situations.

2. Materials and Methods

Tongue pressures at the anterior, medial, and posterior palate were collected from 78 healthy consenting adults in two sex-balanced age groups. The younger participant group ranged in age from 18 to 39 years, with a mean age of 27 years. The older participant group ranged in age from 60 to 87, with a mean age of 70 years. The protocol was approved by the local institutional research ethics board. Exclusion criteria included participant-reported history of type I diabetes, chronic sinusitis, taste disturbance, or any swallowing, motor speech, gastroesophageal, or neurological difficulties. During intake, a brief oral mechanism examination and a water swallow screening were performed by a licensed speech-language pathologist to confirm eligibility to participate.

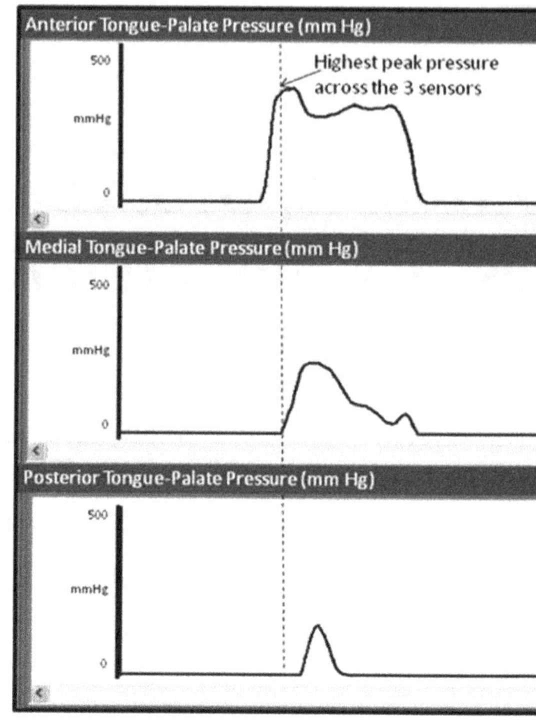

FIGURE 1: Illustration of tongue-palate pressure waveforms on the KayPentax Digital Swallow Workstation. The highest peak pressure (in mm Hg) across the anterior, medial, and posterior sensors was used as the value of peak pressure for each task.

2.1. Data Collection. We used the 3-bulb tongue array of the KayPentax Swallowing Signals Lab to collect tongue pressures, with the bulbs spaced 8 mm apart and adhered to the palate in midline using Stomahesive (Convatec, St-Laurent, Quebec, Canada). The anterior bulb was positioned on the alveolar ridge, immediately behind the upper incisors. Pressure signals were sampled at 250 Hz with the range calibrated to record an upper amplitude limit of 750 mmHg. Five different pressure tasks were included, with each performed in a block of 4 task repetitions. The protocol commenced with the maximum anterior isometric pressure task (AMAX) and then proceeded to one of four randomly assigned sequences for the collection of regular effort saliva swallows (RESS), effortful saliva swallows (ESS), maximum posterior isometric pressures (PMAX), and discrete water swallows (i.e., single sips of ~8–10 mL taken from a cup). The PMAX data have been reported elsewhere and are not used for the calculations reported in this paper.

2.2. Data Processing. Anterior, medial, and posterior palate pressure waveforms were displayed on a computer monitor. The onset, peak, and offset of each pressure event were

TABLE 1: Pearson's correlations between different measures of functional reserve: maximum isometric pressure and age.

Functional reserve measure	Unit of measurement	Maximum isometric pressure (MIP)		Age	
		Pearson's correlation	Significance (2-tailed)	Pearson's correlation	Significance (2-tailed)
MIP minus maximum water swallow pressures	mm Hg	**.814**	.000	−.304	.007
	% MIP	.314	.005	−.104	.368
MIP minus mean water swallow pressures	mm Hg	**.910**	.000	−.359	.001
	% MIP	.320	.005	−.107	.354
MIP minus maximum regular effort saliva swallow pressures	mm Hg	**.796**	.000	−.250	.031
	% MIP	**.453**	.000	−.042	.716
MIP minus mean regular effort saliva swallow pressures	mm Hg	**.899**	.000	−.312	.006
	% MIP	**.493**	.000	−.078	.500
Maximum effortful minus maximum regular effort saliva swallow pressures	mm Hg	.285	.013	n/a	n/a
Maximum effortful minus mean regular effort saliva swallow pressures	mm Hg	.325	.004	n/a	n/a

Correlations with $R > 0.4$ are shown in bold.

indexed by a trained research assistant and pressure amplitudes at each of these timepoints were recorded. Pressure amplitude (in mm Hg) was calculated as the amplitude difference (in mm Hg) between the highest peak pressure amplitude and the lowest baseline pressure amplitude (usually zero mm Hg) seen across all three pressure waveforms (anterior, medial, and posterior) for a given task repetition. Figure 1 provides an illustration of this parameter.

2.3. Analysis. Six different equations were calculated as possible measures of functional reserve as follows.

(a) Maximum peak pressure on the AMAX task minus maximum peak pressure on the water swallowing task.

(b) Maximum peak pressure on the AMAX task minus mean peak pressure on the water swallowing task.

(c) Maximum peak pressure on the AMAX task minus maximum peak pressure on the RESS task.

(d) Maximum peak pressure on the AMAX task minus mean peak pressure on the RESS task.

(e) Maximum peak pressure on the ESS task minus maximum peak pressure on the RESS task.

(f) Maximum peak pressure on the ESS task minus mean peak pressure on the RESS task.

Scatter plots were prepared in IBM SPSS 19.0, plotting each measure of functional reserve, first as a function of maximum isometric pressure (maximum peak pressure on the AMAX task) and second as a function of age. An *a priori* criterion for correlations of interest was established as a Pearson's correlation of $R = 0.4$. Finally, RESS and water swallow pressure values were transformed to a percentage value of each participant's maximum isometric pressures, and scatter plots and correlations were again explored using these transformed data.

3. Results and Discussion

Table 1 provides descriptive statistics for the observed Pearson's correlations between each candidate measure of functional reserve: (a) maximum isometric pressure and (b) age.

As shown in Figure 2(a), when the traditional approach for measuring functional reserve is used (MIP minus water swallowing pressures), there are strong correlations with MIP, regardless of whether mean ($R^2 = 0.85$) or maximum ($R^2 = 0.70$) water swallowing pressure values are used at the bottom of the functional reserve range. Similarly, as shown in Figure 2(b), strong correlations are also seen when either mean ($R^2 = 0.81$) or maximum ($R^2 = 0.64$) saliva swallow pressures are used at the bottom of the functional reserve range. By contrast, as shown in Figure 2(c), measures of swallow reserve, in which effortful saliva swallows are used at the top of the functional reserve range, do not correlate strongly with MIP when either mean ($R^2 = 0.10$) or maximum ($R^2 = 0.07$) saliva swallows are used at the bottom of the range. This suggests that swallow reserve, as proposed by Yeates and colleagues [15], is not sensitive to differences in tongue pressure capacity and is therefore not a good measure of functional reserve.

With respect to the relationship between functional reserve measures and age, Figure 3(a) shows weak but statistically significant negative correlations with age for functional reserve measures comparing MIP to mean ($R = -0.31$, $R^2 = 0.13$) or maximum ($R = -0.25$, $R^2 = 0.10$) water swallowing pressures. Similarly, as shown in Figure 3(b), weak but statistically significant correlations with age are seen when either mean ($R = -0.36$, $R^2 = 0.10$) or maximum ($R = -0.30$, $R^2 = 0.07$) saliva swallow pressures are used at the bottom of the functional reserve range. Age correlations with swallow reserve were not explored given the earlier result showing a lack of sensitivity to changes in strength.

Finally, we explored what happened to the previously observed correlations when we transformed our measures of

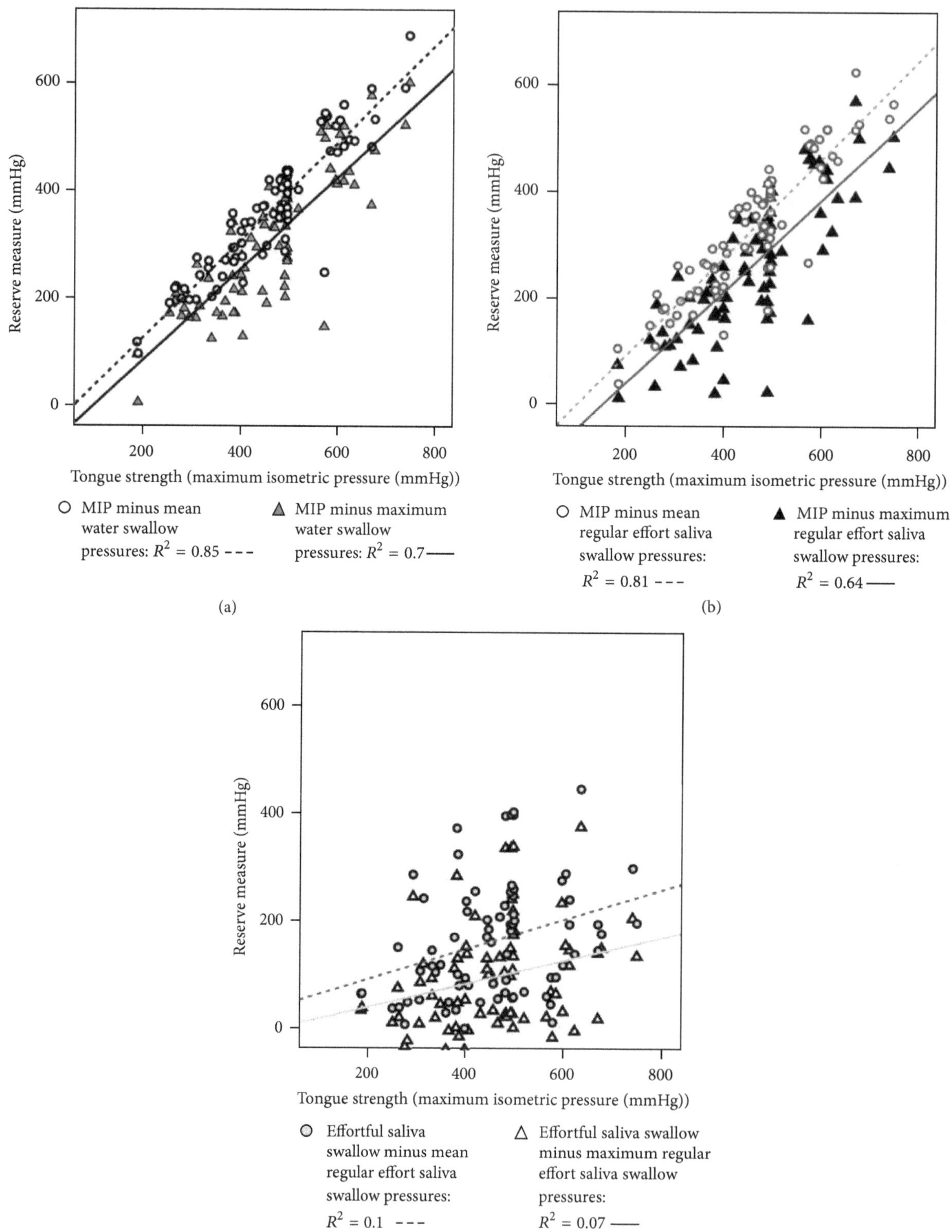

FIGURE 2: (a) Scatter plot showing the relationship between functional reserve measures comparing maximum isometric pressure (MIP) to water swallowing pressures and tongue strength, as measured by MIP. (b) Scatter plot showing the relationship between functional reserve measures comparing maximum isometric pressure (MIP) to regular effort saliva swallowing pressures and tongue strength, as measured by MIP. (c) Scatter plot showing the relationship between functional reserve measures comparing maximum effortful saliva swallowing pressures to regular effort saliva swallowing pressures and tongue strength, as measured by MIP.

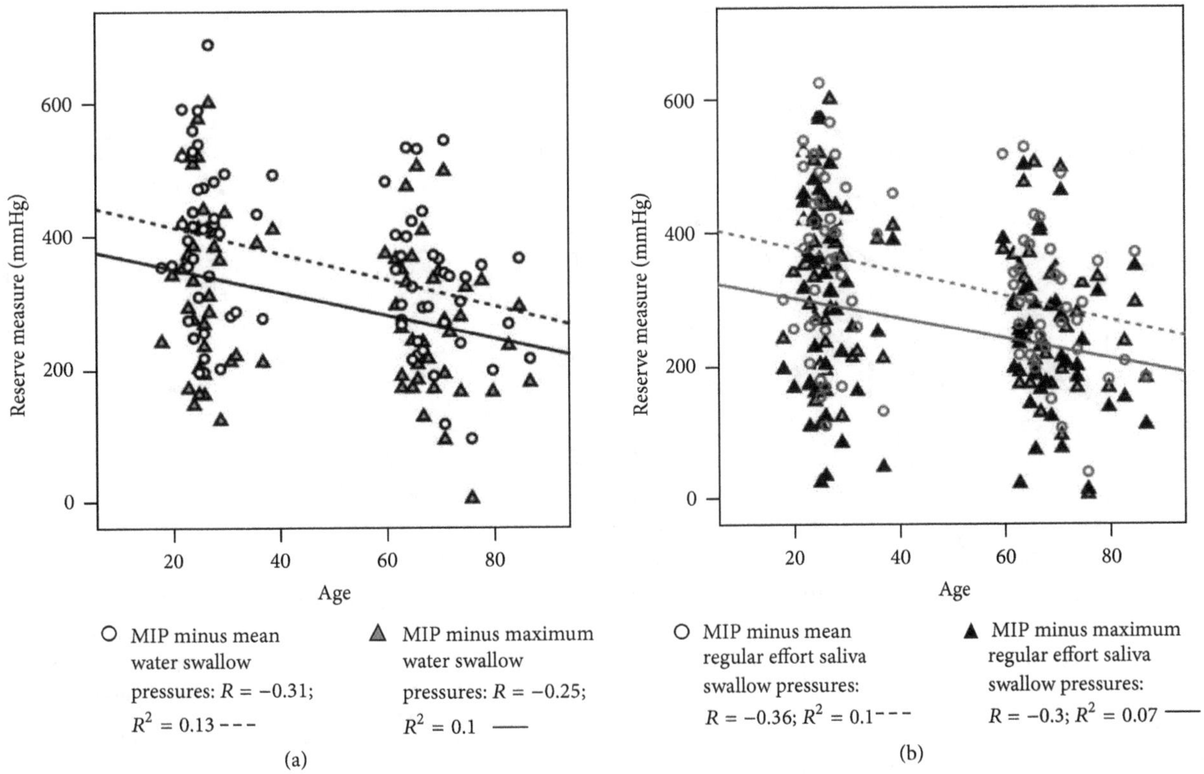

FIGURE 3: (a) Scatter plot showing the relationship between functional reserve measures comparing maximum isometric pressure (MIP) to water swallowing pressures and age. (b) Scatter plot showing the relationship between functional reserve measures comparing maximum isometric pressure (MIP) to regular effort saliva swallowing pressures and age.

swallowing pressure into values normalized to a percentage of each participant's maximum strength measure. As shown in Figure 4(a), strong correlations with MIP are retained with this transformation when saliva swallows are used at the bottom of the functional reserve range. With water swallows, the correlations fall just below the *a priori* criterion of $R = 0.4$, but remain statistically significant (Figure 4(b)). With respect to correlations with age, if a correlation age remains significant after this transformation, we would be able to conclude that functional reserve declines as a function of age, rather than being primarily driven by a person's strength. This, however, was not the case. Figures 5(a) and 5(b) show that the previously observed weak correlations with age are negated by the transformation. No statistically significant correlations with age are seen, regardless of the equation used to calculate functional reserve. This result confirms the previous result reported by Youmans and colleagues [5], suggesting that the appearance of an age-related decline in functional reserve may be an artifact attributable to variability in MIP measures across participants.

4. Conclusions

We conclude that optimally robust measures of functional reserve are those comparing maximum tongue strength (MIPs) to mean water or saliva swallowing pressures. Of these two options, saliva swallows involve less risk of aspiration during data collection. The results of the analysis in this study suggest that it would be reasonably straight forward for clinicians to routinely incorporate the measurement of tongue pressure functional reserve into swallowing assessment, using a short series of MIPs and saliva swallows.

We recommend that functional reserve measures should use a data transformation to account for individual differences in maximum tongue strength measures, by expressing swallowing pressures as a percent of a person's MIP. Using this transformation, functional reserve measures comparing MIP to either mean or maximum saliva swallow pressure retain statistically significant strong correlations with strength. However, this transformation has the effect of negating apparent age-related differences in functional reserve.

When normalized to control individual variations in strength, our data concur with those of Youmans and colleagues [5] in showing that functional reserve does not decline as a function of healthy aging. This finding strongly suggests that older adults should not be assumed to have tongue weakness and reduced functional reserve simply as a function of age. Indeed, our data suggest that the distribution of reduced functional reserve is not age dependent and that individuals with limited functional reserve may be found in the younger population. Certainly, prior studies point to limited functional reserve being a characteristic of dysphagia. The consequences of functional reserve for swallowing function and the ability to benefit from commonly used

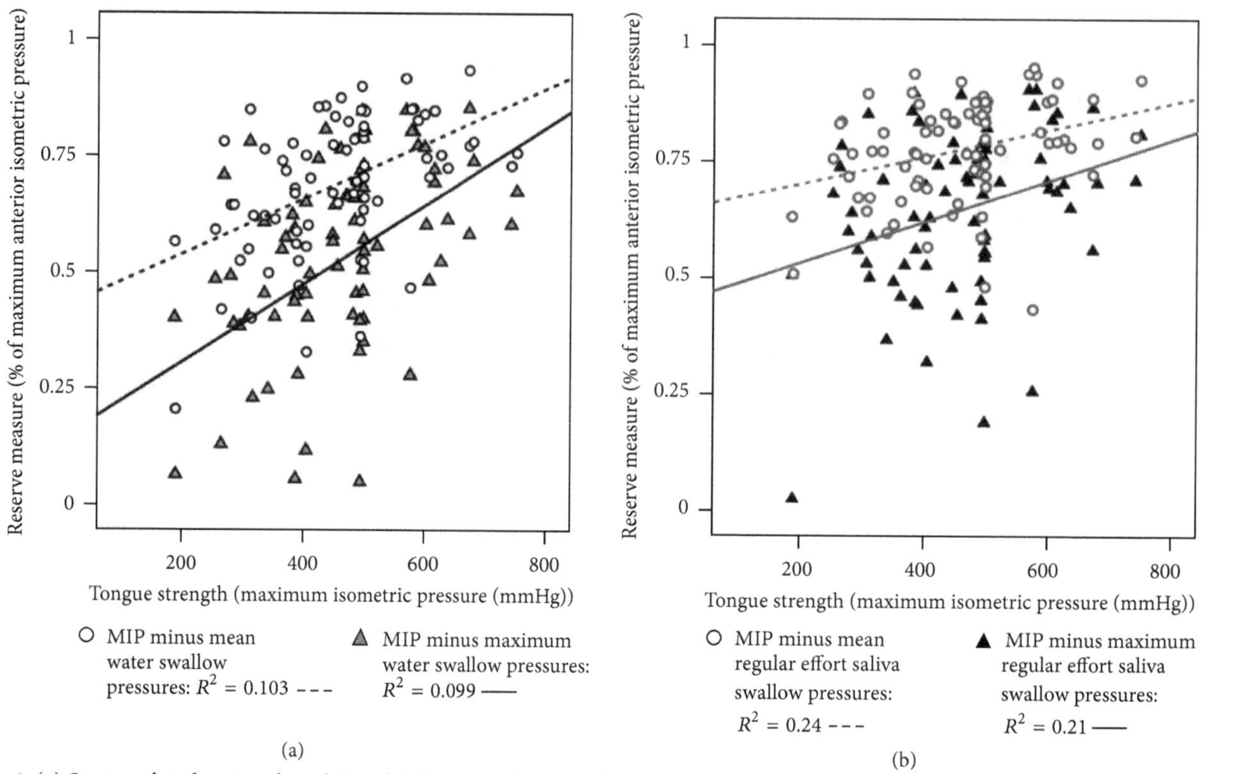

FIGURE 4: (a) Scatter plot showing the relationship between functional reserve measures comparing maximum isometric pressure (MIP) to water swallowing pressures and tongue strength, as measured by MIP, with swallow pressures expressed as a percentage of MIP. (b) Scatter plot showing the relationship between functional reserve measures comparing maximum isometric pressure (MIP) to regular effort saliva swallowing pressures and tongue strength, as measured by MIP, with swallow pressures expressed as a percentage of MIP.

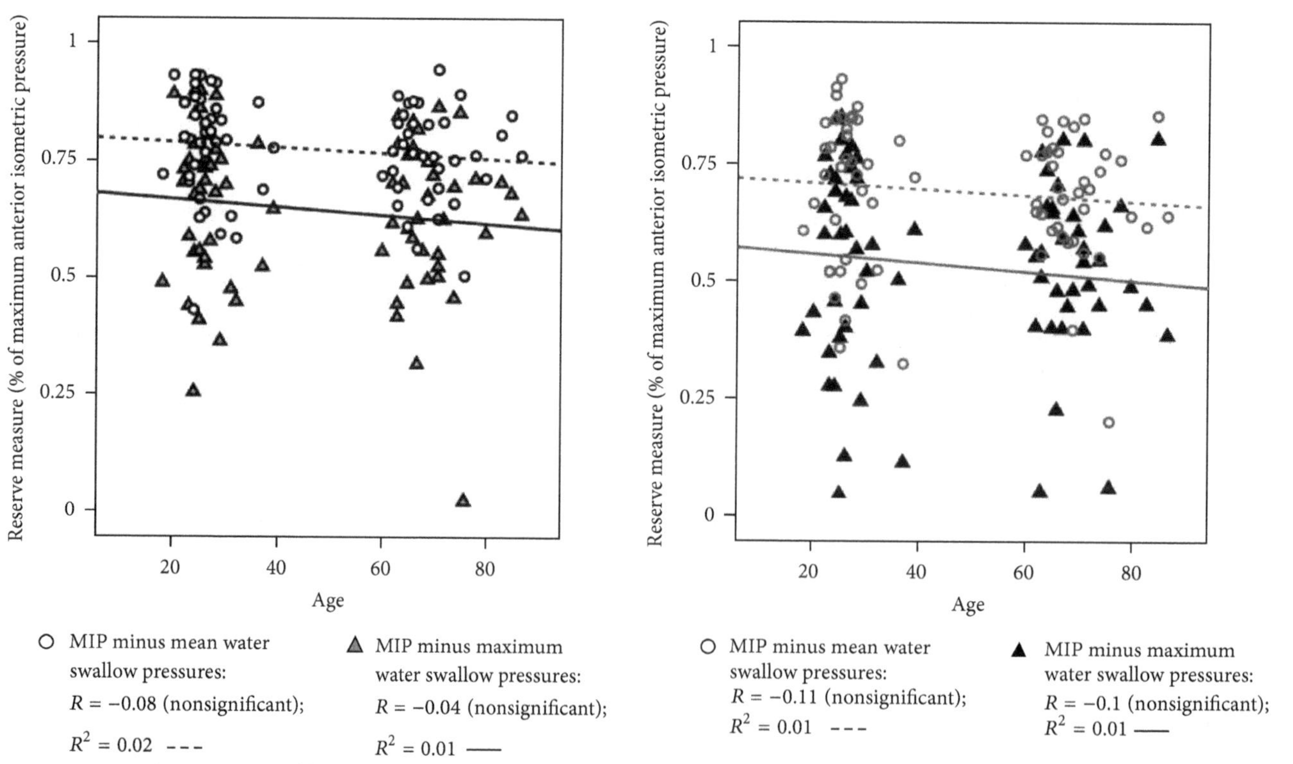

FIGURE 5: (a) Scatter plot showing the relationship between functional reserve measures comparing maximum isometric pressure (MIP) to water swallowing pressures and age, with swallow pressures expressed as a percentage of MIP. (b) Scatter plot showing the relationship between functional reserve measures comparing maximum isometric pressure (MIP) to regular effort saliva swallowing pressures and age, with swallow pressures expressed as a percentage of MIP.

interventions such as texture modification require further elucidation in future studies. Similarly, the benefits of tongue pressure resistance training for building functional reserve and restoring more normal swallowing function are still to be clearly demonstrated.

Acknowledgments

This work was supported by the National Institutes of Health (Grant no. 5R01DC011020 to C. M. Steele); and from the Toronto Rehabilitation Institute, which receives funding under the Provincial Rehabilitation Research Program from the Ontario Ministry of Health and Long-Term Care (MOHLTC). The views expressed do not necessarily reflect those of the ministry. The author would like to thank Drs. Mark Bayley, Cathy Pelletier, and Julie Cichero for their contributions to the study design and interpretation. Assistance from Rebecca Cliffe Polacco, Sarah Hori, Sonja Molfenter, Melanie Peladeau-Pigeon, and Clemence Tsang during data collection and processing is gratefully acknowledged.

References

[1] H. C. Crow and J. A. Ship, "Tongue strength and endurance in different aged individuals," *Journals of Gerontology. Series A*, vol. 51, no. 5, pp. M247–M250, 1996.

[2] M. A. Nicosia, J. A. Hind, E. B. Roecker et al., "Age effects on the temporal evolution of isometric and swallowing pressure," *Journals of Gerontology. Series A*, vol. 55, no. 11, pp. M634–M640, 2000.

[3] S. R. Youmans and J. A. G. Stierwalt, "Measures of tongue function related to normal swallowing," *Dysphagia*, vol. 21, no. 2, pp. 102–111, 2006.

[4] Y. Utanohara, R. Hayashi, M. Yoshikawa, M. Yoshida, K. Tsuga, and Y. Akagawa, "Standard values of maximum tongue pressure taken using newly developed disposable tongue pressure measurement device," *Dysphagia*, vol. 23, no. 3, pp. 286–290, 2008.

[5] S. R. Youmans, G. L. Youmans, and J. A. G. Stierwalt, "Differences in tongue strength across age and gender: is there a diminished strength reserve?" *Dysphagia*, vol. 24, no. 1, pp. 57–65, 2009.

[6] K. Tamine, T. Ono, K. Hori, J. Kondoh, S. Hamanaka, and Y. Maeda, "Age-related changes in tongue pressure during swallowing," *Journal of Dental Research*, vol. 89, no. 10, pp. 1097–1101, 2010.

[7] R. White, S. M. Cotton, J. Hind, J. Robbins, and A. Perry, "A comparison of the reliability and stability of oro-lingual swallowing pressures in patients with head and neck cancer and healthy adults," *Dysphagia*, vol. 24, no. 2, pp. 137–144, 2009.

[8] S. Ball, O. Idel, S. M. Cotton, and A. Perry, "Comparison of two methods for measuring tongue pressure during swallowing in people with head and neck cancer," *Dysphagia*, vol. 21, no. 1, pp. 28–37, 2006.

[9] J. Robbins, S. A. Kays, R. E. Gangnon et al., "The effects of lingual exercise in stroke patients with dysphagia," *Archives of Physical Medicine and Rehabilitation*, vol. 88, no. 2, pp. 150–158, 2007.

[10] N. Hirota, K. Konaka, T. Ono et al., "Reduced tongue pressure against the hard palate on the paralyzed side during swallowing predicts Dysphagia in patients with acute stroke," *Stroke*, vol. 41, no. 12, pp. 2982–2984, 2010.

[11] J. Robbins, R. E. Gangnon, S. M. Theis, S. A. Kays, A. L. Hewitt, and J. A. Hind, "The effects of lingual exercise on swallowing in older adults," *Journal of the American Geriatrics Society*, vol. 53, no. 9, pp. 1483–1489, 2005.

[12] C. L. Lazarus, J. A. Logemann, C. F. Huang, and A. W. Rademaker, "Effects of two types of tongue strengthening exercises in young normals," *Folia Phoniatrica et Logopaedica*, vol. 55, no. 4, pp. 199–205, 2003.

[13] J. Robbins, R. Levine, J. Wood, E. B. Roecker, and E. Luschei, "Age effects on lingual pressure generation as a risk factor for dysphagia," *Journals of Gerontology. Series A*, vol. 50, no. 5, pp. M257–M262, 1995.

[14] T. Fei, R. Cliffe Polacco, S. M. Molfenter, M. Peladeau-Pigeon, C. Tsang, and C. M. Steele, "Age-related differences in tongue-pressure release-slope for saliva and water swallows," in *Proceedings of the 20th Annual Meeting of the Dysphagia Research Society*, Springer, Toronto, Canada, 2012.

[15] E. M. Yeates, C. M. Steele, and C. A. Pelletier, "Tongue pressure and submental surface electromyography measures during noneffortful and effortful saliva swallows in healthy women," *American Journal of Speech-Language Pathology*, vol. 19, no. 3, pp. 274–281, 2010.

6

Is the Cloze Procedure Appropriate to Evaluate Health Literacy in Older Individuals? Age effects in the Test of Functional Health Literacy in Adults

Raymond L. Ownby,[1] Amarilis Acevedo,[2] Drenna Waldrop-Valverde,[3] and Robin J. Jacobs[1]

[1] *Department of Psychiatry and Behavioral Medicine, Nova Southeastern University, Fort Lauderdale, FL 33314, USA*
[2] *Center for Psychological Studies, Nova Southeastern University, Fort Lauderdale, FL 33314, USA*
[3] *Nell Hodgson Woodruff School of Nursing, Emory University, Atlanta, GA 30322, USA*

Correspondence should be addressed to Raymond L. Ownby; ro71@nova.edu

Academic Editor: F. R. Ferraro

Health literacy has received increasing attention because of its importance for older individuals' health, as studies have shown a close relation between older individuals' health literacy and their health. Research also suggests that older individuals have low levels of health literacy, but this finding is variable and may depend on which health literacy test is used. Older individuals assessed with the Test of Functional Health Literacy (TOFHLA) score lower than younger individuals, but a previous study suggested that this may result from age-related differential item functioning (DIF) on the TOFHLA. The study reported here assessed age-related DIF in a sample of community-dwelling volunteers. Twenty-two percent of items were differentially more difficult for older individuals independent of their overall ability, and when these items were eliminated from the total score, age differences were no longer found. Performance on a working memory task predicted older but not younger individuals' performance on the age-related items. At least part of older individuals' apparent deficits in health literacy when assessed by the TOFHLA may be related to DIF on its items. The TOFHLA, and any measure that employs the cloze procedure to evaluate reading comprehension, should be used cautiously in older individuals.

1. Introduction

Over the past several decades, research on health literacy has become increasingly relevant to gerontologists, as studies have shown that older adults' health literacy is an important factor in their health status and service utilization [1–4]. Health literacy has been defined as "... *the degree to which individuals have the capacity to obtain, process, and understand basic health information and services needed to make appropriate health decisions*" [5] and is related to older individuals' ability to use health information for decision making. Studies have shown that level of health literacy is related to use of health services and measures of disease control [1, 6]. It has also been related to increased risk for hospitalization in Medicare beneficiaries [7] and even to greater risk of death [8, 9].

Several studies have found that individuals 65 years of age and older perform at lower levels on measures of health literacy compared to younger individuals [10, 11]. The National Assessment of Adult Literacy (NAAL) was a population-based study of literacy that included a health literacy scale [10]. Age comparisons showed that those 65 years of age and older performed at lower levels compared to participants who were younger. Studies with other measures, including the widely-used Test of Functional Health Literacy in Adults or TOFHLA [12], have also found age-related decrements in performance [13]. On the other hand, some studies with another widely-used measure of health literacy, the Rapid Estimate of Adult Literacy in Medicine, or REALM [14], have not found age-related differences [9, 15–17]. Given the link between health literacy and health, a better understanding of reasons underlying older individuals' poorer performance on some but not all measures of health literacy might yield information that could inform the development of interventions to improve it.

One possible source of age-related differences in performance on tests of health literacy is the type of response required by the measure. The TOFHLA, for example, uses the cloze procedure to evaluate comprehension of health-related written material [18, 19]. With the cloze procedure, the person evaluated is asked to read a text passage and supply words that have been deleted and replaced with a blank (e.g., "The sky is —"). In the case of the TOFHLA the authors deleted every 5th to 7th word from three passages which progressively increased in level of difficulty [12]. Although the cloze procedure was created to assess text readability [19], it has been widely used as a device for measuring comprehension [20] and is incorporated in other health-related measures [21], although it has been criticized as inappropriate for use with low literacy individuals [22, 23] and for routine use in healthcare settings [24].

The cloze format may be difficult for older adults due to its demands on cognitive abilities that decline with age, including verbal fluency and working memory [25]. Studies have shown that cloze performance may depend on working memory and that it modifies the relation between age and general cognitive ability in cognitive task performance [18, 26]. Other authors have also demonstrated that working memory may differentially affect reading comprehension in older individuals [27, 28], still further implicating it as a factor in performance on tests that use the cloze procedure. Finally, a previous study showed age-related differential item functioning (DIF) on several TOFHLA items in individuals over 50 years of age who were treated for HIV infection [29], suggesting that some TOFHLA items may be harder for older individuals than younger individuals even when they have the same overall level of health literacy. This study's small sample size and the existence of disease-related cognitive deficits in study participants, however, make it difficult to generalize its results to other groups.

Using the cloze procedure to assess comprehension may thus inadvertently create a test with items that are differentially more difficult for elders, confounding the assessment of health literacy with age-related changes in cognition. Apparent age-group differences may result that suggest that elders' health literacy skills are lower than they actually are. This possibility can be tested by assessing whether test items display differential item functioning or DIF related to age [30]. A test item is said to exhibit DIF when it is more difficult for a member of one group than another (e.g., men versus women, blacks versus whites, or older versus younger) even though each person's underlying overall ability is the same. If age-related DIF is present in the items of the TOFHLA, some items would be more difficult for older than younger individuals even though they have the same overall ability. This could occur because the DIF-related items make demands on a cognitive ability such as working memory that declines with increasing age. In essence, items with age-related DIF would thus evaluate two abilities in older individuals (health literacy and working memory) while ostensibly assessing only one (health literacy).

The purpose of these analyses was therefore to evaluate whether items on the TOFHLA show age-related DIF using a nonparametric approach to identify DIF due to our sample size. We also chose to explore the possibility that working memory would be related to performance on items showing DIF using standard parametric regression analysis and test whether taking age-related DIF into account would explain age-group differences in performance on the TOFHLA by comparing the performance on age-based groups on the measure with and without items that show age-related DIF.

2. Method

2.1. Overview. In this study we drew on data collected in a larger study whose purpose was to develop and validate a new measure of health literacy [31, 32]. Participants whose ages ranged from 18 to 86 provided demographic information and completed the TOFHLA and a battery of cognitive and academic measures. These data thus provided the basis for an assessment of differences in TOFHLA performance between those 65 years of age and older compared to those who were younger while taking into account potential confounders that included education, general verbal ability, and basic reading skills. Age-related DIF was first assessed in the items of the TOFHLA as described below. As we hypothesized that working memory might be a factor in age-related DIF, the relation of performance on a measure of working memory (digit span backward) to performance on the DIF-related items was evaluated in younger and older individuals. Finally, to evaluate the relevance of DIF to age group differences on total TOFHLA reading scores, differences between groups were tested on the sum of all TOFHLA comprehension items and a recalculated total score with DIF-related items was eliminated.

2.2. Participants. Participants were community-dwelling volunteers aged 18 and older recruited through flyers in community centers, word of mouth, and from previous studies. As the purpose of the parent study was to develop a new measure of health literacy and to provide preliminary norms for it, participants were selected to represent a wide range of ages and educational levels and to be distributed across gender and race [31, 32]. Of the 167 participants who were younger than 65, 70 were white and 97 were black and 75 were men and 92 were women. Of the 69 participants who were 65 years of age or older, 54 were white and 15 were black and 19 were men and 50 were women. It can be seen that the average age of the younger group was approximately 43 while that of the older group was approximately 74 years. Figure 1 shows the number of individuals at each age in the two age groups and additional descriptive information is provided in Table 1.

2.3. Measures. As part of a battery of ability and skill measures, the complete TOFHLA, including 50 reading comprehension items, was administered. The reading comprehension portion of the TOFHLA requires the person assessed to read three paragraphs of health-related material whose difficulties progressively increase. The first paragraph is based

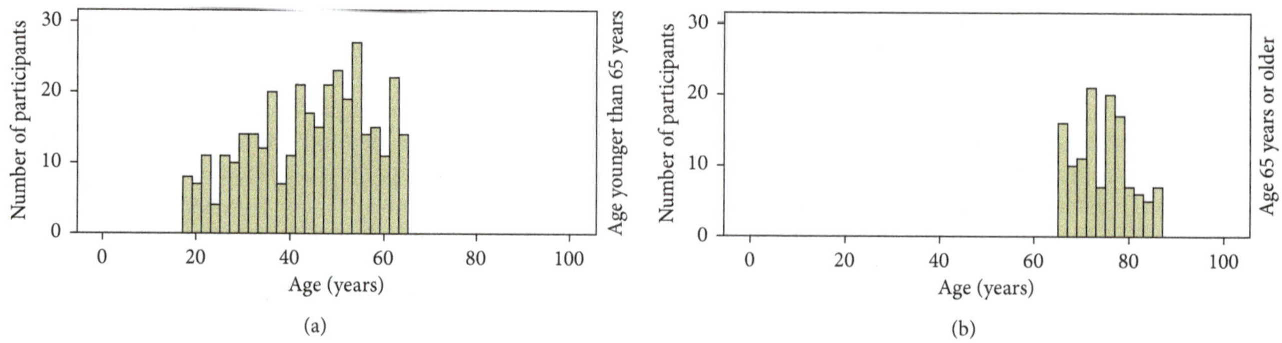

FIGURE 1: Age distribution of participants by group.

TABLE 1: Description of sample.

	Younger than 65 (n = 167)		65 or older (n = 69)		All participants (n = 236)	
	Mean	SD	Mean	SD	Mean	SD
Age (years)	42.81	13.46	73.90	6.01	51.90	18.42
Education (years)	13.01	2.37	13.48	2.54	13.15	2.42
TOFHLA reading[a]	45.83	4.66	45.28	7.21	45.67	5.52
General verbal ability[b]	92.38	10.40	99.22	12.24	94.38	11.38
Reading skills[c]	94.83	9.30	101.43	14.14	96.76	11.32
Digit span backwards[d]	6.72	2.45	6.19	2.05	6.57	2.35

[a]Total number of TOFHLA reading comprehension items answered correctly (range 0–50).
[b]Woodcock-Johnson Psychoeducational Battery Verbal Comprehension composite score (mean = 100; SD = 15).
[c]Woodcock-Johnson Psychoeducational Battery Passage Comprehension subtest standard score (mean = 100; SD = 15).
[d]Wechsler Adult Intelligence Scale, 3rd Ed. Digit Span Backward subtest raw score.

on simple instructions on how to prepare for an X-ray, the second focuses on patient rights and responsibilities in a government-supported health insurance program, and the third is drawn from an informed consent form for a surgical procedure. Every fifth to seventh word is removed from the text and indicated by a line; under the line, several options, one of which is correct, are presented. Participants were tested according to the standard directions for the measure [12] and were allowed 20 minutes to complete the reading comprehension questions. Their responses were categorized as right or wrong according to the test's administration instructions [12].

General verbal ability was assessed using the Verbal Composite score of the Woodcock-Johnson Psycho-Educational Battery [33]. This measure evaluates word knowledge, general information, and verbal reasoning in a series of tasks that yields a single score. Basic reading skills were assessed with the Passage Comprehension subtest of the Woodcock-Johnson Battery. This subtest uses items based on one or two sentences to evaluate a person's ability to understand what is read. Working memory was assessed with the Digit Span Backward subtest of the Wechsler Adult Intelligence Scale, 3rd edition [34].

Participants completed individually-administered cognitive measures in a single session while completing a group of self-report measures in a second session. Sessions were randomized to minimize order effects (i.e., some participants completed self-report measures first and then cognitive measures, while other completed cognitive measures first). The order of test administration within sessions was fixed. The Digit Span test was administered first in the battery because of its simplicity; it was judged as a good warm-up task compared to later measures that included the TOFHLA.

2.4. Analyses

2.4.1. Assessment of DIF. Standard approaches to evaluate DIF typically employ tests of group-based differences based on large-sample parametric statistics [35]. Some experts suggest that the sample size for this type of analysis should be at least 1,000 [30] and a simulation study showed that DIF detection rates may be suboptimal even with a sample of 500 when comparison groups are unequal in size [36]. As the available sample was substantially smaller than required for these techniques, an alternate approach to item assessment was followed using nonparametric item response theory (IRT) techniques. Age-related DIF was assessed with the beta index provided in TestGraf, a free nonparametric IRT program [37]. TestGraf produces item characteristic curves which provide a graphic representation of the probability of individuals in different groups obtaining a correct score on an item in relation to their overall ability. If DIF is not present, the curves for each group should be congruent or nearly so, but if DIF is present, the two curves will diverge

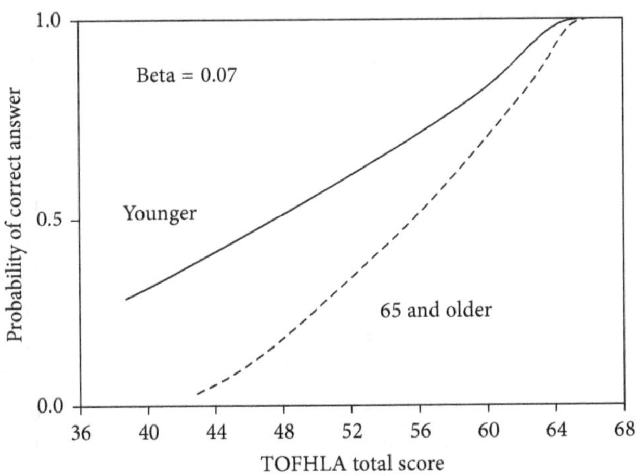

FIGURE 2: Item response curve for TOFHLA item 41 illustrating DIF between younger and older individuals.

(see Figure 2). The beta index is a numeric representation of the area between item response curves for two groups. Cutoff scores for the beta index to identify DIF for small sample sizes have been provided in a simulation study by Zumbo and Witarsa [38], who also showed that standard approaches such as the Mantel-Haenszel chi-square test have inadequate power to reliably detect DIF in small samples. The free software package jMetrik (http://www.itemanalysis.com/) was used to calculate item difficulties, standard deviations, and discriminations (defined as the correlation of each item with the total scale score).

The sample was divided into two groups based on age less than or greater than or equal to 65 years. Age 65 was used for comparison as it has most often been used in research on age-related cognitive abilities and is linked to both age-related changes in working memory [39] and reports of older individuals' lower levels of health literacy [3, 13]. Items that exceeded the critical value of beta for the available sample size [38], thus indicating at a probability of less than 0.05 that DIF was present, were tabulated.

Although we used a nonparametric strategy to evaluate age-related DIF, our sample size was sufficient to allow us to assess the overall effect of DIF on group scores with a standard parametric strategy, analysis of covariance (ANCOVA). This strategy enabled us to correct for between-group differences in important covariates (e.g., education and reading skill) while comparing group mean performances. Each group's scores for all TOFHLA reading items and the corrected total with DIF-related items removed were calculated and compared in analyses that controlled for general verbal ability and reading skills. The possibility that observed age group based differences resulted from older participants' inability to complete all items of the TOFHLA was evaluated using chi-square analyses; we followed up this assessment with a similar analysis of the relation educational achievement less than high school level and failure to complete the TOFHLA. As it was hypothesized that working memory would account for group differences on items, its effect on between-group differences was also evaluated using another parametric strategy by assessing its relation to performance on the DIF-related items in both age groups in regression analyses. As the focus of these analyses was on the possibility that items using the cloze procedure were differentially more difficult for individuals aged 65 and older, TOFHLA Numeracy items were not included as they do not utilize the cloze procedure.

All study procedures were completed under a protocol approved by the Nova Southeastern University Institutional Review Board.

3. Results

Descriptive statistics for participants are presented in Table 1. It should also be noted that each of group's scores on the TOFHLA Reading is similar, in spite of previous reports of significantly lower performance among older individuals. This fact can be attributed to the overall higher levels of education and basic reading skill in the older group, an issue that we addressed in group comparisons (reported below) by taking these factors into account in analysis of covariance (ANCOVA) models.

Item difficulties (percent answering correctly), discriminations (item-total correlations), and DIF analyses (beta values representing the area between item response curves for age groups) are presented in Table 2. Items with beta values greater than the $P < 0.05$ cut point of 0.0421 are in bold font [38]. Eleven of the 50 items (22% of the total) showed evidence of age-related DIF. An example of a nonparametric item characteristic curve for an item with DIF (item 41 in TOFHLA paragraph C) is presented in Figure 2. The figure includes item curves for younger and older individuals; each curve shows the probability of a participant answering the item correctly (left axis, ranging from 0 to 1) in relation to his or her overall ability. As Figure 2 shows, older individuals have a lower probability of answering this item correctly even when their total score was the same as a younger person's total score. Older individuals would thus have lower overall scores on the TOFHLA as a result of age-related DIF on these 11 items.

Table 3 presents regression models assessing factors related to performance on the sum of the DIF-related items for younger and older participants. For younger individuals, general verbal ability, reading skills, and years of education were related to performance on the DIF-related items (model 1). The addition of working memory to the model (model 2) did not significantly improve its relation to performance on the items (change in $R^2 = 0.01$, $F(1, 149) = 1.86$, $P = 0.18$). For individuals 65 or older, reading skills and education, but not general verbal ability, were related to performance on the DIF items. The addition of working memory (model 2) resulted in a significant improvement in the model's relation to performance on the DIF items (change in $R^2 = 0.04$, $F(1, 57) = 5.82$, $P = 0.02$). These results suggest that while working memory may not have been an important determinant of performance on the DIF-related items for younger individuals, it was significant for older participants.

We evaluated the possibility that between-group differences on the TOFHLA resulted from older individuals

TABLE 2: Item difficulties, discriminations, and betas.

Item	Difficulty	SD	Discrimination	Beta[b]
A1[a]	0.99	0.09	0.60	0.03
A2	0.97	0.16	0.53	0.00
A3	0.89	0.31	0.34	0.01
A4	0.97	0.18	0.42	0.04
A5	0.98	0.13	0.35	0.03
A6	0.96	0.20	0.42	0.01
A7	0.97	0.18	0.54	0.01
A8	0.98	0.13	0.34	0.01
A9	0.94	0.24	0.26	0.01
A10	0.97	0.17	0.54	**0.05**
A11	0.98	0.13	0.42	0.02
A12	0.99	0.11	0.54	0.02
A13	0.96	0.20	0.41	0.03
A14	0.95	0.21	0.55	0.01
A15	0.97	0.17	0.38	0.01
A16	0.97	0.16	0.57	0.03
B17	0.98	0.14	0.57	0.01
B18	0.99	0.09	0.60	0.01
B19	0.83	0.37	0.27	0.03
B20	0.97	0.18	0.25	0.00
B21	0.93	0.26	0.65	0.01
B22	0.95	0.22	0.42	0.02
B23	0.96	0.19	0.47	**0.05**
B24	0.84	0.37	0.49	**0.08**[c]
B25	0.92	0.27	0.52	0.04
B26	0.92	0.27	0.52	0.04
B27	0.97	0.16	0.55	0.01
B28	0.97	0.16	0.58	0.02
B29	0.92	0.27	0.53	0.02
B30	0.94	0.24	0.63	0.02
B31	0.89	0.31	0.32	**0.08**[c]
B32	0.92	0.27	0.41	**0.05**[c]
B33	0.97	0.18	0.50	0.03
B34	0.49	0.50	0.19	**0.19**[c]
B35	0.97	0.17	0.65	0.03
B36	0.97	0.17	0.50	0.02
C37	0.97	0.18	0.67	0.02
C38	0.93	0.25	0.68	0.02
C39	0.83	0.38	0.47	**0.10**[c]
C40	0.84	0.37	0.52	0.03
C41	0.81	0.39	0.56	**0.07**
C42	0.92	0.27	0.56	0.02
C43	0.88	0.32	0.63	0.03
C44	0.92	0.27	0.68	0.02
C45	0.55	0.50	0.37	**0.09**[c]
C46	0.83	0.38	0.56	0.02
C47	0.46	0.50	0.32	**0.18**[c]
C48	0.86	0.35	0.57	**0.04**
C49	0.82	0.38	0.54	0.03
C50	0.88	0.32	0.36	0.04

[a]Letter prefixes before items numbers denote in which of the three test paragraphs the item is included.
[b]Items with values greater than the cutoff value of 0.0421 are in bold font, because of rounding some values of 0.04 is less than the cutoff value.
[c]Items that showed age-related DIF in a study of individuals younger and older than 50 treated for HIV infection [29].

TABLE 3: Regression models for performance on DIF items for younger and older participants.

		B	Std. error	t	p	R^2	Adj R^2	Significance of change with working memory
				Models for participants younger than 65				
1	Intercept	−2.95	1.13	−2.61	**0.01**			
	Verbal ability	0.05	0.02	2.93	**0.004**			
	Reading	0.06	0.02	3.69	**<0.001**			
	Education	0.02	0.05	2.55	**0.01**	0.44	0.42	
2	Intercept	−2.70	1.14	−2.37	**0.2**			
	Verbal	0.04	0.02	2.71	**0.001**			
	Reading	0.06	0.02	3.43	**0.001**			
	Education	0.12	0.05	2.49	**0.01**			
	Working memory	0.06	0.05	1.36	0.18	0.44	0.43	0.18
				Models for participants 65 years of age or older				
1	Intercept	0.14	1.28	0.11	0.91			
	Verbal ability	−0.01	0.02	−0.67	0.95			
	Reading	0.06	0.02	3.21	**0.002**			
	Education	0.22	0.08	2.68	**0.009**	0.55	0.52	
2	Intercept	0.30	1.23	0.24	0.81			
	Verbal	−0.003	0.02	−0.16	0.87			
	Reading	0.5	0.02	2.54	**0.01**			
	Education	0.23	0.08	2.87	**0.006**			
	Working memory	0.19	0.08	2.41	**0.02**	0.59	0.56	**0.02**

not completing the test, as the standard directions for the TOFHLA reading section specify a time limit for its completion. Nineteen participants did not finish the TOFHLA because of the time limit, 14 in the younger and 5 in the older groups. We assessed the relation of not completing the TOFHLA to age group and level of education (having completed high school compared to less than high school education) via chi-square analyses. The relation between age group and not completing the TOFHLA was not statistically significant (χ^2 (df = 1) = 0.09, P = 0.77), but the relation between less than high school educational attainment was (χ^2 (df = 1) = 4.46, P = 0.04).

Finally, the impact of DIF on overall performance on the TOFHLA reading scale was evaluated by testing between-group differences on the TOFHLA scores with and without the DIF items. Differences were evaluated in ANCOVA models that included general verbal ability, reading skill, and education as covariates. There was a significant difference between older and younger participants for the score on all 50 reading items (mean score for younger = 46.5; mean for older 43.8 for a mean difference of 2.4 points; $F(1, 231)$ = 17.26, $P < 0.001$). This difference was no longer significant after removal of the 11 items with DIF (mean score for younger = 39.6; mean for older 39.0 for a mean difference of 0.6 points; $F(1, 206) = 2.62$, $P = 0.11$). These results thus suggest that a portion of age-related differences on the TOFHLA reading scale resulted from the older group's performance on DIF-related items.

4. Discussion

These results confirm a previous report of age-related DIF in a potentially clinically relevant number of items of the TOFHLA reading scale [29] and extend this finding by investigating the extent to which working memory may be a factor in age-related DIF and testing its impact on age-related differences in TOFHLA scores. More than 20% of TOFHLA reading items showed age-related DIF; seven of these 11 items also were found to display age-related DIF in a previous study with HIV-infected patients younger or older than 50 years of age [29]. In the present study, working memory as measured by digit span backwards was significantly related to older participants' performance on these items not to that of younger participants. Further, when the 11 DIF-related items were removed from the total TOFHLA reading score, a significant age group difference was no longer present. Since working memory declines with age, an implication is that at least a portion of reported age differences in health literacy, at least for studies that used the TOFHLA, may be the result of its reliance on the cloze procedure that is related to working memory [18] rather than health literacy itself.

The finding of age differences on some health literacy measures while not on others also raises an important issue about how health literacy should be operationally defined. Ownby et al. [40] suggest that health literacy should be defined as a combination of basic cognitive abilities, reading skills, and health knowledge. Within this framework, our findings can be interpreted as showing that working memory may be a more important aspect of health literacy for older than younger individuals. To the extent that working memory is integral to health literacy, individuals 65 and older can be said to have lower levels of health literacy. When health literacy is defined as the ability to read health-related words aloud, however, (as in the REALM) it appears likely that older individuals may not be at a disadvantage. Another study [41] also showed that specific cognitive abilities may have a differential impact on S-TOFHLA performance, similar to the finding reported here. This finding may also reflect the fact that sight word recognition skills such as those assessed in the REALM are often considered resistant to age-related change [42, 43]. The definition of health literacy most commonly used inherently assumes that a patient has necessary basic cognitive abilities and academic skills; these findings emphasize the importance of explicitly recognizing their impact on performance on health literacy measures. A further study is needed to determine which approach to defining and measuring health literacy has the greatest usefulness.

Limitations of these analyses include the relatively small sample size used to assess DIF in the TOFHLA. As discussed above, traditional approaches to assessing DIF may require much larger samples and the approach used in these analyses (nonparametric IRT) is less well established. The selection of working memory as a possible mechanism for observed age-related DIF, while supported by previous work on the cloze procedure [18] and cognitive aging [25], neglects the possibility that some other factors not included in analyses may have been responsible for observed differences in item functioning among older individuals. Still another possibility is that older participants might have become more easily fatigued during assessment activities, thus affecting their responses on the TOFHLA. Since our finding of DIF was not consistent across all items of the TOFHLA, however, this possibility appears unlikely. Our participants completed the study in two sessions, randomized to reduce the possibility of order effects. Since order of administration of the test battery was randomized between mornings and afternoons, we believe that fatigue is an unlikely explanation for the finding of DIF, although it must be acknowledged that the majority of the items that show DIF are in the last third of the test. The finding of age-related DIF on the TOFHLA reading items raises the question as well of alternative explanations for the finding. It is possible, for example, that the content of sections B and C of the TOFHLA Reading scale is less familiar to older compared to younger individuals. We thus acknowledge that other explanations, either instead of or in addition, to age-related cognition might account for these findings.

Another important issue that is raised by these findings is the question of why older individuals perform more poorly on other health literacy tests that do not use the cloze procedure. A study discussed above [17] with the Newest Vital Sign, or NVS [44], found age differences in performance on it but not on the REALM. In the NVS, individuals' health literacy is assessed through their ability to respond to a series of questions about a nutrition label. Perhaps the largest study of health literacy ever done, the National Assessment of Adult Literacy, included items assessing health literacy and found that it was significantly lower in participants 65 and older [10]. One possible explanation for these findings also involves the response format of these measures, all of which require verbal fluency and executive functions in addition to reading and health knowledge for responding correctly. In contrast to the REALM, the NVS and NAAL surveys require the person assessed to produce a new verbal response to questions (compared to the REALM which only requires reading words aloud, a skill that is often highly practiced among older individuals). Since verbal fluency and executive functions, like working memory, may decline with age [45], it can be speculated that findings of age-related decrements on these measures may also reflect at least in part their response formats. In this connection it is also worth noting that others have reported that executive functions are related to performance on the S-TOFHLA [46, 47]. It is thus possible that age-related cognitive changes in addition to working memory may have an impact on older individuals' performance on these measures. It will thus be important to further evaluate the cognitive abilities related to health literacy in individuals across age groups in order to better understand what health literacy tests actually measure. Investigations in this area might also inform efforts to create age-appropriate health education materials for older individuals. For example, cognitive load theory [48, 49] would dictate that taking older individuals' level of working memory into account would be important in the design of instructional materials.

4.1. Practice Implications. These finding have implications for the assessment of health literacy not only in English but also in other languages. The cloze procedure, for example, has been used to assess reading comprehension in languages other than English, such as Japanese [50], and there is considerable interest in measuring health literacy in countries outside North America, for example, Sorensen et al. [51]. These findings may thus be relevant for the assessment of health literacy in languages other than English.

An additional practice implication is that it may be more appropriate to use measures less sensitive to cognitive aging when evaluating health literacy in individuals 65 and older, especially as other analyses have shown that performance on the TOFHLA is closely related to cognitive abilities that show age-related cognitive decline [40], such as fluid cognitive abilities like nonverbal reasoning [52]. In this study, the REALM was shown to be less dependent on general cognitive abilities and more closely related to reading and health knowledge. This suggests that the REALM may be a better tool than the TOFHLA for assessing the skills needed to understand health-related material. A new measure of health literacy, FLIGHT/VIDAS (developed as part of the study reported here), was created to explicitly exclude items that showed age-related DIF during initial development and testing [31].

Several other approaches are available that allow for an approximation of older individuals' health literacy while not requiring the same cognitive skills as does the TOFHLA. The Brief Health Literacy Screen [53] allows an assessment of a person's health literacy skills by self-report; the individual to be assessed is asked about the degree of difficulty he or she experiences with several forms of written health information. While this approach has the advantage of providing an estimate of an individual's subjective perception of his or her health literacy, it is not a direct assessment of an individual's performance with health-related materials and does not take into account factors beyond health literacy that might affect a patient's self-report. It should be noted that the correlation between standard measures of health literacy and the Brief Health Literacy Screen questions is substantially smaller than that between direct assessments of health literacy [31, 54]. The Demographic Assessment for Health Literacy [55] provides an estimate of a person's score on the short version of the TOFHLA [56] based on his or her demographic characteristics. This measure's regression-based approach may be useful in large group analyses (as was intended by its developers) but it is not a direct individual assessment of a person's performance.

It may be reasonable to conclude, as have others, that it is important to consider cognitive task demands and purpose when selecting a health literacy measure [54]. These results thus further support others' observations of the variable relations of common measures of health literacy with age and the importance of specific cognitive abilities for performance on measures of health literacy [41]. Given the evidence of age-related DIF on a substantial number of items in the reading comprehension subtest of the TOFHLA, it may be incorrect to interpret findings from it alone as proof that older individuals have lower levels of health literacy. The TOFHLA and any measure using the cloze procedure to assess comprehension should be used cautiously in older individuals; the REALM or FLIGHT/VIDAS may be more appropriate.

Conflict of Interests

The authors declare that there is no conflict of interests regarding the publication of this paper.

Acknowledgment

The authors were supported by Grant R01HL096578 from the National Heart, Lung, and Blood Institute provided to Dr. Ownby.

References

[1] N. D. Berkman, S. L. Sheridan, K. E. Donahue, D. J. Halpern, and K. Crotty, "Low health literacy and health outcomes: an updated systematic review," *Annals of Internal Medicine*, vol. 155, no. 2, pp. 97–107, 2011.

[2] N. D. Berkman, D. A. Dewalt, M. P. Pignone et al., "Literacy and health outcomes," *Evidence Report/Technology Assessment*, no. 87, pp. 1–8, 2004.

[3] S. White, *Assessing the Nation's Health Literacy*, AMA Foundation, Chicago, Ill, USA, 2008.

[4] R. L. Sudore, K. M. Mehta, E. M. Simonsick et al., "Limited literacy in older people and disparities in health and healthcare access," *Journal of the American Geriatrics Society*, vol. 54, no. 5, pp. 770–776, 2006.

[5] Department of Health and Human Services, *Healthy People 2020: Topics and Objectives*, Department of Health and Human Services, Washington, DC, USA, 2011.

[6] D. A. Dewalt, N. D. Berkman, S. Sheridan, K. N. Lohr, and M. P. Pignone, "Literacy and health outcomes: a systematic review of the literature," *Journal of General Internal Medicine*, vol. 19, no. 12, pp. 1228–1239, 2004.

[7] D. W. Baker, J. A. Gazmararian, M. V. Williams et al., "Functional health literacy and the risk of hospital admission among Medicare managed care enrollees," *The American Journal of Public Health*, vol. 92, no. 8, pp. 1278–1283, 2002.

[8] D. W. Baker, M. S. Wolf, J. Feinglass, and J. A. Thompson, "Health literacy, cognitive abilities, and mortality among elderly persons," *Journal of General Internal Medicine*, vol. 23, no. 6, pp. 723–726, 2008.

[9] R. L. Sudore, K. Yaffe, S. Satterfield et al., "Limited literacy and mortality in the elderly: the health, aging, and body composition study," *Journal of General Internal Medicine*, vol. 21, no. 8, pp. 806–812, 2006.

[10] S. White and S. Dillow, *Key Concepts and Features of the 2003 National Assessment of Adult Literacy (NCES 2006-471)*, Department of Education, National Center for Educational Statistic, Washington, DC, USA, 2005.

[11] C. Y. Osborn, M. K. Paasche-Orlow, T. C. Davis, and M. S. Wolf, "Health literacy: an overlooked factor in understanding HIV health disparities," *The American Journal of Preventive Medicine*, vol. 33, no. 5, pp. 374–378, 2007.

[12] R. M. Parker, D. W. Baker, M. V. Williams, and J. R. Nurss, "The test of functional health literacy in adults: a new instrument for measuring patients'literacy skills," *Journal of General Internal Medicine*, vol. 10, no. 10, pp. 537–541, 1995.

[13] D. W. Baker, J. A. Gazmararian, J. Sudano, and M. Patterson, "The association between age and health literacy among elderly persons," *Journals of Gerontology B: Psychological Sciences and Social Sciences*, vol. 55, no. 6, pp. S368–374, 2000.

[14] P. W. Murphy, T. C. Davis, S. W. Long, R. H. Jackson, and B. C. Decker, "Rapid estimate of adult literacy in medicine (REALM): a quick reading test for patients," *Journal of Reading*, vol. 37, no. 2, pp. 124–130, 1993.

[15] J. A. Green, M. K. Mor, A. M. Shields et al., "Prevalence and demographic and clinical associations of health literacy in patients on maintenance hemodialysis," *Clinical Journal of the American Society of Nephrology*, vol. 6, no. 6, pp. 1354–1360, 2011.

[16] L. D. McGowan, M. S. Goodman, and K. A. Kaphingst, *Using SAS/STAT Software to Validate a Health Literacy Prediction Model in a Primary Care Setting*, SAS Global Forum, 2014.

[17] C. L. Shigaki, R. L. Kruse, D. R. Mehr, and B. Ge, "The REALM versus NVS, A comparison of health literacy measures in patients with diabetes," *Annals of Behavioral Science and Medical Education*, vol. 18, 9, p. 13, 2012.

[18] P. L. Ackerman, M. E. Beier, and K. R. Bowen, "Explorations of crystallized intelligence: completion tests, cloze tests, and knowledge," *Learning and Individual Differences*, vol. 12, no. 1, pp. 105–121, 2000.

[19] W. L. Taylor, "Cloze procedure: a new tool for measuring readability," *Journalism Quarterly*, vol. 30, no. 4, pp. 415–433, 1953.

[20] C. G. Robinson, "Cloze procedure: a review," *Educational Research*, vol. 23, no. 2, pp. 128–133, 1981.

[21] A. Luk and P. Aslani, "Tools used to evaluate written medicine and health information: document and user perspectives," *Health Education and Behavior*, vol. 38, no. 4, pp. 389–403, 2011.

[22] C. C. Doak, L. G. Doak, and J. H. Root, *Teaching Patients with Low Literacy Skills*, Lippincott, Philadelphia, Pa, USA, 2nd edition, 1996.

[23] L. B. Trifiletti, W. C. Shields, E. M. McDonald, A. R. Walker, and A. C. Gielen, "Development of injury prevention materials for people with low literacy skills," *Patient Education and Counseling*, vol. 64, no. 1–3, pp. 119–127, 2006.

[24] T. C. Davis, R. Michielutte, E. N. Askov, M. V. Williams, and B. D. Weiss, "Practical assessment of adult literacy in health care," *Health Education and Behavior*, vol. 25, no. 5, pp. 613–624, 1998.

[25] D. C. Park and A. H. Gutchess, "Cognitive aging and everyday life," in *Aging and Communication*, D. C. Park, B. Sabel, and N. A. Charness, Eds., pp. 217–232, Springer, New york, NY, USA, 2000.

[26] P. L. Ackerman, M. E. Beier, and M. O. Boyle, "Individual differences in working memory within a nomological network of cognitive and perceptual speed abilities," *Journal of Experimental Psychology: General*, vol. 131, no. 4, pp. 567–589, 2002.

[27] D. Caplan, G. Dede, G. Waters, J. Michaud, and Y. Tripodis, "Effects of age, speed of processing, and working memory on comprehension of sentences with relative clauses," *Psychology and Aging*, vol. 26, no. 2, pp. 439–450, 2011.

[28] R. de Beni, E. Borella, and B. Carretti, "Reading comprehension in aging: the role of working memory and metacomprehension," *Aging, Neuropsychology, and Cognition*, vol. 14, no. 2, pp. 189–212, 2007.

[29] R. L. Ownby and D. Waldrop-Valverde, "Differential item functioning related to age in the reading subtest of the test of functional health literacy in adults," *Journal of Aging Research*, vol. 2013, Article ID 654589, 6 pages, 2013.

[30] S. E. Embretson and S. P. Reise, *Item Response Theory for Psychologists*, Lawrence Erlbaum, Mahwah, NJ, USA, 2000.

[31] R. L. Ownby, A. Acevedo, D. Waldrop-Valverde, R. J. Jacobs, A. M. Homs, and S. J. Czaja, "Development and initial validation of a computer-administered health literacy assessment in Spanish and English: FLIGHT/VIDAS," *Patient Related Outcome Measures*, vol. 4, pp. 1–15, 2013.

[32] R. L. Ownby, A. Acevedo, R. J. Jacobs, J. Caballero, and D. Waldrop-Valverde, "Quality of life, health status, and health service utilization related to a new measure of health literacy: FLIGHT/VIDAS," *Patient Education and Counseling*, 2014.

[33] R. W. Woodcock, K. S. McGrew, and N. Mather, *Woodcock-Johnson III Normative Update*, Riverside, Rolling Meadows, Ill, USA, 2007.

[34] D. Wechsler, *Manual for the Wechsler Adult Intelligence Scale*, Pearson Assessment, San Antonio, Tex, USA, 3rd edition, 1997.

[35] G. Camilli and L. A. Shepard, *Methods for Identifying Biased Test Items*, Sage, Thousand Oaks, Calif, USA, 1994.

[36] A.-N. Herrera and J. Gómez, "Influence of equal or unequal comparison group sample sizes on the detection of differential item functioning using the Mantel-Haenszel and logistic regression techniques," *Quality and Quantity*, vol. 42, no. 6, pp. 739–755, 2008.

[37] J. O. Ramsay, "TestGraft 98 Manual," McGill University, Montreal, Canada, 2000, http://www.psych.mcgill.ca/faculty/ramsay/TestGraf.html.

[38] B. D. Zumbo and P. M. Witarsa, "Nonparametric IRT methodology for detecting DIF in moderate-to-small scale measurment: Operating characteristics and a compartions with the Mantel Haenszel," in *Proceedings of the Annual Meeting of the American Educational Research Association*, 2004.

[39] D. C. Park, G. Lautenschlager, T. Hedden, N. S. Davidson, A. D. Smith, and P. K. Smith, "Models of visuospatial and verbal memory across the adult life span," *Psychology and Aging*, vol. 17, no. 2, pp. 299–320, 2002.

[40] R. L. Ownby, A. Acevedo, D. Waldrop-Valverde, R. J. Jacobs, and J. Caballero, "Abilities, skills and knowledge in measures of health literacy," *Patient Education and Counseling*, vol. 95, no. 2, pp. 211–217, 2014.

[41] J. Chin, D. G. Morrow, E. A. L. Stine-Morrow, T. Conner-Garcia, J. F. Graumlich, and M. D. Murray, "The process-knowledge model of health literacy: evidence from a componential analysis of two commonly used measures," *Journal of Health Communication*, vol. 16, no. 3, pp. 222–241, 2011.

[42] P. Bright, E. Jaldow, and M. D. Kopelman, "The National Adult Reading Test as a measure of premorbid intelligence: a comparison with estimates derived from demographic variables," *Journal of the International Neuropsychological Society*, vol. 8, no. 6, pp. 847–854, 2002.

[43] J. R. Crawford, I. J. Deary, J. Starr, and L. J. Whalley, "The NART as an index of prior intellectual functioning: a retrospective validity study covering a 66-year interval," *Psychological Medicine*, vol. 31, no. 3, pp. 451–458, 2001.

[44] B. D. Weiss, M. Z. Mays, W. Martz et al., "Quick assessment of literacy in primary care: the newest vital sign," *Annals of Family Medicine*, vol. 3, no. 6, pp. 514–522, 2005.

[45] S. Kemper and J. McDowd, "Dimensions of cognitive aging: executive function and verbal fluency," in *Handbook of Cognitive Aging: Interdisciplinary Perspectives*, S. M. Hofer and D. F. Alwin, Eds., pp. 181–92, Sage, Thousand Oaks, Calif, USA, 2008.

[46] R. L. Ownby and D. Waldrop-Valverde, "Health literacy is related to problem solving," in *Proceedings of the Health Literacy Research Conference*, Washington, DC, USA, October 2009.

[47] S. S. Sequeira, L. H. Eggermont, and R. A. Silliman, "Limited health literacy and decline in executive function in older adults," *Journal of Health Communication*, vol. 18, supplement 1, pp. 143–157, 2013.

[48] F. Paas, A. Renkl, and J. Sweller, "Cognitive load theory: instructional implications of the interaction between information structures and cognitive architecture," *Instructional Science*, vol. 32, no. 1-2, pp. 1–8, 2004.

[49] J. Sweller, "Cognitive load during problem solving: effects on learning," *Cognitive Science*, vol. 12, no. 2, pp. 257–285, 1988.

[50] M. Kobayashi, "Cloze tests revisited: exploring item characteristics with special attention to scoring methods," *The Modern Language Journal*, vol. 86, no. 4, pp. 571–586, 2002.

[51] K. Sorensen, S. van den Broucke, J. Pelikan et al., "Measuring health literacy in populations: illuminating the design and development process of the european health literacy survey questionnaire (HLS-EU-Q)," *BMC Public Health*, vol. 13, no. 1, article 948, 2013.

[52] J. L. Horn and R. B. Cattell, "Refinement and test of the theory of fluid and crystallized general intelligences," *Journal of Educational Psychology*, vol. 57, no. 5, pp. 253–270, 1966.

[53] K. A. Wallston, C. Cawthon, C. D. McNaughton, R. L. Rothman, C. Y. Osborn, and S. Kripalani, "Psychometric properties of the brief health literacy screen in clinical practice," *Journal of General Internal Medicine*, vol. 29, no. 1, pp. 119–126, 2014.

[54] J. Haun, S. Luther, V. Dodd, and P. Donaldson, "Measurement variation across health literacy assessments: implications for assessment selection in research and practice," *Journal of Health Communication*, vol. 17, supplement 3, pp. 141–159, 2012.

[55] A. D. Hanchate, A. S. Ash, J. A. Gazmararian, M. S. Wolf, and M. K. Paasche-Orlow, "The Demographic Assessment for Health Literacy (DAHL): a new tool for estimating associations between health literacy and outcomes in national surveys," *Journal of General Internal Medicine*, vol. 23, no. 10, pp. 1561–1566, 2008.

[56] D. W. Baker, M. V. Williams, R. M. Parker, J. A. Gazmararian, and J. Nurss, "Development of a brief test to measure functional health literacy," *Patient Education and Counseling*, vol. 38, no. 1, pp. 33–42, 1999.

7

Effect of Caloric Restriction on Hepatic Sinusoidal System and Stellate Cells in Mice

Jian Chen,[1] Kara King,[2] and Jian X. Zhang[2]

[1] *School of Human Kinetics, Laurentian University, 935 Ramsey Lake Road, Sudbury, ON, Canada P3E 2C6*
[2] *Biology Department, University of North Carolina, 9201 University City Bulevard, Charlotte, NC 28223, USA*

Correspondence should be addressed to Jian Chen; jchen@laurentian.ca

Academic Editor: Barbara Shukitt-Hale

Aging associated changes in liver include reduced hepatic blood flow, increased number of stellate cells, and collagen deposits in perisinusoidal space. We tested the possibility of mitigating these changes with caloric restriction. Two-month-old mice were subjected to 30 percent caloric restriction for 12 months and then examined for the effect of caloric restriction on the sinusoidal network, collagen deposition, and the number of stellate cells. Using intravital fluorescence microscopy, assessments were made on sinusoidal diameter, density, volumetric flow, perfusion index, and autofluorescence of vitamin A that was primarily stored with lipid droplets in stellate cells. A significant effect was observed in the vitamin A autofluorescence of stellate cells; stellate cell associated fluorescence was diminished in terms of number and size of fluorescent spots. Caloric restriction reduced collagen deposits in liver sections and lowered the gene expression of α1-(I) collagen but not α-smooth muscle actin. No differences were detected in sinusoidal dimension measurements. Our results showed that caloric restriction was effective in ameliorating the increase in stellate cells and the mild fibrosis in old mice. However, caloric restriction had no impact on stellate cell activity level as indicated by the unaffected α-smooth muscle actin expression.

1. Introduction

Aging liver exhibits metabolic alteration, slower hepatic clearance [1], fibrosis [2], reduced blood flow, and perfusion [3]. Ultrastructure of the sinusoids also undergoes changes that are characterized with narrowing of sinusoidal diameter [17], reduced fenestration, and thickening of the endothelial wall of the capillary [4, 5]. Such changes may contribute to disorder of liver lipid metabolism [6]. Aging liver has heightened susceptibility to fibrogenic agents due to altered immune response [7]. Hepatic fibrogenic response is elevated in older patients with primary liver diseases [8, 9]. Stellate cells that store most vitamin A in the liver are primarily responsible for hepatic fibrosis [10]. There is an increase in nonactivated lipid laden stellate cells and hyperplasia in aged animals [11]. Older rats display increased autoflorescence due to accumulation of vitamin A derived metabolites in stellate cells [12].

Caloric restriction mitigates or delays many aging related alterations in gene expression that impact inflammation, cellular stress, and fibrosis in mammals [13]. However, there is very limited research into the impact of caloric restriction on sinusoidal system and stellate cells in aged animals. This study was undertaken to examine the effect of caloric restriction on fibrogenic gene expression, stellate cell, and sinusoidal dimension and perfusion.

2. Methods and Materials

2.1. Experimental Design, Caloric Restriction, and Sample Collection. The animal protocol was approved by the Institutional Animal Care and Use Committee at the University of North Carolina at Charlotte. C57BL/6J mice were placed into one of two groups at 8 weeks of age: 30% caloric restriction ($N = 10$) or ad libitum feeding (control; $N = 10$). The animals were maintained on their respective diets for 12 months. The amount of food allotted and consumed was recorded daily. The amount of food given to the individual animals in the caloric restriction group was 30% less than the recorded average food consumption by the ad libitum fed group during the week just before the start of the experiment. After the duration of the study, the microcirculation of each animal was evaluated via intravital microscopy. Subsequently, the animals were sacrificed via cardiac puncture. Liver samples were snap-frozen in liquid nitrogen immediately after collection and were stored at −80°C till use. For tissue staining, frozen tissue sections (10 μm) were cut in the cryostat chamber at a temperature of −18 to −20°C and stored at −80°C until further processing. Liver sections were formalin fixed and paraffin embedded.

2.2. Masson's Trichrome Staining. Slides of liver sections were deparaffinized to deionized water and mordant in preheated Bouin's solution at 56°C for 15 minutes. Slides were subsequently cooled in tap water (18–26°C) in a Coplin jar. They were washed in running tap water to remove yellow color from sections and stained in working Weigert's Iron Hematoxylin Solution for 5 minutes. Next, they were washed in running tap water for 5 minutes and rinsed in deionized water. They were stained in Biebrich Scarlet-Acid Fucshin for 5 minutes, rinsed in deionized water, and placed in working Phosphotungstic/Phosphomolybdic Acid Solution for 5 minutes. Finally, slides were placed in Aniline Blue Solution, for 5 minutes and placed in 1% acetic acid for 2 minutes. The solution was discarded and the slides were rinsed, dehydrated through alcohol and xylene, and mounted. All reagents were obtained from Sigma Aldrich.

2.3. Intravital Microscopy. For sinusoidal epi-illumination preparation, mice fasted for 12 hours before the procedure and were allowed free access to water. They were anesthetized intraperitoneally using sodium pentobarbital (50 mg/kg body weight). After the surgery, liver lobes were examined under an Olympus IX70 inverted fluorescence microscope. For visualization of sinusoids, carboxyfluorescein diacetate succinimidyl ester (CFSE, 50 μM in 0.1 mL saline) was injected intravenously. The liver surface was epi-illuminated with a 100 W mercury lamp and a filter set consisting of an excitation filter band pass 485 nm, dichroic mirror 510 nm, and barrier filter 515–565 nm. The images were processed by an ARGUS-20 image processor (Hamamatsu Photonics, Japan) at specimen-monitor ratios of ×840-2500 and projected onto a Hamamatsu C2400-08 SIT camera and viewed on a high resolution video monitor. Fields were recorded onto a VCR tape for offline analysis. Assessment of sinusoidal parameters for sinusoidal flow dynamics was done off-line from the video-recorded images using digitized frame-by-frame analysis with MetaMorph image analysis system (Universal Imaging Co., West Chester, PA, USA).

2.4. Quantitative Video Analysis. Sinusoid diameter and number of perfused sinusoids: for sinusoid diameter (D), using MetaMorph image analysis software, 5 random lines were vertically drawn across each visible sinusoid within the field. Subsequently these values were averaged to yield an average sinusoid diameter for each field. Five fields were then averaged together to yield an average diameter for each animal. Animals examined then are combined to yield a group average. The number of perfused sinusoids (P_s) within a given microscopic field (150 μm in diameter) was counted and averaged in the same way to ascertain a group average.

White blood cell velocity measurement: for white blood cell velocity (VWBC) measurements, neutrophils were labeled with carboxyfluorescein diacetate succinimidyl ester (CFSE) and tracked from the time they first appeared in the field to the time they disappeared. The velocities for each field were averaged as described for sinusoid diameter. Rolling and adhered neutrophils were excluded.

Calculation of volumetric flow and perfusion index: using the measurement of white blood cell velocity (VWBC) and sinusoidal diameter (D), the volumetric flow (VF) in each sinusoid was calculated based on the formula: VWBC $\times \pi(D/2)^2$. The volumetric flow was then used to generate the perfusion index by multiplying it with the number of perfused sinusoids in each group: $P_s \times$ VF. Intravital microscopy measurements were derived and measured as previously described [12].

Retinyl ester (vitamin A) fluorescence measurement: vitamin A within hepatic stellate cells was detected using 366 nm excitation and 450 nm emission band pass filters [14].

2.5. RT-PCR Analysis of α-Smooth Muscle Actin (α-SMA) and α1-(I) Collagen. Reverse transcriptase-polymerase chain reaction was used to determine the mRNA levels of α-SMA and α1-(I) collagen. Total RNA was isolated using TRIzol reagent (Gibco-BRL, Invitrogen, Carlsbad, CA, USA) with approximately 50 mg of whole liver tissue. Reverse transcription was performed using 1 μg/μL of RNA and SuperScript reverse transcriptase II. For RT-PCR, a master mix was created containing 5 μL of 10x PCR buffer without $MgCl_2$, 5 μL 25 mM $MgCl_2$, 0.5 μL of 20 mM dNTP, 0.5 μL of forward primer, 0.5 μL of reverse primer, and 0.5 μL of Taq polymerase per reaction. The sense and antisense primer sequences were for mouse α-SMA, SMA 5′-GCTGGACTCTGGAGATGGCCGTGAC, and 5′-CCCGAGAGGACGTTGTTAGCATAG; for mouse α1-(I) collagen 5′-AAACCCGAGGTATGCTTGATCTGTA, and 5′-GTCCCTCGACTCCTACATCTTCTGA, for mouse glyceraldehyde-3-phosphate dehydrogenase, GAPH 5′-CCATCACCATCTTCCAGGAGCGAG, and 5′-CAC-AGTCTTCTGGGTGGCAGTGAT, respectively. Hot start RT-PCR was used. cDNA was heated for 3 minutes at 75°C. The master mix was added and the subsequent reaction took place in a thermocycler. Denaturation temperature: 94°C, annealing temperature: 55°C, and extension temperature: 72°C. The housekeeping gene, glyceraldehyde-3-phosphate dehydrogenase (GADPH) was amplified to serve as an internal control for sample loading amount. The PCR products were separated by electrophoresis on a 2% agarose gel and visualized by ethidium bromide staining. All reagents were obtained from Sigma Aldrich and Fisher Scientific (Hampton, NH, USA).

2.6. Statistical Analysis. Data are presented as mean ± SEM. Statistical analysis was performed using either a 1-way analysis of variance (1-way ANOVA) or a 2-Way ANOVA for

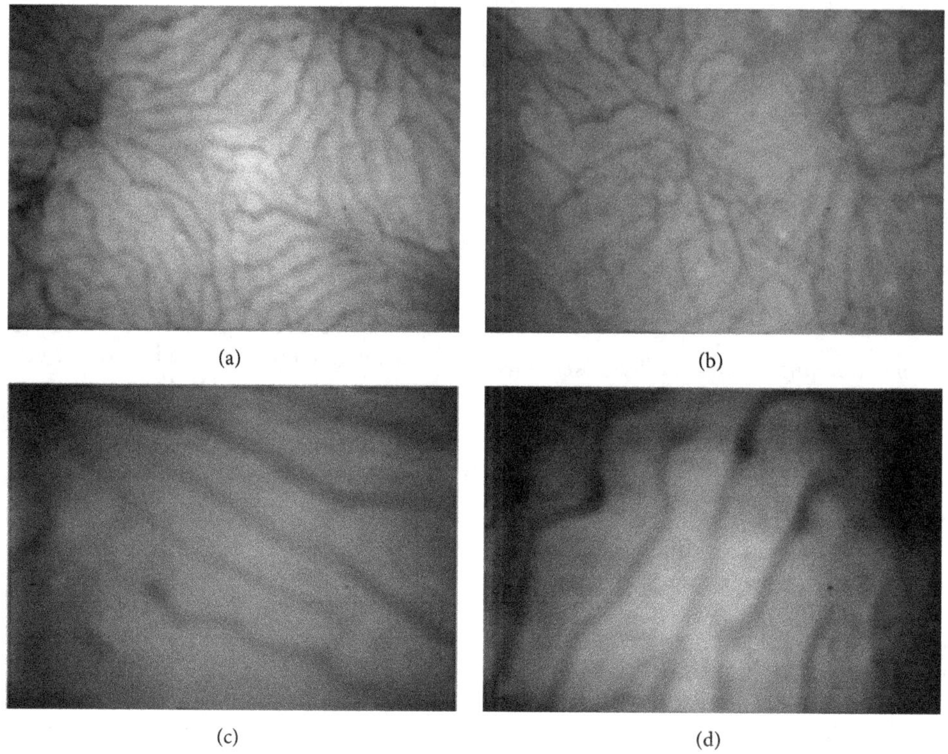

FIGURE 1: Representative intravital fluorescence microscopic images of the retinyl ester auto-fluorescence ((a) and (b)) and sinusoidal architecture ((c) and (d)). Liver from calorically restricted mice (a) shows diminished spots and intensity of vitamin A auto-fluorescence compared with control liver (b); the calorically restricted liver also has homogenous sinusoids (c) while the unrestricted liver contains more torturous sinusoids (d). Animal age is 14 months. The magnification is 20x ((a), (b)) or 100x ((c), (d)).

the caloric restriction. Statistical significance was set at $P < 0.05$. The Tukey post hoc test was used to evaluate all pairwise comparisons. Statistical analysis was performed using SigmaStat (San Jose, CA, USA).

3. Results

3.1. Caloric Restriction Reduces Hepatic Collagen Deposition and Stellate Cell Population. The visualization of in vivo autofluorescence of intracellularly stored vitamin A provided an indirect way of assessing stellate cell population [12].

Figure 1 shows representative intravital fluorescence microscopic images of livers from control mice and calorically restricted mice. With CR, the number and size of fluorescence spots decreased in 14-month-old mice. Masson's Trichrome stain for collagen showed less collagen deposits in the liver sections of calorically restricted mice (Figure 2). The representative images were randomly selected sections of the liver. Compared with the control mice, there was less collagen staining in hepatic perivenular regions of the calorically restricted group ($N = 7$).

3.2. Effect of Caloric Restriction on α-SMA Induction and Fibrogenic Gene Expression. The induction of α-SMA is the single most reliable marker of stellate activation since no other cell types express α-SMA in liver [15]. Caloric restriction had no effect on the activation and level of stellate cells in this study. The expression of α-SMA was not affected by caloric restriction (Figure 3). However, the expression of α-1(I) collagen was lower in calorically restricted mice (Figure 3). The lowered expression of α-1(I) collagen provided further support for the caloric restriction effect on fibrosis, the observed decrease in collagen deposits that were identified by Masson's Trichrome stain.

3.3. Effect of Caloric Restriction on Sinusoids and Microcirculation. The view of intravital microscopic field revealed different appearances of sinusoidal systems between the calorically restricted animals and their unrestricted controls. The sinusoidal network of calorically restricted liver is more homogenous and less tortuous while control animals have more nonperfused areas (Figure 1).

The average sinusoidal diameters in livers of caloric restriction and control animals is $4.54 \pm 0.5\,\mu$m and $4.31 \pm 0.3\,\mu$m, respectively (Figure 4). The sinusoidal perfusion rate, expressed as the average number of perfused sinusoids per microscopic examining field, is 4.6 ± 0.4 for caloric restriction and 4.3 ± 0.3 for control groups. The volumetric flow was 3015 ± 335 picoliters per second in calorically restricted group and 2770 ± 274 picoliters per second in the control group. The calculated perfusion indexes are 13871 ± 1928 (caloric restriction) versus 12361 ± 1510 (control). Although all measurements associated with caloric restriction are higher than

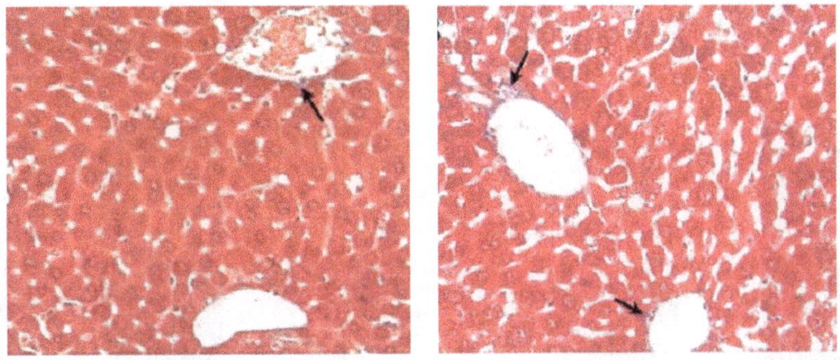

(a) (b)

FIGURE 2: Representative images of Masson's Trichrome Stain. Collagen deposits (→) are examined on liver sections at 60x magnifications. Calorically restricted liver (a) exhibits less collagen deposits than liver of ad libitum fed animal (b); animal age is 14 months.

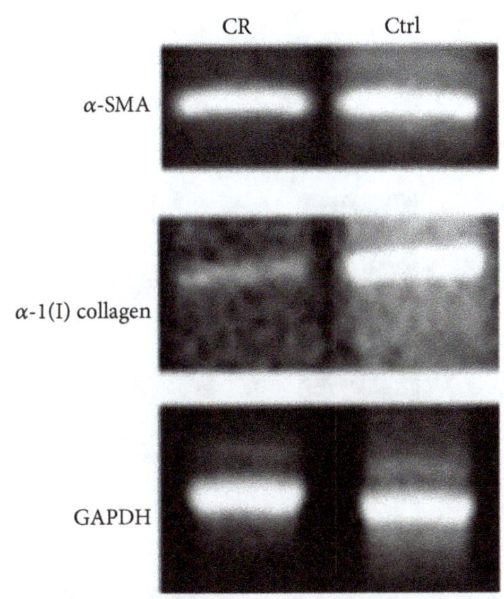

FIGURE 3: RT-PCR of profibrogenic proteins. Gene expressions of α-Smooth Muscle Actin (α-SMA, product size = 446 bp) and α-1(I) collagen (product size = 174 bp). The house keeping gene, glyceraldehyde-3-phosphate dehydrogenase (GAPDH, product size = 346 bp) was used to establish equal loading. The calorically restricted (CR) mice ($N = 7$) has decreased expression of α-1(I) collagen as compared with mice fed ad libitum (Ctrl, $N = 7$).

the control, these differences did not achieve statistical significance.

4. Discussion

Age associated increases in hepatic collagen deposition have been reported in several species including rat [4, 15], mouse [16, 17], and human [18, 19]. Aged liver also exhibits accumulation of stellate cells without apparent activation of these cells. Immunological staining of desmin, a stellate specific protein, revealed an increase in desmin positive cells in older mouse liver [11]. Vollmar et al. [12] reported a rise in stellate cell population in aged rats as indicated by the increased number and intensity of vitamin A autofluorescence spots. Our data demonstrated that caloric restriction ameliorated the aging related increases in hepatic stellate cell number and mild fibrosis.

The vitamin A rich stellate cells are the predominant producer of collagen fibers in liver. Once activated by injury of any etiology, they lose their storage of lipid droplets and vitamin A, transform into fibroblast-like cells, and dramatically escalate expression of fibrogenic genes [20]. Despite its well established role as a major fibrogenic cell type in liver, stellate cells may not have a significant influence on normal aging-related fibrosis. In old mice, the level of α-SMA expression was unchanged indicating no activation of stellate cells despite a rise of collagen content in liver [11]. In our study, even though both collagen deposits and stellate cell population were reduced by caloric restriction, α-SMA expression was unaffected. Therefore, the effects of normal aging and caloric restriction on fibrosis appear to be mediated by factors other than stellate cells.

Changes in collagen degradation and production of collagen by other cell types in liver may be responsible for the elevated collagen deposits. Old age was associated with increased levels of proinflammatory cytokines and inhibition of collagen degradation that can lead to fibrosis in liver [21]. Similarly, caloric restriction lowered many of the proinflammatory cytokines [13] and ameliorated age associated fibrosis [15]. Other liver cells may also contribute partly to the collagen content change in the aging liver. Liver sinusoidal endothelial cells (LSEC) play an important role in promoting inflammatory and fibrogenic milieu in liver [22]. These collagen producing cells exhibit functional changes and structural abnormality that are part of sinusoidal alteration referred as pseudocapillarization in old liver [5]. In fibrotic liver, LSEC hold several hold increases in type I collagen production [23].

Caloric restriction did not have significant impact on sinusoidal dimension and perfusion index in this study. At the end of the dietary intervention period, the mice in this study were 14 months old and were considered middle aged. It may be difficult to demonstrate a significant effect of caloric restriction on sinusoidal perfusion in the middle aged mice. Hepatic sinusoidal system of middle aged mice displayed certain functional alterations of endothelial cells and

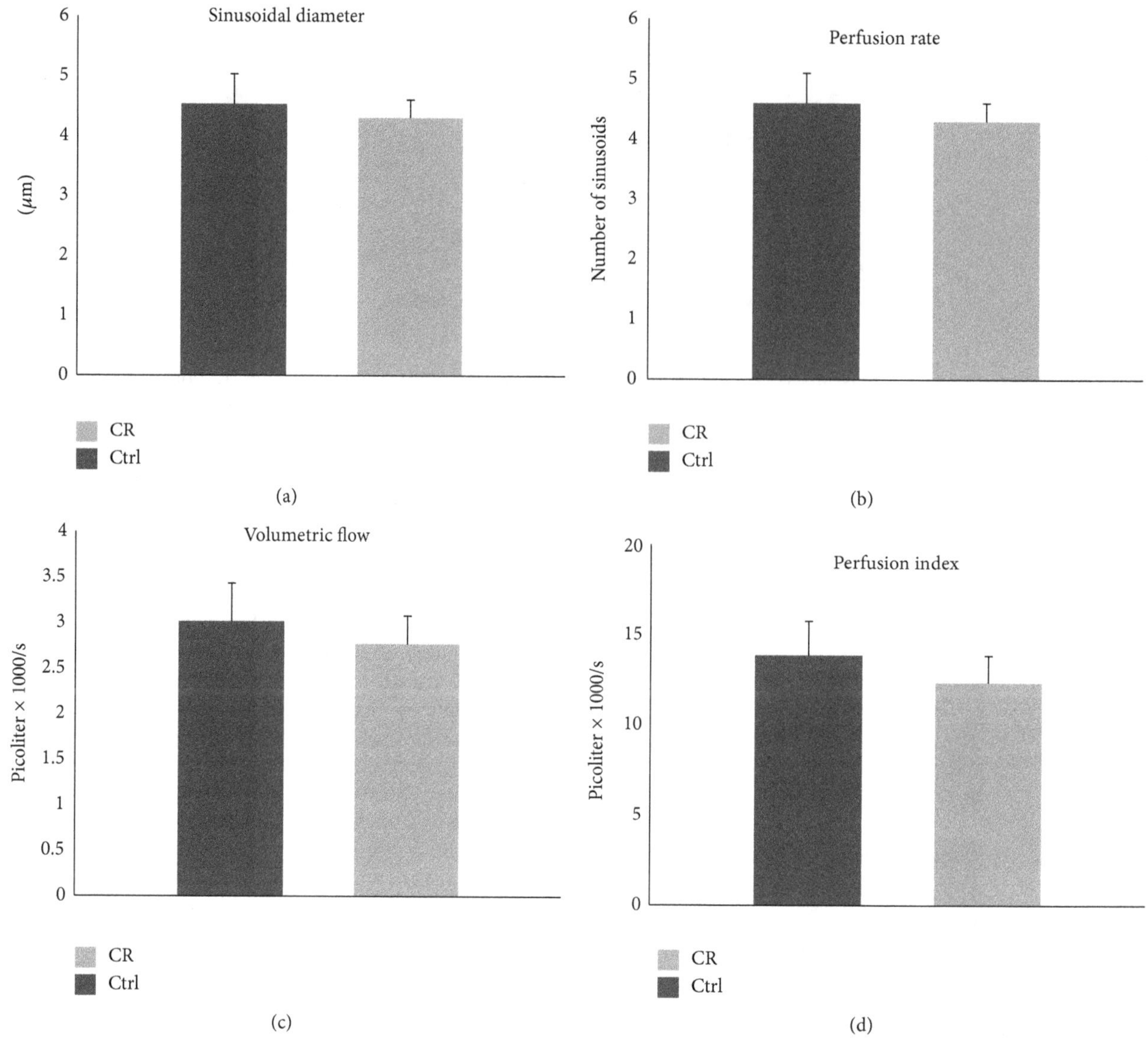

FIGURE 4: Intravital fluorescence microscopic examination of sinusoids of calorically restricted mice (CR) and control mice (Ctrl). Between the CR mice ($N = 7$) and NR mice ($N = 7$), there were so significant differences in the diameter of sinusoids (a), the perfusion rate expressed as the number of perfused sinusoids per field (b), the volumetric flows (c), and the perfusion index (d). Bars represent mean ± SEM. The mice were 14 months old.

Kupffer cell phagocytic activity but had no overt changes in sinusoidal dimension and perfusion when compared with three-months-old mice [17]. In the same study [17], however, significant reduction in sinusoidal perfusion and blood flow was present in 27-month-old mice. It remains to be investigated if caloric restriction will be able to prevent or reduce alterations of sinusoidal structure and function in senescent animals.

5. Conclusion

The age associated increases in hepatic collagen deposition and stellate cells can be attenuated in mice by caloric restriction. However, caloric restriction had no effect on the level of stellate cell activities since the expression of α-SMA was unchanged in comparison with the control. Changes in LSEC collagen production and in collagen degradation may be responsible for the diminished collagen production and hepatic deposits in livers of calorically restricted animals. The caloric restriction induced reduction in stellate cells and fibrosis may lessen the fibrogenic response to pathological stimuli in old liver.

Conflict of Interests

The authors declare they have no competing financial interests.

References

[1] C. Durnas, C. M. Loi, and B. J. Cusack, "Hepatic drug metabolism and aging," *Clinical Pharmacokinetics*, vol. 19, no. 5, pp. 359–389, 1990.

[2] D. E. Hinton and W. L. Williams, "Hepatic fibrosis associated with aging in four stocks of mice," *The Journal of Gerontology*, vol. 23, no. 2, pp. 205–211, 1968.

[3] H. A. Wynne, L. H. Cope, E. Mutch, M. D. Rawlins, K. W. Woodhouse, and O. F. W. James, "The effect of age upon liver volume and apparent liver blood flow in healthy men," *Hepatology*, vol. 9, no. 2, pp. 297–301, 1989.

[4] D. G. Le Couteur, V. C. Cogger, A. M. A. Markus et al., "Pseudocapillarization and associated energy limitation in the aged rat liver," *Hepatology*, vol. 33, no. 3, pp. 537–543, 2001.

[5] D. G. Le Couteur, A. Warren, V. C. Cogger et al., "Old age and the hepatic sinusoid," *The Anatomical Record*, vol. 291, no. 6, pp. 672–683, 2008.

[6] S. N. Hilmer, V. C. Cogger, R. Fraser, A. J. McLean, D. Sullivan, and D. G. le Couteur, "Age-related changes in the hepatic sinusoidal endothelium impede lipoprotein transfer in the rat," *Hepatology*, vol. 42, no. 6, pp. 1349–1354, 2005.

[7] M. Mahrouf-Yorgov, A. C. de L'Hortet, C. Cosson et al., "Increased susceptibility to liver fibrosis with age is correlated with an altered inflammatory response," *Rejuvenation Research*, vol. 14, no. 4, pp. 353–363, 2011.

[8] T. Poynard, P. Bedossa, and P. Opolon, "Natural history of liver fibrosis progression in patients with chronic hepatitis C," *The Lancet*, vol. 349, no. 9055, pp. 825–832, 1997.

[9] T. Poynard, P. Mathurin, C. L. Lai et al., "A comparison of fibrosis progression in chronic liver diseases," *Journal of Hepatology*, vol. 38, no. 3, pp. 257–265, 2003.

[10] R. K. Moreira, "Hepatic stellate cells and liver fibrosis," *Archives of Pathology and Laboratory Medicine*, vol. 131, no. 11, pp. 1728–1734, 2007.

[11] A. Warren, V. C. Cogger, R. Fraser, L. D. Deleve, R. S. McCuskey, and D. G. le Couteur, "The effects of old age on hepatic stellate cells," *Current Gerontology and Geriatrics Research*, vol. 2011, Article ID 439835, 7 pages, 2011.

[12] B. Vollmar, S. Pradarutti, S. Richter, and M. D. Menger, "In vivo quantification of ageing changes in the rat liver from early juvenile to senescent life," *Liver*, vol. 22, no. 4, pp. 330–341, 2002.

[13] S. X. Cao, J. M. Dhahbi, P. L. Mote, and S. R. Spindler, "Genomic profiling of short- and long-term caloric restriction effects in the liver of aging mice," *Proceedings of the National Academy of Sciences of the United States of America*, vol. 98, no. 19, pp. 10630–10635, 2001.

[14] M. Suematsu, M. Oda, H. Suzuki et al., "Intravital and electron microscopic observation of Ito cells in rat hepatic microcirculation," *Microvascular Research*, vol. 46, no. 1, pp. 28–42, 1993.

[15] H. A. Jamieson, S. N. Hilmer, V. C. Cogger et al., "Caloric restriction reduces age-related pseudocapillarization of the hepatic sinusoid," *Experimental Gerontology*, vol. 42, no. 4, pp. 374–378, 2007.

[16] A. Warren, P. Bertolino, V. C. Cogger, A. J. McLean, R. Fraser, and D. G. le Couteur, "Hepatic pseudocapillarization in aged mice," *Experimental Gerontology*, vol. 40, no. 10, pp. 807–812, 2005.

[17] Y. Ito, K. K. Sørensen, N. W. Bethea et al., "Age-related changes in the hepatic microcirculation in mice," *Experimental Gerontology*, vol. 42, no. 8, pp. 789–797, 2007.

[18] A. J. McLean, V. C. Cogger, G. C. Chong et al., "Age-related pseudocapillarization of the human liver," *Journal of Pathology*, vol. 200, no. 1, pp. 112–117, 2003.

[19] K. M. Mak, E. Chu, K. H. V. Lau, and A. J. Kwong, "Liver fibrosis in elderly cadavers: localization of collagen types I, III, and IV, α-smooth muscle actin, and elastic fibers," *The Anatomical Record*, vol. 295, pp. 1159–1167, 2012.

[20] S. L. Friedman, F. J. Roll, J. Boyles, and D. M. Bissell, "Hepatic lipocytes: the principal collagen-producing cells of normal rat liver," *Proceedings of the National Academy of Sciences of the United States of America*, vol. 82, no. 24, pp. 8681–8685, 1985.

[21] D. Horrillo, N. Gallardo, N. Lauzurica et al., "Development of liver fibrosis during aging: effects of caloric restriction," *Journal of Biological Regulators and Homeostatic Agents*, vol. 27, no. 2, pp. 377–388, 2013.

[22] M. K. Connolly, A. S. Bedrosian, A. Malhotra et al., "In hepatic fibrosis, liver sinusoidal endothelial cells acquire enhanced immunogenicity," *Journal of Immunology*, vol. 185, no. 4, pp. 2200–2208, 2010.

[23] J. J. Maher and R. F. McGuire, "Extracellular matrix gene expression increases preferentially in rat lipocytes and sinusoidal endothelial cells during hepatic fibrosis in vivo," *Journal of Clinical Investigation*, vol. 86, no. 5, pp. 1641–1648, 1990.

8

Active Aging: Exploration into Self-Ratings of "Being Active," Out-of-Home Physical Activity, and Participation among Older Australian Adults Living in Four Different Settings

Rosemary L. Aird and Laurie Buys

School of Design, Queensland University of Technology, Brisbane, QLD 4001, Australia

Correspondence should be addressed to Rosemary L. Aird; r.aird@qut.edu.au

Academic Editor: Patrik Eklund

We examined whether self-ratings of "being active" among older people living in four different settings (major city high and lower density suburbs, a regional city, and a rural area) were associated with out-of-home participation and outdoor physical activity. A mixed-methods approach (survey, travel diary, and GPS tracking over a one-week period) was used to gather data from 48 individuals aged over 55 years. Self-ratings of "being active" were found to be positively correlated with the number of days older people spent time away from home but unrelated to time traveled by active means (walking and biking). No significant differences in active travel were found between the four study locations, despite differences in their respective built environments. The findings suggest that additional strategies to the creation of "age-friendly" environments are needed if older people are to increase their levels of outdoor physical activity. "Active aging" promotion campaigns may need to explicitly identify the benefits of walking outdoors to ambulatory older people as a means of maintaining their overall health, functional ability, and participation within society in the long-term and also encourage the development of community-based programs in order to facilitate regular walking for this group.

1. Introduction

Together, the World Health Organization's [1] policy framework for active aging and its guide for the development of "age-friendly" cities [2] have set a policy and research agenda in which the built environment is conceived to play a crucial role as a facilitator or inhibitor of older people's capacity to age "actively." This theoretical standpoint assumes that built environments which are conducive to the outdoor mobility of older people will help provide them with ongoing opportunities for both participation within society and maintenance of their health through the gaining of physical exercise as they move around their neighborhoods. It remains unclear, however, whether or not older people's self-assessments of "being active" are linked to either their levels of participation within society or their engagement in outdoor physical activity, and, to date, there is no convincing evidence of a direct relationship between the built environment and older people's walking behavior.

"Active aging" is defined by the WHO [1, page 12] as "the process of optimizing opportunities for health, participation, and security in order to enhance quality of life as people age." This concept presents both opportunities and challenges to policy makers and researchers alike. In terms of policy, active aging has been acknowledged as providing a sound basis for responding to the challenges posed by population aging in industrialized nations by linking a number of key policy domains including employment, pensions, retirement, health, and citizenship [3, page 121]. Yet within Europe, for example, the focus on active aging has so far been largely limited to a "crude reduction in terms of working longer" [4, page S117]. Walker [3, page 124] noted more than a decade ago that active aging "does not amount to a coherent strategy and is sometimes just a slogan used to cover anything that seems to fit under it." More recently, he has stressed that this concept is more of an aspiration for both individuals and collectivities than it is a process that exists in practice [4, page S126]. The usefulness of the active aging concept for policy makers aiming to comprehensively address issues associated with the growing aging population will necessarily rest on their capacity to devise a coherent set of strategies that effectively deal with all of the three key determinants of active aging identified by the WHO—participation, health, and security. The sheer scope of this concept makes this a difficult task.

One key opportunity presented to researchers by the development of the active aging concept is its potential to act as a driver for greater attention on the older person-macroenvironment relationship. Indeed, there has been unprecedented research interest in this area since the release of the WHO's [1] policy framework; prior to the early 2000s, it was the microenvironments of older people which predominated as the main focus of investigations into the older person-environment relationship (see [5]). Nevertheless, the complex, multifaceted nature of the active aging concept is problematic, especially since it effectively encompasses dimensions covered by a number of earlier concepts. These include "successful ageing" which Walker [3] traces back to the early 1960s (a concept emphasizing the importance of maintaining activity patterns and values of middle age into old age) and "productive aging" which emerged in the 1980s (mostly focused on removing barriers to older persons engaging in work—paid or unpaid—and thereby extending their productive capacity beyond retirement age). Walker [3, page 123-124] notes that "active aging" emerged in the 1990s, giving recognition to both the connection between activity and health and the importance of "healthy aging." His account of the development of the active aging concept clearly demonstrates that active aging is much broader in scope than all of these earlier concepts. Nevertheless, a review of empirical literature recently undertaken by Hung and colleagues [6] grouped "active aging" with "successful," "productive," "positive," and "robust" aging as cognates of "healthy aging"—despite the fact that the active aging concept encompasses more dimensions than any of these other concepts (including continued participation in society; the maximization of social, mental, and physical health; the maintenance of dignity, self-efficacy, and human rights; and the creation of age-friendly physical environments to facilitate autonomy and independence) (see [3, 7]). Coherency of the accumulating evidence on active aging may well be undermined by both the overlap between this concept and its predecessors and the treatment of them as interchangeable terms. It is also noteworthy that "successful aging" has now been a focus of research for around half a century and there is still no widely agreed definition for this term or consistency between studies in the measures used to investigate this subject area, and the first rigorous analysis of measures was only undertaken recently (see [8]). There would seem to be much greater potential for disagreement about how "active aging" is operationally defined by researchers given the broad scope of this concept. This is not only an issue for the research community. If active aging objectives are to be met, it would seem crucial that laypersons ascribe meanings to this term that are in line with the WHO's [1] policy framework and fully grasp the nature and importance of all of the constituents of active aging as laid out in this framework.

To date, only a few studies have explored older people's perceptions of active aging. Research undertaken in the United Kingdom by Bowling [7] found this term was most commonly conceived by a sample of older people aged 60 years and over, to involve having/maintaining physical health and functioning (43%), leisure and social activities (34%), mental functioning and activity (18%), and social relationships and contacts (15%). Comparison with academic conceptualizations of active aging showed that there was overlap between lay perceptions of the constituents of active ageing and those used in theoretical models within the literature, although the latter entailed additional components (productivity, empowerment, human rights, and dignity) to those identified by laypersons. Multiple regression analyses revealed that health status, longstanding illness, and quality of life (all based on self-report) explained 41% of the variance in self-ratings of active aging, while sociodemographic and economic variables were not significantly associated with this outcome [7, page 298]. Comparison of data gathered on the perceived constituents of active aging in this particular study with data obtained from an earlier survey of older people's perceptions of successful aging, also administered in the United Kingdom but with adults aged 50 years and over (for further details see [9]), showed that there was considerable overlap in the meanings ascribed to "active" and "successful" aging. A later study by Bowling [10] compared the perceptions of minority ethnic groups with those of the general population in the United Kingdom, revealing that ethnically diverse respondents were less likely to define active aging in terms of good physical health and fitness (and exercise to promote these two aims) and also less likely to rate themselves as aging actively than respondents within the general population. From Bowling's [7] research, it would seem that individual factors such as health status and longstanding illness impact on older people's self-assessments of aging actively, but we currently have little understanding of whether or not there is any relationship between these self-assessments and the actual behaviors of older persons with respect to their actual levels of participation and physical activity outside of the home domain.

Older people's participation in the wider community necessarily relies on their capacity for remaining mobile in their out-of-home environments. The accumulated body of evidence suggests that individual factors as well as multiple aspects of the built environment affect older people's potential out-of-home mobility and thus their capacity to participate in society. Driving status [11, 12], quality and availability of public transport [13, 14], and numerous other features of the built environment (see [15, 16]) are all implicated in this regard. Walkable environments are particularly important, given that neighborhood walking increases not only older people's opportunities for physical exercise but also social interaction [17]. Engagement in outdoor physical activity by older people is crucial to them remaining ambulatory and also provides numerous other health benefits [18].

In the United States, lack of physical activity among older people has been described as a major public health issue; the release of Surgeon-General's Report in 1996 indicated that less than one-third of adults aged 65 years and over met health recommendations of moderate intensity exercise (e.g., brisk walking) for 30 minutes, five or more days per week [19, S267]. More recent research conducted in New Jersey shows a similar pattern, with just 28.6 percent of 50- to

74-year-olds being found to meet exercise recommendations [20]. The proportion of older people who meet exercise guidelines has been shown to be highly variable, however, both within and between different countries. A systematic review of studies investigating physical activity among older adults (limited to those studies which reported their findings in terms of older people meeting exercise guidelines) revealed that this proportion ranges between 2.4 and 83.0 percent, with the majority of the 53 studies reviewed being found to report proportions of between 20 and 60 percent [21]. Only 6 of these studies (undertaken in the United States, Australia, the United Kingdom, Brazil, China, Canada, New Zealand, Columbia, South Africa, Greece, Cyprus, Sweden, and Switzerland) used an objective measure of physical activity (i.e., accelerometer), with the remainder being based on self-reported activity.

Research efforts over the past decade have provided insight into many features of the built environment that encourage or constrain older people's walking decisions. Yet, the extent to which older people's walking behavior actually differs as a function of the particular built environment in which they live remains unclear. Much of the research literature related to the built environment and walking activity is based on random samples, with findings being largely representative of those living in urbanized areas (i.e., similar built environments) [22]. In addition, the vast majority of available studies of walking behavior among older people are based on self-report, making the findings subject to bias (e.g., participant recall and selection of socially acceptable responses). A recent review of empirical literature that examined mobility or disability among older people and also utilized objective measures of the built environment [15] identified 17 studies published between 1990 and 2010 that met these criteria. Of these, 14 studies investigated walking behavior, with all but one [23] being based on self-reports of walking. Rosso et al. [15] concluded that although evidence of a direct relationship between the built environment and elderly walking behavior was lacking, of all of the features of the built environment investigated, high density of intersections, street and traffic conditions, proximity to destinations, and green space were the factors most likely to have a direct effect on older people's out-of-home mobility. Nevertheless, a study of the consumption patterns and mode of travel used by older people (via GPS tracking) for accessing goods and services within two different countries (suburbs of Canada and France) showed that older people in both locations were highly reliant on travel by motor vehicle, despite substantial differences in the built environment and availability of public transport in the two study sites [24]. This raises questions about the assumption that levels of walking outdoors among the older segment of the population will naturally follow modifications to the built environment that make them more "age-friendly," without a shift away from sedentary lifestyles and a change in the propensity of the elderly to rely predominantly on motor vehicles for movement outside of the home domain.

Older people have identified particular urban design features such as green and open spaces [25, 26] as being conducive to walking. Other features like poorly maintained pedestrian infrastructure and traffic, however, heighten their fears about personal safety [27]. Evidence suggests that these fears about safety are well grounded, given that most falls occur outside of the home domain with the majority taking place on curbs, sidewalks, and streets [28] and that older people are the most likely group to present at hospital for injuries sustained from pedestrian-cyclist collisions [29]. Unfortunately, however, fear of moving outdoors also increases older people's risk of diminished capacity to walk outdoors in the longer term. Longitudinal research has shown that older people who fear walking outdoors are 4.6 times more likely than those without this fear to develop difficulties in walking a distance of 0.5 kms [30]. Older people's personal expectations about aging also influence their walking behavior. A pilot test of a behavioral intervention aimed at altering belief in the inevitability of becoming sedentary as a consequence of the aging process demonstrated that older people not only increased their walking after intervention but also experienced multiple other benefits including ease in performing daily life tasks and improvements in mental health-related quality of life, pain, energy, and quality of sleep [31].

Meeting the objective of maximising people's opportunities for ongoing participation within society as they proceed into older age is likely to be a major challenge for policy makers in industrialized nations. Cross-country analyses (of Canada, Finland, Germany, Italy, Japan, the Netherlands, Sweden, the United Kingdom, and the United States) indicate that there is a remarkably similar pattern in the age profile of work and passive and active leisure activities across countries [32]. Despite considerable variation in hours spent doing paid work between countries for adults in the 45–54 age group, intercountry differences seem to vanish by the age of 75 years and over, with time that was previously spent doing paid work being predominantly reallocated to passive rather than active leisure activities [32]. Much of older people's time also appears to be spent at home. Research undertaken in Berlin with community-based and institutionalized adults aged 70 years and over, for example, indicates that older people spent the majority of their day alone at home (80% of awake time) and less than a fifth of their day outdoors (18.7%) [33]. Similarly, more recent Australian research indicates that only a small proportion of time is spent away from home (90.2% spent at home) by community-based adults aged 65 years and over, with the mean number of episodes spent away from home in the previous week being 6.3 (SD = 4.5; range 0–19) [34]. In addition, the average daily time spent away from home by older people who have had a stroke and those who have not appears to very similar (0.9 versus 1.1 hours, resp.) [34]. Age- and/or health-related issues are implicated, however, in a substantial difference observed in older Australians' engagement in volunteering. Twice as many current drivers (66%) as retired drivers (30%) reported involvement in this particular form activity [35].

The current study used a mixed-methods approach to explore areas of interest within the area of active aging that are currently underresearched, including (1) the connection between older people's self-perceptions of "being active" and indicators of their health and participation (domains which are proposed by the WHO to be two of the three key determinants of "active aging"); (2) older people's perceptions of characteristics of their respective communities, which are generally conceived to facilitate aging in place; and (3) the extent to which older people's out-of-home physical activity differs across different built environments, based on high quality objective measures of active travel (walking and biking).

2. Materials and Methods

2.1. Participants and Study Locations. A convenience sampling method was used to recruit a total sample of 48 adults aged 55 years and over, comprising 4 subsamples of equal numbers ($n = 12$) of individuals living in (1) inner city suburbs and (2) suburbs outside the inner city area of a capital city, (3) a regional city, and (4) a rural town in Queensland, Australia. Recruitment took place via two methods. The first involved residents of inner city suburbs of Brisbane (within 5 kms of the central business district) who had participated in a previous project (Living in the City) and also indicated their willingness to be contacted for future research being invited to participate as representatives of high density living environments. Eleven were recruited. The second recruitment method involved key community organisations and groups being approached to assist in identifying potential participants living in Brisbane suburbs situated outside the inner city, Toowoomba (a regional city), and Roma (a rural town), as well as one individual to complete the Brisbane inner city subsample. Each individual was subsequently contacted via phone and/or email and invited to participate in the study. The total sample comprised 24 males and 24 females with each of the four subsamples being comprised of equal numbers of males and females (a thirteenth individual from Roma who volunteered to participate in the study jointly with her spouse was excluded from the study to ensure both an equal gender ratio and subsample size).

All participants were ambulatory and the age range for the whole sample was 56 to 93 years (average age of 72.02 years; SD = 8.46). Table 1 provides a demographic profile of the sample across the four study locations with respect to age, income, marital status, and current housing (derived from survey data). The population density for each of the four study locations is reported in the footnotes of the same table. The mean age for three of the subsamples was almost identical, but the mean age of the regional city (RC) subsample was between 2.5 and 2.7 years higher than the inner city (IC), city suburban (CS), and rural town (RT) groups. Nearly all of those from the IC group had high incomes, while the majority living in the CS, RC, and RT locations had incomes that fell in the low range. The most common source of income across the whole sample was the old age pension (33.3%), but superannuation also provided whole or part of the annual incomes of one-third of the sample. Only a small proportion of the whole sample was engaged in full- or part-time work (15.2%). The majority of participants in each subsample were married and also owned the homes in which they resided. All members of the IC group were living in a flat or unit (interview data revealed that most lived in a unit), while the majority of the other three subsamples were living in a house. Most of the older people in each of the four study locations owned their own dwelling.

2.2. Data Collection. Quantitative data were gathered from a GPS device (which captured one logged position every one minute and was used to track all out-of-home travel over seven consecutive days) as well as responses to a brief survey contained in the front section of a travel diary. The GPS device, GPS charger, and diary were posted to each participant, which they returned to the project site by post or courier at the end of the tracking period. Qualitative data were obtained from daily travel diary entries made by each participant (documenting all out-of-home travel, activities undertaken outside the environment, and the mode of transport used for each trip). In a few cases, participants forgot to either recharge their GPS device or take the device when they left home on one or two days and so were asked to continue completing their travel diaries and using the GPS to ensure that their out-of-home travel was monitored for the required seven days. Following the return of the completed diaries, GPS device, and charger, the GPS data were converted into individual time/space maps for each participant using Google Earth software. Diary entries were used to color-code each trip line shown on the maps to indicate the means of travel used for each trip made (by car, bus, ferry, train, taxi, and bicycle and on foot). These maps were subsequently used to direct discussion and verify correspondence between the GPS data and diary entries during in-depth, semistructured interviews held with each participant approximately two weeks after the tracking period. Interviews lasted approximately 90 minutes on average. Approval for this study was given by the QUT Human Research Ethics Committee.

2.3. Measures

2.3.1. Survey Data. Survey items tapped demographic characteristics (see Table 1) as well as attributes of the built environment in which participants lived. The latter were assessed from endorsement of statements that represented reasons for them living in their current community and included proximity to destinations (it is close to shops, etc., and close to my family/friends) and safety (it is a safe area). Participants' perceptions of the age-friendliness and disability-friendliness of their communities were captured by responses to two separate items with a shared lead-in question ("Do you think your community is: (1) "age-friendly"; and (2) "disability-friendly". Available options were the same for each item ("yes", "no", "do not know", and "never thought about it"). Self-perceptions of being healthy and being active were tapped from responses to two single-item, five-level Likert scales (options and coding for these variables are reported in Table 3). Survey forms also included a question asking about all modes of transport normally used for moving around one's neighbourhood (for details of survey item and available options, see footnotes of Table 4).

2.3.2. GPS and Travel Diary Data. Travel diary entries were used in conjunction with GPS data for determining the

TABLE 1: Demographic profile of participants by study location.

	Inner city[a] ($n = 12$)	City suburban[b] ($n = 12$)	Regional city[c] ($n = 12$)	Rural town[d] ($n = 12$)	Totals (%)
Age (in years)					
Range	56–80	57–87	68–93	59–88	N/A
Mean	72.3	72.3	75.0	72.4	N/A
Annual income					
Low ($40k and below)	1	9	8	8	26 (54.2)
Mid ($40k–$70k)	1	2	3	—	6 (12.5)
High ($70k and over)	7	1	—	—	8 (16.7)
No response	3	—	1	4	8 (16.7)
Source of income					
Wage	3	1	1	1	6 (12.5)
Superannuation	3	3	1	—	7 (14.6)
Part superannuation	—	—	1	—	1 (2.1)
Pension	4	5	7	—	16 (33.3)
Part pension	1	—	—	1	2 (4.2)
Part super/part pension	3	3	2	—	8 (16.7)
Self-funded	2	1	1	—	4 (8.3)
Self-employed	—	—	—	3	3 (6.3)
No response	—	—	1	—	1 (2.1)
Employment					
Full-time	2	—	1	1	4 (8.3)
Part-time	1	1	1	—	3 (6.3)
Not employed	9	10	10	10	39 (81.3)
No response	—	1	—	1	2 (4.2)
Marital status					
Married	7	6	9	10	32 (66.7)
Separated	—	—	—	1	1 (2.1)
Widowed	2	1	—	1	4 (8.3)
Not married	3	5	3	—	11 (22.9)
Dwelling type					
Flat/unit	12	2	1	1	16 (33.3)
Duplex	—	—	1	1	2 (4.2)
Townhouse	—	—	—	1	1 (2.1)
House	—	10	10	8	28 (58.3)
Room	—	—	—	1	1 (2.1)
Owns current dwelling					
Yes	11	9	10	11	41 (85.4)
No	1	3	2	1	7 (14.6)

[a] IC location includes six statistical local areas (SLAs) in the capital city of Brisbane (total population in 2010 = 1,067,290); average population density of the six SLAs = 4,193.6 persons per km^2.
[b] CS location includes 12 SLAs in Brisbane; average population density (in 2010) = 1,912.7 persons per km^2.
[c] RC location is 127 kms west of Brisbane; total population in 2010 = 131,258; population density = 236.8 persons per km^2 (based on statistical subdivision of Toowoomba).
[d] RT location is 420 kms west of Brisbane; total population in 2010 = 7,156; population density = 96.6 persons per km^2 (based on SLA known as Maranoa, Roma, under statistical subdivision South West in Queensland).

number of days when participants ventured out of home, their use of public transport, time spent travelling on foot and by bicycle outside of the home environment, and the total time spent traveling outside home over the seven-day tracking period. In combination, travel diary entries and GPS tracking produce high quality data on travel behavior [36]. A new variable was created which measured the total time spent travelling on foot and by bicycle to ensure that all of participants' travel by active means over the tracking period was captured.

The continuous variables for time spent walking and travelling by active means were converted into a six-level

TABLE 2: Participants' perceptions of their respective communities.

	Inner city ($n = 12$)	City suburban ($n = 12$)	Regional city ($n = 12$)	Rural town ($n = 12$)	Totals (%)
Age-friendliness of community					
Yes	7	6	8	10	31 (64.6)
No	—	2	2	1	5 (10.4)
Do not know	—	2	2	—	4 (8.3)
Never thought about it	4	2	—	1	7 (14.6)
No response	1	—	—	—	1 (2.1)
Disability-friendliness of community					
Yes	3	3	6	8	20 (41.4)
No	2	4	1	1	8 (16.7)
Do not know	3	3	3	—	9 (18.8)
Never thought about it	2	1	—	2	5 (10.4)
No response	2	1	2	1	6 (12.5)
Community features					
It is close to my family/friends	3	3	7	3	16 (33.3)
It is close to shops, etc.	4	3	4	3	14 (29.2)
It is a safe area	5	2	4	5	16 (33.3)

measure of 30-minute intervals (ranging from zero to a maximum of over 2 hours) for the purpose of correlational analysis because of the wide variation in minutes travelled on foot and walking/biking by those who walked or used active means for a period of more than two hours. Travel time captured by GPS in off-road open spaces (such as parks and golf courses) was included, but any time spent inside buildings (such as shopping centers) was excluded from travel calculations.

2.4. Analysis. All of the analyses were undertaken using SPSS 21.0. Cross tabulations were run for individual categorical and ordinal variables for descriptive purposes. Results are reported in tables in the form of cell counts due to the small size of each subsample, with percentages being shown in the totals column of each table. Missing values are reported in the tables (as "no response") and are included in the row totals.

Pearson correlation analyses were performed to identify relationships between select variables for the entire sample for exploratory purposes to determine relationships between self-perceptions of being active and being healthy and objective measures of participation (number of days when participants travelled out of their homes) and travel by active means outside the home environment. Comparative analyses of the four study locations were undertaken using a nonparametric approach, the Kruskal-Wallis test of significance, due to its appropriateness for three or more independent, small, and nonrandom samples. The statistical significance of differences between groups determined by this test is based on ordinal information only, with observations being ranked and the mean rankings of the various groups being compared [37]. The original continuous variable minutes spent walking and minutes spent walking/biking were used for these analyses to ensure true ranking of data (actual minutes) and minimization of tied ranks.

3. Results and Discussion

3.1. Results

3.1.1. Older People's Perceptions of Their Communities Being Age- and/or Disability-Friendly. Table 2 shows that the majority (64.6%) of the whole sample believed that their communities were "age-friendly" but less than half (41.4%) agreed that they were "disability-friendly." Interestingly, a similar proportion (41.7% in total) neither agreed nor disagreed about the disability-friendliness of their communities and either "did not know" (18.8%), had "never thought about it" (10.4%), or did not respond to the question (12.5%). More individuals within the RC and RT subsamples rated their communities as being age- and disability-friendly than the two capital city subsamples (IC and CS).

3.1.2. Perceived Attributes of the Community. Participants' reasons for living in their current community are shown in the lower part of Table 2. One-third of the whole sample identified their respective communities as being safe areas (33.3%) and similar proportions reported proximity as a factor that contributed to their reasons for living in their current communities ("close to family/friends" = 33.3%; "close to shops, etc.," = 29.2%). More older people living in the RC location identified being close to family/friends than those in the IC, CS, and RT groups (7 versus 3) as a reason for living in their current community, while similar numbers selected "being close to shops, and so forth." Only two older people living in the CS area agreed that safeness of the area was a reason for them living in their communities (compared to 4 or 5 in the other three groups).

3.1.3. Self-Perceptions of Being Healthy and Active and Participation outside Home. The patterns of self-ratings of being

Table 3: Self-ratings of being healthy and of being active and days ventured out of home over a seven-day period.

	Inner city (n = 12)	City suburban (n = 12)	Regional city (n = 12)	Rural town (n = 12)	Totals (%) (N = 48)
Being active[a]					
Very inactive	1	—	—	—	1 (2.1)
Inactive	1	—	—	—	1 (2.1)
Somewhat active	3	4	4	3	14 (29.2)
Active	6	4	6	7	23 (47.9)
Very active	1	4	2	2	9 (18.8)
Being healthy[b]					
Very unhealthy	—	—	—	—	—
Unhealthy	1	3	2	1	7 (14.6)
Okay	2	2	—	5	9 (18.8)
Healthy	5	4	8	5	22 (45.8)
Very healthy	4	3	2	1	10 (20.8)
Number of days ventured out of home[*]					
Two	1	1	—	—	2 (4.2)
Four	1	1	—	1	3 (6.3)
Five	—	2	4	1	7 (14.6)
Six	4	2	5	4	15 (31.3)
Seven	6	6	3	6	21 (43.8)
Mean (overall mean = 6.00)	6.00	5.83	5.92	6.25	N/A
Median (overall median = 6.00)	6.50	6.50	6.00	6.50	N/A

[a]Survey item: "think about the things you do during an average week. How active would you describe yourself to be?"; coding: 1 = very inactive; 2 = inactive; 3 = somewhat active; 4 = active; 5 = very active.
[b]Survey item: "how healthy are you?"; coding: 1 = very unhealthy; 2 = healthy; 3 = okay; 4 = healthy; 5 = very healthy.
[*]Number of days ventured out of home significantly related to self-ratings of being active at $P = <0.05$.

active and of being healthy were each found to follow a normal distribution with a left skew (prone to being healthy and active), results that are to be expected for a community-based older sample. The majority rated themselves as being either "very active" (18.8%) or "active" (47.9%), and just under one-third of the sample considered themselves to be "somewhat active" (29.2%). Only two identified themselves with inactivity (one selected "inactive" and the other "very inactive"). A majority also perceived themselves to being either "very healthy" (20.8%) or "healthy" (45.8%). Less than one-fifth rated themselves as "unhealthy" (14.6%) and none of the participants reported being "very unhealthy" (see Table 3).

No relationship was found to exist between self-ratings of being active and self-rated health status (r = 0.24; P = 0.098). Self-perceptions of being active were also found to be unrelated to age (r = −0.15; P = 0.317), but a statistically significant, negative correlation was found between self-rated health status and age (r = −0.32; P = 0.027).

Only five of the total sample of 48 travelled outside of their home in four days or less over the monitored week. The number of days on which participants ventured out of home was positively associated with their self-ratings of being active (r = 0.36; P = 0.011) but was unrelated to both self-ratings of health (r = 0.11; P = 0.468) and age (r = −0.26; P = 0.072), and the subsample means and medians for days travelled outside home were remarkably similar (see Table 3).

3.1.4. Out-of-Home Travel Using Active Means. The first part of Table 4 summarizes self-report travel-related information derived from survey to provide context to the GPS tracking results for time actually spent walking and walking/biking combined. The vast majority (81.3%) reported being drivers of a motor vehicle. Most drove cars but one person drove a motorcycle and another two drove both a car and a motorcycle. Another six (12.5%) travelled by motor vehicle as a passenger, and only three reported that they did not travel by motor vehicle (as either drivers or passengers). Less than half (41.7%) of the whole sample reported ever using public transport, and all but one of this group were from the IC and CS locations. None of the RC sample reported using public transport even though bus services are available in their location. Both the RC and RT locations only have access to train travel for the purpose of traveling outside of their local areas (rail link extends eastbound to Brisbane and westbound to Charleville), and only one participant from the RT group reported ever using the train. GPS data showed that only a quarter (25.0%) of the sample actually used public transport during the tracking period.

The actual time spent walking and time spent walking and biking combined by individuals living within the four study locations (based on GPS data) are shown in the lower section of Table 4. With respect to walking, one-third of the whole sample did not travel on foot out of their home environments at all over the tracking period. Considering this group and the

TABLE 4: Self-reported travel modes ever used and time spent walking and using active means of travel over a seven-day period.

	Inner city ($n = 12$)	City suburban ($n = 12$)	Regional city ($n = 12$)	Rural town ($n = 12$)	Totals (%)
Self-reported modes of travel ever used[a]					
Walking	10	8	6	10	34 (70.8)
Bicycling	1	2	—	1	4 (8.3)
Public transport	9	10	—	1	20 (41.7)
Motor vehicle					
Car as driver only	7	7	5	5	24 (50.0)
Car as driver or passenger	3	2	4	3	12 (25.0)
Car as passenger only	2	1	2	1	6 (12.5)
Driver of motorcycle	—	—	1	—	1 (2.1)
Driver of car and motorcycle	—	—	—	2	2 (4.2)
Neither driver nor passenger	—	2	—	1	3 (6.3)
Actual travel by public transport over seven days					
Bus	2	5	1	1[b]	9 (18.8)
Train	—	2	—	—	2 (4.2)
Ferry	3	1	N/A	N/A	4 (8.3)
Total number using public transport[c]	4	6	1	1[b]	12 (25.0)
Time walked over seven days in categories					
Nil	3	6	3	4	16 (33.3)
1–30 mins	—	1	3	1	5 (10.4)
31–60 mins	2	1	1	2	6 (12.5)
61–90 mins	1	1	1	—	3 (6.3)
91–120 mins	2	—	1	—	3 (6.3)
>2 hrs	4	3	3	5	15 (31.3)
Actual minutes walked					
Range	0–586	0–790	0–293	0–590	N/A
Mean rankings (Kruskal-Wallis test)[d]	26.38	21.92	23.46	26.25	N/A
Time spent walking/biking over seven days					
Nil	3	3	2	3	11 (22.9)
1–30 mins	—	2	4	2	8 (16.7)
31–60 mins	2	1	1	2	6 (12.5)
61–90 mins	1	1	1	—	3 (6.3)
91–120 mins	2	1	1	—	4 (8.3)
>2 hrs	4	4	3	5	16 (33.3)
Actual minutes using active means of travel					
Range	0–960	0–1562	0–293	0–590	N/A
Mean rankings (Kruskal-Wallis test)[d]	25.67	25.42	22.04	24.88	N/A
Proportion of total time travelled by active means					
Range	0–83.0	0–100.0	0–77.0	0–76.3	N/A
Mean rankings (Kruskal-Wallis test)[b]	26.08	24.83	22.33	24.75	N/A

[a]Survey item: "how do you get around? Tick all that apply"; options: I walk; I use a bicycle; I drive myself with a ... [car, motorcycle, motored wheelchair, or mobility scooter]; someone else drives me: [my partner, my children/grandchildren, community members, social or senior services, or taxi]; I use public transport [bus, train, or ferry].

[b]Travelling by private bus, as there is no public bus service in Roma.

[c]Only 12 individuals used public transport as some used more than one mode during the tracked seven days.

[d]No statistically significant difference between groups at $P = <0.05$.

next two categories (1–30 mins and 31–60 mins), more than half (56.2%) of the whole sample travelled out of home on foot for an hour or less during the monitored week. Just under one-third (31.3%) travelled on foot for more than two hours over the seven days. No correlation was found between time spent walking and self-perceptions of being active ($r = 0.12$; $P = 0.401$) and being healthy ($r = 0.12$; $P = 0.414$) or age ($r = -0.06$; $P = 0.688$).

In Table 4, it can also be seen that the number of nonwalkers in the lower density suburbs of Brisbane was

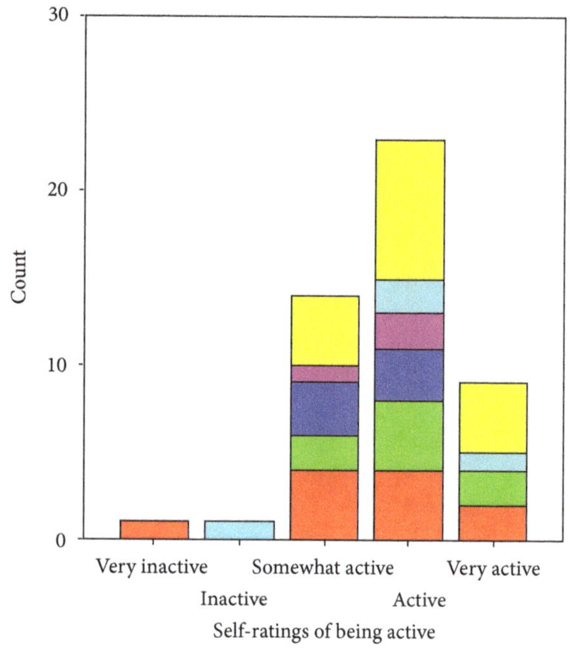

FIGURE 1: Active travel time by self-perceptions of "being active."

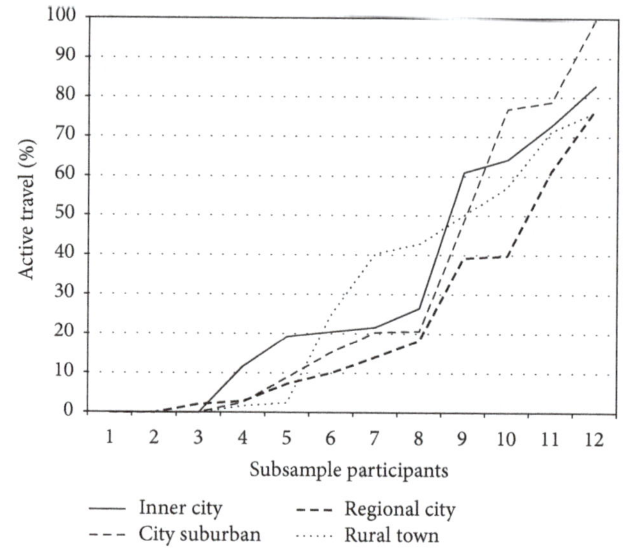

FIGURE 2: Proportion of total time travelled using active means over seven days by study location.

twice that of their counterparts living in the inner city suburbs of Brisbane, with the numbers of nonwalkers in the IC group being similar to both the RC and RT groups. Considering the actual time spent walking (in minutes) by each individual across each of the four groups, however, the Kruskal-Wallis test indicated there was no significant difference in the mean rankings by study location ($H(3) = 0.892$; $P = 0.827$).

Once time spent traveling by bicycle was taken into account, only three individuals in the CS group were found to have spent no time using active means of travel (on foot or biking), but the remainder of the findings were similar to those observed for walking. Time spent travelling by active means was found to be unrelated to both self-ratings of being active ($r = 0.16$; $P = 0.279$) and healthy ($r = 0.18$; $P = 0.216$) and to age ($r = -0.16$; $P = 0.284$). No significant difference between the four study locations was identified in the mean rankings of active travel (based on actual minutes) either ($H(3) = 0.520$, $P = 0.915$).

A visual representation of the lack of correlation between self-perceptions of being active and use of active means of travel is shown in Figure 1. Note, for example, that self-ratings of being active among those who spent no time walking or biking are distributed across four categories, from "very inactive" to "very active." A visual representation of the proportion of all time travelled over the tracking period spent using active forms of transport is shown in Figure 2. The similarity in the overall pattern that emerged for each of the four study locations is clearly evident and the Kruskal-Wallis test confirmed that there was no significant difference in the mean rankings of the proportion of overall time spent travelling by active means across the four study locations ($H(3) = 0.457$, $P = 0.928$).

4. Discussion

Overall, the findings contribute to a relatively small but growing empirical literature focused on active aging, by way of whole sample analysis and equal-sized subsample comparison. They add value to this body of evidence in five main ways. Firstly, the whole sample analyses enabled determinations to be made about the distribution of self-ratings of being active among community-based adults living in Australia. Like Bowling's [7] study undertaken in the United Kingdom (based on a larger sample than the current study), the most common self-rating for being active was the fourth level of a five-level single-item Likert scale ("active" in this study and "fairly actively" in Bowling's study). However, while the second most common rating in Bowling's [7] study was the fifth-level option "very actively," our research found the third-level option "somewhat active" to be the second most common, followed by "very active." This difference may be attributable in part to the wording and response options used by each study but may reflect either true difference in activity levels between older people in the United Kingdom and Australia or difference in the benchmark used by older people in these two nations when making this form of self-assessment. Replication studies of Bowling's [7, 10] research are needed in Australia and elsewhere in order to further understand older people's perceptions about the key constituents of active aging from their own perspective if we are to gauge similarities and differences across different cultures and countries.

Secondly, the current study was able to investigate correlates of self-ratings of being active beyond those examined by previous studies. Our finding that age was unrelated to self-ratings of "being active" is consistent with Bowling's [7] study. Our finding that self-rated health status was unrelated to self-perceptions of being active differs however. Bowling [7] found a strong positive association between them. This inconsistency may rest on the nature of the sample used in the current study, whereby three-quarters were recruited through community organisations (and thus were actively participating in community activities) and around two-thirds reported being "healthy" or "very healthy" or differences in the measure of health status used in each study (Bowling's study used presence of a "limiting longstanding condition or disability" while this study used self-rated health status). The negative correlation we found between age and self-rated health is consistent with previous research showing an association between increasing age and more chronic health problems and declining functional ability [8].

Thirdly, this study had the capacity to explore whether self-ratings of "being active" were connected with actual behavior. The fact that these self-ratings were positively correlated with the number of days when time was spent out of home but unrelated to levels of out-of-home physical activity raises the possibility that older people in this study have embraced the idea that "active aging" is primarily about one's current participation within society. Future research efforts need to be directed at exploring the degree that self-assessments of being active as people age correspond with objective measures of both participation and outdoor physical activity. Active aging objectives are unlikely to be met if a gap exists between the meanings ascribed to active aging by older people and their actual behavior with respect to the latter. More than half of the sample (all ambulatory and mostly healthy) spent a daily average of between zero and 8.6 minutes walking outside of home over seven days. If this level of outdoor physical activity is representative of these participants' normal pattern of walking outdoors, their long-term prospects of remaining ambulatory and capable of performing daily life activities could potentially be compromised, with this in turn eventually undermining their capacity for living independently, aging in place, and participating in society. Our finding that less than one-third of older people in this study had walked for more than 2 hours over seven days is consistent with findings from studies undertaken in the United States [19, 20], where a similar car culture to Australia's prevails. Given the accumulated evidence about barriers to walking (see [16, 27]) and the difficulties associated with using public transport [14] experienced by older people, as well as this group's reliance on cars [12, 24], it may be that the developments of community-based programs that encourage walking behavior among older people with a specific focus on recreational walking in spaces where pedestrian infrastructure is in good condition and free of traffic (e.g., parks and cyclist-free pedestrian walkways) are needed. These programs could target individuals as well as groups (such as senior citizens organizations) and may require the use of motorized transport (e.g., private motor vehicles and public or private bus) for gaining access to well-maintained, safe walking tracks. This approach could potentially create opportunities for older people to overcome their fears about moving outdoors, increase their number of social interactions [17], maintain or improve their overall health and well-being through the gaining of regular exercise [18, 31], and also change expectations that an increasingly sedentary life is a natural part of the aging process [31].

Fourthly, this study was able to explore whether different built environments (with varying public transport services and population densities) were associated with higher or lower levels of active travel. While the lack of difference in time spent walking (or walking/biking combined) between locations observed in this study could potentially be due to the size of the groups in the subsample, there is no reason to suspect that this particular finding is simply spurious in nature. We were able to gather a range of information about each location, including older people's perceptions of the age- and disability-friendliness of their respective communities, their safeness and closeness to amenities and family/friends, and differences in public transport services. Interestingly, similar numbers of participants in each location identified being "close to shops, and so forth" as a reason for living in their current communities. Thus this particular feature of the environment was not one that differentiated the inner city subsample from the other three lower density areas, even though higher density areas are often touted to be places that provide greater and easier access to amenities, goods, and services than lower density areas. Previous research indicates that it is proximity to particular destinations (especially shopping malls, retail outlets, and places of employment) and not population density that is associated with the walking behavior of older people (see [15]). Despite differences in public transport services in each study location and in older residents' perceptions of the age- and disability-friendliness of their respective communities, the emergent pattern of the proportion of time traveled by active means over seven days by older people was remarkably similar. This along with the finding from the whole sample analysis that only one-third engaged in active travel for more than two hours, a proportion that is consistent with findings from large population studies of older people's walking behaviour [19, 20], raises the possibility that variability in the walking behavior of older people has more to do with normal variation within populations (as a consequence of numerous factors) than it does to features of the surrounding environment. Together with the absence of any convincing evidence that there is a direct relationship between the built environment and older people's walking behavior [15] and the many barriers identified in the extant empirical literature which deter older people from venturing out of home on foot, our study's findings give grounds for questioning any taken-for-granted assumption that older people will walk outdoors more frequently if the surrounding environment is made more "walkable." A universal approach may need to be taken with respect to the provision of community-based walking programs for older people (discussed earlier) to ensure they are widely available, irrespective of the nature of the surrounding built environment of their homes, if a substantial increase in the outdoor physical activity of this segment of the population is to be achieved.

Fifthly, the mixed-methods approach used in this study provided the opportunity to explore connections between self-ratings of being active and objective measures of physical activity outside of the home domain via GPS tracking, as well as comparison of physical activity across four different settings that differ by population density and built environment (including public transport services). This combination of methods represents a major strength of our study. The capturing of time spent biking is an additional strength of this study, since research that relies on walking behavior alone ignores physical activity undertaken through alternative means. By instructing participants to document all modes of transport used for their out-of-home travel in combination with GPS tracking, this research avoided the circumstance where the research process itself leads participants to modify their walking behavior. This is a limitation of studies based on accelerometer-based information, the results of which do not necessarily reflect people's usual pattern of walking, because participation procedures (i.e., wearing an accelerometer) potentially prompt individuals to walk more frequently than normal for the monitored period.

Finally, further research based on objective measures of walking (as well as larger samples recruited from urban and rural settings) is needed if evidence-based determinations are to be made about the extent to which particular built environments foster greater levels of walking among older people (as proposed by Giles-Corti et al. [22]). The constraints imposed on the size of this study's sample by the nature of its methodological approach may be averted by future studies, given that technological advancements in recent years are making this approach increasingly feasible for larger samples. The developments of digital diaries, which are able to be used by participants at the same time and on the same device as GPS tracking takes place, hold great promise in their capacity to streamline data collection of movement and activity information, as well as data management and analysis, and may also reduce participant burden (see Draijer et al. [36]). Whether or not these new devices are useful for older samples (who may resist making diary entries in a technological device in place of paper and pencil diaries) remains to be seen however. The high quality of data produced by GPS/travel diary methods suggests significant benefits could accrue from the trialing of these new technologies with older samples. If successful, substantial headway could be made in expanding the body of evidence on the relationship between the built environment and older people's walking behavior gathered from high quality measures of walking.

5. Conclusions

Given that "active aging" is being promoted as a key policy agenda for dealing with the growing aging populations in industrialized nations, this particular subject area warrants much greater attention than it has attracted to date. It is imperative that older people understand the nature of all the constituents of the active aging concept as outlined by the WHO [1] if the objectives of its policy framework are to be met. Currently, evidence related to the meanings older people ascribe to this concept as well as the particular constituents of active aging that inform this group's self-ratings of being active is limited. More research is needed to determine if older populations are prone to connect "active aging" with "getting out and about and doing things" in the present more than they do behaviors such as walking outdoors as a means to maintain their health into the future. "Active aging" is extremely broad in scope compared to its conceptual predecessors ("successful," "healthy," and "productive" aging). It may therefore be necessary for messages communicated to the public under the banner of "active aging" to clearly articulate and emphasize the need for physical activity as a means to maintain health and prolong older people's participation within society. Furthermore, the flurry of research interest in the relationship between the built environment and older people's walking behavior that appears to have been sparked by the WHO's [2] Global Age-Friendly Cities publication has not been matched by similar interest in other areas pertaining to active aging. Researchers and policy makers alike need to remain mindful that the built environment is just one of many factors affecting older people's opportunities to age actively and that modifications to the built environment may be insufficient to the task of overturning older people's unwillingness to move outdoors on foot through fear of falls and injuries from traffic and poorly maintained pedestrian infrastructure, their expectations about aging, or the perceived comfort and convenience of the motor vehicle.

Conflict of Interests

The authors declare that there is no conflict of interests regarding the publication of this paper.

Acknowledgments

The authors extend their thanks to the Australian Research Council for funding this research (Grant no. LP0883447), all study participants, and Kimberley van Megen and Steve Snow for their valuable contributions to this study (data collection and GPS data management, resp.).

References

[1] World Health Organization, *Active Ageing: A Policy Framework*, WHO, Geneva, Switzerland, 2002.

[2] World Health Organization, *Global Age-Friendly Cities: A Guide*, WHO, Geneva, Switzerland, 2007.

[3] A. Walker, "A strategy for active ageing," *International Social Security Review*, vol. 55, no. 1, pp. 121–139, 2002.

[4] A. Walker and T. Maltby, "Active ageing: a strategic policy solution to demographic ageing in the European Union," *International Journal of Social Welfare*, vol. 21, no. 1, pp. S117–S130, 2012.

[5] H. Kendig, "Directions in environmental gerontology: a multidisciplinary field," *The Gerontologist*, vol. 43, no. 5, pp. 611–615, 2003.

[6] L.-W. Hung, G. I. J. M. Kempen, and N. K. De Vries, "Cross-cultural comparison between academic and lay views of healthy ageing: a literature review," *Ageing and Society*, vol. 30, no. 8, pp. 1373–1391, 2010.

[7] A. Bowling, "Enhancing later life: how older people perceive active ageing?" *Aging and Mental Health*, vol. 12, no. 3, pp. 293–301, 2008.

[8] R. A. Pruchno, M. Wilson-Genderson, and F. Cartwright, "A two-factor model of successful aging," *Journals of Gerontology Series B: Psychological Sciences and Social Sciences*, vol. 65, no. 6, pp. 671–679, 2010.

[9] A. Bowling and P. Dieppe, "What is successful ageing and who should define it?" *British Medical Journal*, vol. 331, no. 7531, pp. 1548–1551, 2005.

[10] A. Bowling, "Perceptions of active ageing in Britain: divergences between minority ethnic and whole population samples," *Age and Ageing*, vol. 38, no. 6, pp. 703–710, 2009.

[11] H. Mollenkopf, A. Hieber, and H.-W. Wahl, "Continuity and change in older adults' perceptions of out-of-home mobility over ten years: a qualitative-quantitative approach," *Ageing and Society*, vol. 31, no. 5, pp. 782–802, 2011.

[12] H. Mollenkopf, F. Marcellini, I. Ruoppila, Z. Szeman, M. Tacken, and M. Kaspar, "The role of driving in maintaining mobility in later life: a European view," *Gerontechnology*, vol. 1, no. 4, pp. 231–250, 2002.

[13] D. Banister and A. Bowling, "Quality of life for the elderly: the transport dimension," *Transport Policy*, vol. 11, no. 2, pp. 105–115, 2004.

[14] K. Broome, K. McKenna, J. Fleming, and L. Worrall, "Bus use and older people: a literature review applying the Person-Environment-Occupation model in macro practice," *Scandinavian Journal of Occupational Therapy*, vol. 16, no. 1, pp. 3–12, 2009.

[15] A. L. Rosso, A. H. Auchincloss, and Y. L. Michael, "The urban built environment and mobility in older adults: a comprehensive review," *Journal of Aging Research*, vol. 2011, Article ID 816106, 10 pages, 2011.

[16] D. Vine, L. Buys, and R. Aird, "Experiences of neighbourhood walkability among older Australians living in high density inner city areas," *Planning Theory and Practice*, vol. 13, no. 3, pp. 421–444, 2012.

[17] K. M. Leyden, "Social capital and the built environment: the importance of walkable neighborhoods," *American Journal of Public Health*, vol. 93, no. 9, pp. 1546–1551, 2003.

[18] R. L. Heikkinen, *The Role of Physical Activity in Healthy Ageing*, WHO, Geneva, Switzerland, 1998.

[19] T. Prohaska, E. Belansky, B. Belza et al., "Physical activity, public health, and aging: critical issues and research priorities," *The Journals of Gerontology Series B: Psychological Sciences and Social Sciences*, vol. 61, no. 5, pp. S267–S273, 2006.

[20] R. Pruchno and M. Wilson-Genderson, "Adherence to clusters of health behaviors and successful aging," *Journal of Aging and Health*, vol. 24, no. 8, pp. 1279–1297, 2012.

[21] F. Sun, I. J. Norman, and A. E. While, "Physical activity in older people: a systematic review," *BMC Public Health*, vol. 13, article 449, 2013.

[22] B. Giles-Corti, A. Timperio, F. Bull, and T. Pikora, "Understanding physical activity environmental correlates: increased specificity for ecological models," *Exercise & Sport Sciences Reviews*, vol. 33, no. 4, pp. 175–181, 2005.

[23] K. S. Hall and E. McAuley, "Individual, social environmental and physical environmental barriers to achieving 10 000 steps per day among older women," *Health Education Research*, vol. 25, no. 3, pp. 478–488, 2010.

[24] S. Lord and N. Luxembourg, "The mobility of elderly residents living in suburban territories," *Journal of Housing for the Elderly*, vol. 20, no. 4, pp. 103–121, 2007.

[25] S. Alves, P. A. Aspinall, C. W. Thompson, T. Sugiyama, R. Brice, and A. Vickers, "Preferences of older people for environmental attributes of local parks: the use of choice-based conjoint analysis," *Facilities*, vol. 26, no. 11-12, pp. 433–453, 2008.

[26] J. Maas, R. A. Verheij, P. P. Groenewegen, S. de Vries, and P. Spreeuwenberg, "Green space, urbanity, and health: how strong is the relation?" *Journal of Epidemiology & Community Health*, vol. 60, no. 7, pp. 587–592, 2006.

[27] R. Day, "Environmental justice and older age: consideration of a qualitative neighbourhood-based study," *Environment and Planning A*, vol. 42, no. 11, pp. 2658–2673, 2010.

[28] W. Li, T. H. M. Keegan, B. Sternfeld, S. Sidney, C. P. Quesenberry Jr., and J. L. Kelsey, "Outdoor falls among middle-aged and older adults: a neglected public health problem," *American Journal of Public Health*, vol. 96, no. 7, pp. 1192–1200, 2006.

[29] S. Chong, R. Poulos, J. Olivier, W. L. Watson, and R. Grzebieta, "Relative injury severity among vulnerable non-motorised road users: Comparative analysis of injury arising from bicycle-motor vehicle and bicycle-pedestrian collisions," *Accident Analysis and Prevention*, vol. 42, no. 1, pp. 290–296, 2010.

[30] M. Rantakokko, M. Manty, S. Iwarsson et al., "Fear of moving outdoors and development of outdoor walking difficulty in older people," *Journal of the American Geriatrics Society*, vol. 57, no. 4, pp. 634–640, 2009.

[31] C. A. Sarkisian, T. R. Prohaska, C. Davis, and B. Weiner, "Pilot test of an attribution retraining intervention to raise walking levels in sedentary older adults," *Journal of the American Geriatrics Society*, vol. 55, no. 11, pp. 1842–1846, 2007.

[32] A. H. Gauthier and T. M. Smeeding, "Time use at older ages: cross-national differences," *Research on Aging*, vol. 25, no. 3, pp. 247–274, 2003.

[33] A. L. Horgas, H.-U. Wilms, and M. M. Baltes, "Daily life in very old age: everyday activities as expression of successful living," *The Gerontologist*, vol. 38, no. 5, pp. 556–568, 1998.

[34] K. Mckenna, J. Liddle, A. Brown, K. Lee, and L. Gustafsson, "Comparison of time use, role participation and life satisfaction of older people after stroke with a sample without stroke," *Australian Occupational Therapy Journal*, vol. 56, no. 3, pp. 177–188, 2009.

[35] J. Liddle, L. Gustafsson, H. Bartlett, and K. Mckenna, "Time use, role participation and life satisfaction of older people: impact of driving status," *Australian Occupational Therapy Journal*, vol. 59, no. 5, pp. 384–392, 2012.

[36] G. Draijer, N. Kalfs, and J. Perdok, "Global positioning system as data collection method for travel research," *Transportation Research Record*, no. 1719, pp. 147–153, 2000.

[37] A. Agresti and B. Finlay, *Statistical Methods for the Social Sciences*, Prentice Hall, Upper Saddle River, NJ, USA, 3rd edition, 1997.

9

Is There Successful Aging for Nonagenarians? The Vitality 90+ Study

Lily Nosraty,[1] Tytti Sarkeala,[2] Antti Hervonen,[1] and Marja Jylhä[1]

[1] *Gerontology Research Center and School of Health Sciences, 33014 University of Tampere, Tampere, Finland*
[2] *Finnish Cancer Registry, Institute of Statical and Epidemiological Cancer Research, Pieni Roobertinkatu 9, 00130 Helsinki, Finland*

Correspondence should be addressed to Lily Nosraty, lily.nosraty@uta.fi

Academic Editor: Loretta DiPietro

Objectives. This study was designed (1) to estimate the prevalence of successful aging among nonagenarians based on six different models and (2) to investigate whether successful aging is associated with socio-demographic factors. *Methods.* A mailed survey was conducted with people aged 90+ in Tampere in 2010. Responses were received from 1283 people. The prevalence of successful aging was measured by six multidimensional models including physical, social, and psychological components. Age, sex, marital status, level of education, and place of living were studied as factors associated with successful aging. *Results.* The prevalence of successful aging varied from 1.6% to 18.3% depending on the model applied. Successful aging was more prevalent in men, and also more prevalent among community-living people. In most models, successful aging was also associated with younger age, being married, and a higher level of education. *Discussion.* Models which emphasize the absence of disease and activity as criteria for successful aging may not be the most relevant and applicable in oldest old. Instead, preference should be given to models that focus more on autonomy, adaptation and sense of purpose. Age-sensitive approaches would help us better understand the potential of successful aging among individuals who already have success in longevity.

1. Introduction

Increasing longevity is one of the great achievements of our civilization, but it has also given rise to discussion about good and successful aging. The concept of successful aging has attracted much debate, but there is still no universally accepted definition or standard measurement tool for it. The Encyclopedia of Aging defines successful aging as survival (longevity), health (lack of disabilities), and life satisfaction (happiness) [1]. It appears that the main sources of difficulty lay in the ambiguity of the meaning of "success," in the complexity of the aging process, the rapid changes taking place in society, and the changing characteristics of the older population.

Discussions on successful aging have taken two main perspectives: one defines successful aging as a state of being, while the other understands it as a process of adaptation, described as doing the best with what one has [2]. Studies taking the adaptation approach have often found that older people themselves feel they are aging successfully, even though traditional quantitative models say otherwise [3, 4]. Successful aging as a state of being, then, is an objective measurable condition at a certain point in time, demonstrating the positive extreme of normal aging. The most influential model of successful aging as a state of being was introduced by Rowe and Kahn [5–8], who characterize "success" as absence of disease and disability, maintained physical and mental functioning, and active engagement with life. Many studies and definitions take the view that successful aging is possible only among individuals without disease and impairment. Obviously such categorizations are likely to exclude most older people, typically the oldest-old, from the possibility of successful aging [9].

Successful aging is of course impossible in the absence of aging. Still, according to Bowling [3], longevity is only rarely mentioned in lay or biomedical definitions. In studies using quantitative measures, younger age is one of the most regular predictors of successful aging [10, 11], and the rate of "success" drops dramatically in very old age. This may largely be due to the usual focus on physical deficits.

Indeed, several researchers have emphasized the need to use multidimensional models and to adopt different conceptual approaches to studying different age groups [3, 12]. Recently, Young et al. [13] suggested that successful aging may coexist with diseases and functional limitations if compensatory psychological and social mechanisms are used. Their model considers three important principles: the heterogeneity of aging, multiple pathways to successful aging, and individual compensation mechanisms to adjust for age-related changes.

The oldest-old group of nonagenarians meets the key biomedical criterion of successful aging that is longevity. They are also a rapidly growing age group that is heterogeneous in terms of health and functioning: a large majority have some health problems but are independent in basic everyday activities [14].

In this study, we investigate successful aging in an unselected population of nonagenarians, applying several different models that include physical, social, and psychological dimensions. The models differ with respect to the threshold for "success" on the physical, social, and psychological dimensions. Our aim is not to introduce an ideal or universal model, but rather to demonstrate the variation in the prevalence of successful aging by applying different criteria. The first objective of this study was to construct six different models of successful aging and to use these models to estimate the prevalence of successful aging among nonagenarians. The second objective was to investigate whether successful aging in nonagenarians, defined in several different ways, is associated with sociodemographic factors.

2. Methods

2.1. Data. The Vitality 90+ study is a population-based multidisciplinary research program on nonagenarians in the city of Tampere, Finland. In the context of this program, mailed surveys were conducted with all community-dwelling people in 1996 and 1998, and with both community-dwelling and institutionalized people four times since 2001. This study used the data from the mailed survey in 2010. A questionnaire was sent to all individuals aged 90 or over in Tampere ($N = 1630$). Responses were received from 1283 people, giving a response rate of 79%. Proxy responses were obtained from 22% of the subjects who were themselves unable to answer the questions. For additional 20%, the respondent chose the answers but someone else helped in reading the questions or writing down the answers.

The research protocol was approved by the City of Tampere Ethics Committee. Informed consent was obtained from all respondents or their legal representatives.

2.2. Independent Variables. We explored the associations of five sociodemographic factors with successful aging: age, sex, marital status, level of education, and place of living. Age was categorized into three groups: 90-91, 92-93, and 94–107. Marital status was classified as currently married and currently unmarried, including never married, divorced, and widowed. Education was categorized into four groups as low (no more than elementary schooling), middle (lower secondary school), high (vocational school, folk high school, or upper secondary school), and highest (college and academic education). Place of living was dichotomized as community (private and service housing) and institution (residential care, service housing with 24-hour assistance, and hospitals).

2.3. Components of Successful Aging. Our dependent variable was successful aging. It was described by six different models that were constructed using psychical, social, and psychological indicators.

The physical component included three elements: diseases, functioning, and senses. The participants were asked whether they had been told by a doctor that they had (1) a heart problem, (2) stroke, (3) circulatory problems in the brain, (4) diabetes, (5) arthritis, (6) Parkinson's diseases, (7) hip fracture, or (8) dementia or memory problems. For the measurement of functional ability, the participants were asked whether they were able to perform independently (a) three mobility activities: moving about indoors, walking 400 meters, using stairs and (b) two ADL activities: getting in and out of bed and dressing and undressing. The response options, (1) yes, without difficulty; (2) yes, with difficulty; (3) only with help; (4) not at all, were categorized as independent (1 + 2) and dependent (3 + 4). The participants were also asked whether they were able to read the newspaper, with glasses if they used glasses (vision), and to hear what another person was saying when they were alone with them, with hearing aid if they used a hearing aid (hearing).

The psychological component was described by three variables. The participants were asked whether they suffered from depression or had depressive feelings (yes, no). Present self-rated health was categorized as average or good (very good, fairly good, and average) and poor (fairly poor and poor). Self-rated health was included in the psychological components because it is a subjective measure with no predetermined criteria: it reflects not only the more objective components of health, but also and importantly the age-related way in which the individual adjusts and adapts to different health problems [15]. The participants were also asked whether they thought it was good for people to live to be 100 years (yes, no).

The social component was measured by two questions: the frequency of meetings with children (six categories from today or yesterday to several years ago) and the frequency of talking on the phone with family members or friends (six categories from today or yesterday to several years ago). One-fifth (20.1%) of the respondents had no children. If these participants had had telephone contacts during the past two weeks, they were categorized as having had contact with children.

The percentage of missing data varied between the different variables. The highest figures were recorded for two psychological variables. Part of the reason for this was that these questions were not asked of proxy respondents. Most of these participants lived in institutions and had multiple health problems. To avoid reducing the number of participants in the analyses, we categorized both proxy responses and other missing values in these two variables at the negative extreme (poor self-rated health and thinking

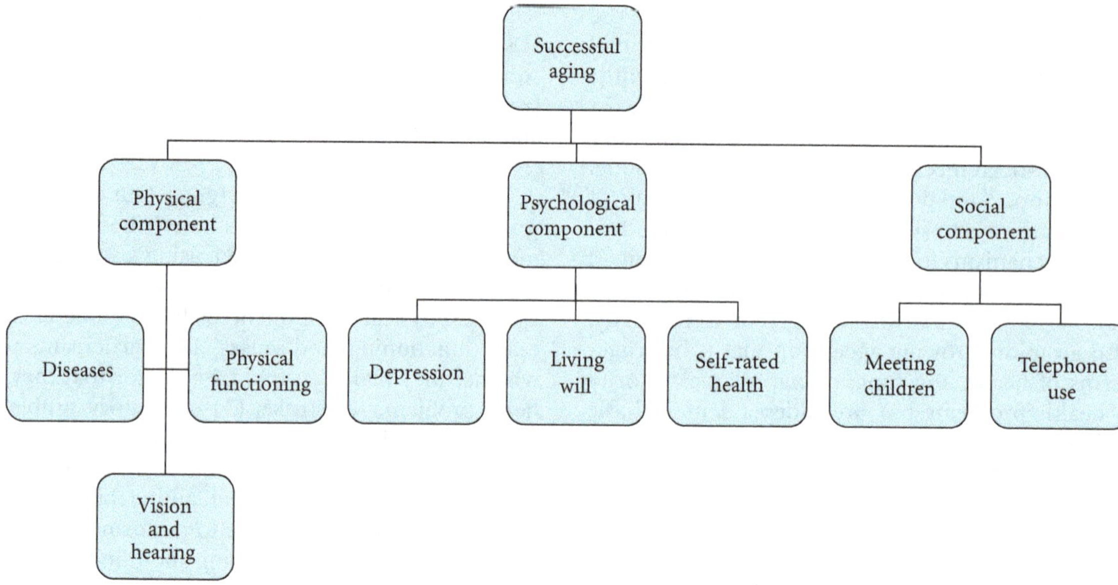

FIGURE 1: Three components of successful aging.

that it is not good to live to be 100). This imputation was done to avoid overestimation of the prevalence of successful aging, which would happen if the frailest participants were lost from the analyses.

2.4. Constructing Six Models of Successful Aging. Following Rowe and Kahn [6] and Young et al. [13], we defined successful aging as consisting of three components as shown in Figure 1. Six different models were constructed with different thresholds. The main differences between the models are in the physical component, where we defined four alternative criteria for "success," ranging from most to least demanding as follows:

Criterion 1: absence of disease + good vision and hearing + independence in all five activities.

Criterion 2: less than three diseases, no dementia, good vision and hearing, and independence in ADL and moving about indoors (independent in 3 easier activities).

Criterion 3: no dementia, good vision and hearing, and independence in all five activities.

Criterion 4: good vision and hearing, and independence in all five activities.

In the psychological component, "success" was defined as absence of depressiveness, average or good self-rated health, and agreement with the view that it is good to live to be 100. In the social component, "success" was defined as having met one's children and having talked on the phone with family members or friends during the past two weeks.

The six models of successful aging were constructed as follows:

Model 1: Physical component criterion 1 and psychological component & social component.

Model 2: Physical component criterion 2 and psychological component & social component.

Model 3: Physical component criterion 3 and psychological component & social component.

Model 4: Physical component criterion 4 and psychological component & social component.

Model 5: Physical component criterion 3 and psychological component.

Model 6: Physical component criterion 3 and social component.

2.5. Analysis. The prevalence of successful aging in different sociodemographic categories was compared by cross tabulation using the Chi-square test. Logistic regression models were used to assess the independent associations of different models of successful aging with sociodemographic factors. Odds ratios (ORs) and 95% confidence intervals (95% CI) were calculated. These analyses were performed using the SPSS Package 16.

3. Results

Most of the participants (85.9%) were under 95 years of age, and more than 80% were women. These figures well reflect the distributions in the general population. Only 12.1% were still married and 37.5% lived in an institution. The majority had no more than elementary schooling (Table 1). Heart problems, arthritis, and dementia were the most frequent diseases, and only 14.7% of men and 10.2% of women did not have any of the eight conditions listed in the questionnaire. Four in ten respondents were independent in all five activities, and seven in ten were independent in ADL and moving about indoors. According to different criteria, 5.3 to 25.2% were aging successfully if only the physical

Table 1: Population characteristics.

Characteristic	Frequency %
Age	(N = 1283)
90–91	44.5
92–93	25.5
94+	30.0
Gender	(N = 1283)
Women	81.2
Men	18.8
Marital status	(N = 1267, missing 16)
Unmarried	87.9
Married	12.1
Education	(N = 1234, missing 49)
Low	56.4
Middle	9.9
High	22.7
Higher	11.0
Place of living	(N = 1278, missing 5)
Community	62.5
Institution	37.5

component was considered. In the psychological component, the prevalence of successful aging was 20%, in the social component the figure was markedly higher at 75%. Men had better scores than women in both the physical component (most criteria) and the psychological component (Table 2).

The prevalence of successful aging varied between the six models (Table 3). It was lowest (1.6%) for Model 1, which required absence of all diseases, independence in all five activities, and good vision and hearing, in addition to the psychological and social components, and highest (18.3%) for Model 6, which differed from Model 1 in that diseases other than dementia were allowed, and the psychological component was not included. Successful aging was significantly more prevalent in men than women and among community-living than institutionalized individuals, regardless of the model. According to most models, successful aging was more frequent among those aged 90–93 than those aged 94+, among married people, and among those with a higher education.

Finally, logistic regression models were calculated to examine the independent association of different sociodemographic indicators with the six models of successful aging (Table 4).

In four models, higher age was independently associated with less successful aging. Gender was another predictive variable, and in all models except model 6, men were significantly more successful in aging than women. Higher education was a significant predictor in two models, and in Model 6 both those with a high and the highest educational level differed significantly from those with the lowest level of education. Marital status did not play an independent role, but place of living was a significant determinant of successful aging in all but Model 1.

4. Discussion

This paper examined one the most prominent concepts in aging research, successful aging, by constructing six different models to measure it among nonagenarians. The models were based on work by Rowe and Kahn, Rowe, and Young et al. [6–8, 13, 16], although not the exact same indicators were used. According to Young et al. [13] and Rowe and Khan [6], successful aging is typically understood as comprising three main domains: physical (in Young et al.: physiological), psychological, and social (in Young et al.: sociological). The results showed that the prevalence of successful aging varies markedly from one model to another, standing at 1.6% for Model 1 that required the absence of any disease, independence in functioning, and the ability to hear and read, as well as meeting the psychological and social criteria, and at 18.3% for Model 6, which required the absence of dementia, independence in functioning, the ability to hear and read, and meeting the social criteria. However, the main socioeconomic predictors remained largely the same across the models.

It is obvious that the absence of disease is the most demanding criterion for measuring successful aging. Disease and at least some functional deterioration are almost inevitable in very old age. Only 11% of the nonagenarians in our study had no major disease, and only 5.3% were both free of disease, able to hear and see, and independent in five daily activities (physical dimension criterion 1). Very few earlier studies have attempted to estimate the prevalence of successful aging in nonagenarians or in very old age in general. von Faber et al. [2] classified only 10% of community-dwelling and 1.9% of institutionalized participants aged 85 or over as successful agers. In the NonaSantfeliu study by Formiga et al. [17], the figure was 12% with community-dwelling nonagenarians. These studies emphasized the role of health and physical functioning, but also included some social or quality-of-life measures. It is clear that especially when the focus is on the physical dimension, successful aging will be very rare among people experiencing longevity.

Rowe and Kahn [6] included productive activities in their model of successful aging but these can hardly be expected from nonagenarians. Horgas et al. [18] showed that the daily activities of individuals aged 90 or over differed from other age groups, and in all categories this age group was engaged in significantly less activity than others. This implies that the social dimension of successful aging among the oldest old should be measured using different criteria and against different activities than in the case of the younger old and should be seen in relation to the situation of the best performers in the same age group.

In cross-sectional analysis, we limited our examination to socioeconomic predictors that at least potentially have played a role in the lives of the individuals for a longer time, and, with the exception of place of living, are not supposed to be influenced by factors that were thought to be components of successful aging. In most studies age has emerged as one of the strongest predictors of successful aging [18]. In our study, persons aged 94 or over were less likely to meet the successful aging criteria than the younger age groups. The difference

Table 2: Frequency (%) of the variables composing three components of successful aging in men and women.

Variables	Men (N = 226–238) %	Women (N = 1006–1038) %	P value	All (N = 1227–1283) %
Physical component				
No heart problem	42.4	47.1	0.192	46.2
No stroke	96.2	94.4	0.250	94.7
No circulatory problems in brain	78.6	79.3	0.798	79.2
No diabetes	85.7	88.8	0.178	88.2
No arthritis	69.7	54.3	<0.001	57.2
No Parkinson's disease	99.6	98.3	0.148	98.6
No hip fracture	89.2	81.3	0.003	82.8
No dementia	66.4	59.2	0.033	60.6
No disease	14.7	10.2	0.045	11.0
2 or less diseases with no dementia	39.5	29.8	0.004	31.6
Able to see	72.8	59.9	<0.001	62.3
Able to hear	68.1	71.5	0.299	70.9
Able to see and hear	53.2	48.2	0.170	49.2
Independent in five activities	58.3	34.9	<0.001	39.2
Independent in 3 easier activities	83.0	72.5	<0.001	74.5
Criterion 1*	7.7	4.8	<0.001	5.3
Criterion 2*	28.3	26.1	0.500	26.5
Criterion 3*	24.8	19.1	0.050	20.2
Criterion 4*	33.9	23.2	<0.001	25.2
Psychological				
No depressiveness	87.8	79.6	0.004	81.2
Self-rated health average or good	72.3	61.4	0.002	63.4
Willing to live up to 100 years	42.4	24.8	<0.001	28.1
Psychological component	34.0	16.7	<0.001	20.0
Social engagement				
Met children during past 2 weeks	92.7	93.5	0.644	93.4
Phone contacts	84.6	79.4	0.070	80.4
Social component	78.8	74.4	0.166	75.2

* Criterions. Criterion 1: No disease, and able to hear and read, and independent in all five activities. Criterion 2: Less than 3 diseases, no dementia, able to hear and read, and independent in three easier activities. Criterion 3: No dementia, able to hear and read, and independent in 5 activities. Criterion 4: Able to hear and read, independent in 5 activities.

TABLE 3: Prevalence of successful aging (%) according to the six models in different socioeconomic categories.

	Models of successful aging*					
	1	2	3	4	5	6
Total prevalence	1.6	6.3	5.7	6.8	6.3	18.3
Age						
90–91	1.9	7.9	6.5	7.5	7.5	23.8
92–93	2.5	6.8	7.1	8.6	7.7	21.2
94+	0.5	3.4	3.2	4.2	3.4	7.8
P value	0.104	0.021	0.042	0.048	0.022	<0.001
Gender						
Men	4.7	12.4	11.1	13.2	12.4	22.3
Women	1	5	4.5	5.5	5.1	17.5
P value	<0.001	<0.001	<0.001	<0.001	<0.001	0.095
Marital status						
Married	3.3	11.8	11.8	14.5	12.5	24.2
Not married	1.4	5.6	4.9	5.9	5.6	17.6
P value	0.095	0.003	0.001	<0.001	0.001	0.03
Place of living						
Community	2.3	8.4	7.6	9.1	8.2	25.9
Institution	0.6	2.9	2.5	3.1	2.5	6.1
P value	0.026	<0.001	<0.001	<0.001	<0.001	<0.001
Education						
Low	1.3	4.7	4.6	6	5.8	14.4
Middle	1.6	7.4	4.9	4.9	5.7	20.5
High	2.1	7.5	7.1	8.2	7.2	22.6
Higher	3	12.5	9.6	11.9	9.6	29.1
P value	0.51	0.005	0.093	0.058	0.377	<0.001

*Models of successful aging. Model 1. Health and functioning criterion 1 + psychological + social. Model 2. Health and functioning criterion 2 + psychological + social. Model 3. Health and functioning criterion 3 + psychological + social. Model 4. Health and functioning criterion 4 + psychological + social. Model 5. Health and functioning criterion 3 + psychological. Model 6. Health and functioning criterion 3 + social.

between the age groups was significant for all except Model 1, and it was greatest in Model 6 where the overall prevalence of successful aging was highest. After adjusting for other sociodemographic variables, a significant age difference still persisted in four models.

In our study, the prevalence of successful aging was consistently higher for men, and in all except the last model the differences were also significant after the adjustments. Earlier studies [10] show no consistent patterns of gender differences, but the results seem to be dependent on the model used. McLaughlin et al. [11] found no gender difference in prevalence, but higher odds of successful aging in women after controlling for sociodemographic variables. Our findings among nonagenarians are only partly explained by the high prevalence of disabilities and disease in women, as men had clearly better scores in the psychological component as well. These disparities are likely to reflect differential survival, lifelong differences in biological, health, and social conditions.

Marital status was associated with successful aging in unadjusted analysis but not in the adjusted models, where the uneven age and gender distribution of the variable was controlled for.

Education is known to have an impact on health and life style, and it reflects socioeconomic status; therefore, it can also be considered a potential predictor of successful aging. Most of the studies reviewed by Depp and Jeste [10] found no differences according to educational level, but the analysis by McLaughlin et al. [11] in the Health and Retirement Study showed that the prevalence of successful aging was higher in groups with a higher education and household income. The study of Pruchno et al. [19] revealed that a higher level of formal education is associated with successful aging. Our findings with an older group than in these studies showed a graded increase in the prevalence of successful aging with higher education, although the difference was not significant for all models. The discrepancy between the findings may at least partly be due to sampling bias. In several studies institutionalized people and those of lower social position were less likely to participate [10], while our study represents the whole age group in the region.

Place of living is not usually considered a predictor of successful aging and in many (but not all, see e.g., von Faber et al. [2]) studies samples only include community-dwelling individuals. In our study, we wanted to take account of the possibility of successful aging even in an institution.

Table 4: Associations of successful aging, according to the six models, with socioeconomic characteristics. A multivariate logistic regression model, all the predictors included in the model simultaneously. Odds ratios (OR) and 95% confidence intervals (CI).

	Models of successful aging					
	1	2	3	4	5	6
Age						
90–91	2.74 (0.59–12.76)	1.93 (0.99–3.78)	1.68 (0.83–3.4)	1.43 (0.76–2.66)	1.82 (0.93–3.57)	2.85 (1.81–4.49)
92–93	3.93 (0.82–18.89)	2.15 (1.02–4.53)	1.76 (0.91–3.42)	1.93 (1.0–3.73)	2.14 (1.05–4.40)	2.90 (1.79–4.73)
94+	1	1	1	1	1	1
Gender						
Men	1	1	1	1	1	1
Women	0.20 (0.07–0.54)	0.46 (0.26–0.82)	0.53 (0.29–0.96)	0.54 (0.31–0.94)	0.47 (0.27–0.83)	0.98 (0.06–1.50)
Marital status						
Unmarried	1	1	1	1	1	1
Married	0.85 (0.26–2.73)	1.17 (0.61–2.26)	1.60 (0.82–3.12)	1.71 (0.92– 3.16)	1.42 (0.74–2.7)	1.11 (0.69–1.81)
Education						
Low	1	1	1	1	1	1
Middle	1.64 (0.34–7.88)	1.77 (0.81–3.85)	1.16 (0.47–2.87)	0.89 (0.37–2.18)	1.10 (0.47–2.54)	1.57 (0.94–2.63)
High	1.14 (0.39–3.33)	1.28 (0.72–2.3)	1.23 (0.68–2.22)	1.10 (0.64–1.91)	0.95 (0.54–1.69)	1.45 (1.00–2.11)
Higher	1.35 (0.38–4.6)	2.03 (1.06–3.89)	1.48 (0.73–2.99)	1.45 (0.76–2.76)	1.14 (0.57–2.28)	2.00 (1.26–3.17)
Place of living						
Community	3.11 (0.89–10.8)	2.48 (1.36–4.53)	2.66 (1.39–5.05)	2.64 (1.48–4.72)	3.18 (1.68–6.0)	4.30 (2.83–6.53)
Institution	1	1	1	1	1	1

However, the results showed that the prevalence of successful aging was clearly lower for those living in institutions, and this was also true for the adjusted models. Our earlier analyses (not shown here) indicated that disease, disability, and problems with hearing and seeing are more prevalent in institutions, as is self-rated health, which partly explains this finding.

4.1. Strengths and Limitations. The major strength of this study is that it covers the whole population aged 90 or over in the area concerned, including institutionalized people as well as proxy responses. The response rate was high. Our earlier and ongoing analyses suggest that the information on health and functioning collected by mailed questionnaires among nonagenarians is sufficiently valid and reliable [20, 21]; particularly as for a majority for those suffering from dementia, the answers were given by a proxy respondent.

In order to gain a broad and thorough understanding of successful aging, we included both physical, psychological, and social components in our analyses. Unlike most other studies, we also included the ability to see and hear as an important contributing factor to independence and quality of life. The main limitations of our study have to do with the measures used to assess the social and psychological components. Our only information about meeting with other people concerned meetings with children; no data were available about other family members or friends. One fifth of the respondents had no children, and we decided to give them a positive score for social contacts if they had made or received any telephone calls during the past two weeks. One-fifth of our responses were from proxies, who were not asked about self-rated health or living to be 100. Therefore, we had a high percentage of missing or proxy answers to two questions regarding the psychological dimension of successful aging. In order not to overestimate the prevalence of successful aging, we scored this missing data and proxy answers as negative. These kinds of problems are unavoidable in unselected samples of very old people, but they nonetheless add some uncertainty to our findings. Another obvious limitation of our study is that we had no direct questions designed to capture our respondents' self-evaluations of their life.

4.2. Implications. Our study in a nonselected population of persons aged 90 or over supports earlier findings that the prevalence of successful aging is highly dependent on the model applied, but in every case successful aging is associated with age, gender, and socioeconomic status. However, it is apparent that with any model that defines successful aging as a state of being and that uses criteria commonly used for younger age groups, successful aging remains a rare situation among the oldest old. An increased likelihood of health and functional problems, often followed by reduced opportunities for active social engagement, is normative consequences of biological aging and typical of extreme longevity. Therefore, in very old age, rather than models emphasizing the absence of disease and activity, emphasis should be given to approaches focusing on autonomy, adaptation, and sense of purpose [3, 22, 23]. These age-sensitive approaches would help us better understand the potential of successful aging among those individuals who have already had success in longevity.

Acknowledgments

Gerontology Research Center is a joint effort between the Universities of Jyväskylä and Tampere. This study was supported by Grants from the CIMO Fund to L. Nosraty and from the Competitive Research Funding of Tampere University Hospital (9M025) to M. Jylhä. The authors wish to thank Anna-Maija Koivisto, M.S. dgree, for her statistical help and advice.

References

[1] E. B. Palmore, "Successful ageing," in *The Encyclopedia of Aging*, G. L. Maddox, S. W. Sussman, R. C. Atchley et al., Eds., pp. 914–915, Springer, New York, NY, USA, 1995.

[2] M. von Faber, A. Bootsma-van der Wiel, E. van Exel et al., "Successful aging in the oldest old: who can be characterized as successfully aged?" *Archives of Internal Medicine*, vol. 161, no. 22, pp. 2694–2700, 2001.

[3] A. Bowling, "Aspirations for older age in the 21st century: what is successful aging?" *International Journal of Aging and Human Development*, vol. 64, no. 3, pp. 263–297, 2007.

[4] A. Bowling, "Erratum: Lay perceptions of successful ageing: Findings from a national survey of middle aged and older adults in Britain (European Journal Ageing (2006) vol. 3 (123-136) 10.1007/s10433-006-0032-2)," *European Journal of Ageing*, vol. 4, no. 1, pp. 57–58, 2007.

[5] J. W. Rowe and R. L. Kahn, "Human aging: usual and successful," *Science*, vol. 237, no. 4811, pp. 143–149, 1987.

[6] J. W. Rowe and R. L. Kahn, "Successful aging," *Gerontologist*, vol. 37, no. 4, pp. 433–440, 1997.

[7] J. W. Rowe and R. L. Kahn, "Successful aging," *Aging—Clinical and Experimental Research*, vol. 10, no. 2, article 142, 1998.

[8] J. W. Rowe, *Successful Ageing*, Dell, New York, NY, USA, 1999.

[9] M. Minkler and P. Fadem, "Successful aging," *Journal of Disability Policy Studies*, vol. 12, no. 4, pp. 229–235, 2002.

[10] C. A. Depp and D. V. Jeste, "Definitions and predictors of successful aging: a comprehensive review of larger quantitative studies," *American Journal of Geriatric Psychiatry*, vol. 14, no. 1, pp. 6–20, 2006.

[11] S. J. McLaughlin, C. M. Connell, S. G. Heeringa, L. W. Li, and J. S. Roberts, "Successful aging in the United States: prevalence estimates from a national sample of older adults," *Journals of Gerontology—Series B*, vol. 65, no. 2, pp. 216–226, 2010.

[12] R. A. Pruchno, M. Wilson-Genderson, and F. Cartwright, "A two-factor model of successful aging," *Journals of Gerontology—Series B*, vol. 65, no. 6, pp. 671–679, 2010.

[13] Y. Young, K. D. Frick, and E. A. Phelan, "Can successful aging and chronic illness coexist in the same individual? A multidimensional concept of successful aging," *Journal of the American Medical Directors Association*, vol. 10, no. 2, pp. 87–92, 2009.

[14] T. Sarkeala, T. Nummi, M. Vuorisalmi, A. Hervonen, and M. Jylhä, "Disability trends among nonagenarians in 2001–2007: vitality 90+ study," *European Journal of Ageing*, vol. 8, no. 2, pp. 87–94, 2011.

[15] M. Jylhä, "What is self-rated health and why does it predict mortality? Towards a unified conceptual model," *Social Science and Medicine*, vol. 69, no. 3, pp. 307–316, 2009.

[16] Y. Young, M. Y. Fan, J. M. Parrish, and K. D. Frick, "Validation of a novel successful aging construct," *Journal of the American Medical Directors Association*, vol. 10, no. 5, pp. 314–322, 2009.

[17] F. Formiga, A. Ferrer, D. Chivite, M. Rubio-Rivas, S. Cuerpo, and R. Pujol, "Predictors of long-term survival in nonagenarians: the NonaSantfeliu study," *Age and Ageing*, vol. 40, no. 1, Article ID afq127, pp. 111–116, 2011.

[18] A. L. Horgas, H. U. Wilms, and M. M. Baltes, "Daily life in very old age: everyday activities as expression of successful living," *Gerontologist*, vol. 38, no. 5, pp. 556–568, 1998.

[19] R. A. Pruchno, M. Wilson-Genderson, M. Rose, and F. Cartwright, "Successful aging: early influences and contemporary characteristics," *Gerontologist*, vol. 50, no. 6, pp. 821–833, 2010.

[20] S. Goebeler, M. Jylhä, and A. Hervonen, "Self-reported medical history and self-rated health at age 90. Agreement with medical records," *Aging—Clinical and Experimental Research*, vol. 19, no. 3, pp. 213–219, 2007.

[21] M. Vuorisalmi, *Examining Self-Rated Health in Old Age Methodological Study of Survey Questions*, Tampere University Press, Tampere, Finland, 2007.

[22] P. B. Baltes and M. M. Baltes, *Successful Aging: Perspectives from the Behavioral Sciences*, Cambridge University Press, Cambridge, UK, 1990.

[23] M. M. Baltes and L. L. Carstensen, "The process of successful ageing," *Ageing and Society*, vol. 16, no. 4, pp. 397–422, 1996.

10

The Effect of Three Months of Aerobic Training on Stroop Performance in Older Adults

David Predovan,[1,2] Sarah A. Fraser,[1,2] Mélanie Renaud,[1,2] and Louis Bherer[1,3]

[1] *Centre de Recherche, Institut universitaire de gériatrie de Montréal, Montréal, QC, Canada H3W 1W5*
[2] *Département de Psychologie, Université du Québec à Montréal, Montréal, QC, Canada H3C 3P8*
[3] *PERFORM Centre and Department of Psychology, Concordia University, Montréal, QC, Canada H4B 1R6*

Correspondence should be addressed to David Predovan, predovan.david@courrier.uqam.ca

Academic Editor: Kirk Erickson

Growing evidence supports the use of physical training interventions to improve both physical and cognitive performances in healthy older adults. Few studies have examined the impact of aerobic exercise on Stroop task performance, a measure of executive functions. In the current 3-month aerobic training study, 50 older adults (mean age = 67.96 ± 6.25 years) were randomly assigned to either a three-month physical training group or to a control group (waiting list). Training sessions were 3 times per week for 60 minutes. All participants completed pre- and post-test measures of cognitive performance using the modified Stroop task and physical performance (Rockport one-mile test). Compared to controls, the training group showed significant improvements in physical capacity ($P < 0.001$) and enhanced Stroop performance, but only in the inhibition/switching condition ($P < 0.03$). Furthermore, the increase in aerobic capacity induced by the training regimen correlated negatively with reaction time in the inhibition/switching condition of the Stroop task at posttest ($r = -0.538$; $P = 0.007$). Importantly, the reported gains in cognitive performance were observed after only three months of physical training. Taken together, the results suggest that even short-term physical interventions can enhance older adults' executive functions.

1. Introduction

A variety of executive function processes sustained by the prefrontal cortex decline over time [1] (e.g., response preparation [2] and task switching [3]). Recent accounts of executive functions suggest that they rely on distinct basic mechanisms [4], namely, updating (of new information), inhibition (suppressing prepotent responses) and shifting (from one mental set to another), that could be differentially altered as we age. The variability in the trajectories of cognitive decline [5] suggests that compensatory mechanisms [6] and individual factors (i.e., involvement in physical activity and cognitive reserve) [7] could minimize these deficits.

Physical activity, defined as any activity that involves bodily movements, is one individual factor that can reduce the impact of aging on executive functions [8, 9]. In goal-directed research, physical activity that was planned, structured, and repetitive improves physical fitness, defined as the ability to function efficiently and effectively in work and leisure activities and to meet unforeseen emergency situations [10]. Theoretically, the "selective improvement" hypothesis [11] argues that aerobic exercise known to increase cardiorespiratory fitness as indexed by direct measures or estimations of $V_{O_2\,max}$ (i.e., capacity of the body to transport and use oxygen during incremental exercise) should present the largest benefit in tasks requiring executive control processes [12, 13] (but also see [14] for the effect of resistance training).

A recent review [15] found evidence that long-term physical activity interventions have consistent effects on tasks requiring inhibition or requiring dual-task coordination, compared to tasks requiring shifting which suggests that basic executive function mechanisms may be differentially affected by physical activity. However, the consistency of the effect on dual-task coordination remains precarious as it is based on only two results [16, 17]. In the current study, we explore the effect of aerobic exercise on a complex task requiring both inhibition and shifting (dual executive function condition), compared to a task requiring only inhibition.

One task commonly used to explore age differences in inhibitory control processes is the Interference condition of the Stroop color-word task [18]. In this condition, the Stroop effect occurs when naming the color of the ink in which a word is written, and this happens faster and more accurately when the color denoted by the name is congruent (e.g., blue written in blue), rather than incongruent (e.g., blue written in red). When compared to younger adults, older adults demonstrate longer reaction times (RTs) and higher error rates in the incongruent condition (i.e., interference condition) [19–22].

The present study targeted sedentary older adults (i.e., no or irregular physical activity) and examined if the benefits of aerobic exercise extend to different executive processes measured by using a modified version of the Stroop task [23]. This modified version includes a switching condition in addition to the classic interference or inhibition condition. The executive component of shifting, or the ability to switch between different task sets, has demonstrated the most robust age-related deficits [24] and has been identified as an important predictor of the maintenance of independent living in elderly [25]. In accordance with Barenberg et al. [15], the aerobic exercise training benefit on executive functions should be observed in the inhibition condition. In comparison to the inhibition condition, we expect the dual executive function condition to demonstrate smaller training benefits, since the existing findings of long-term physical activity benefits on tasks requiring shifting are less consistent [15].

2. Methods

2.1. Participants. Through advertisement in community centers in the Montreal area, 77 older adults were recruited. All participants completed a phone screening evaluating their physical health prior to admission in the study. The level of risk when engaging in intense physical activity and the level of physical activity over the 12 past months were assessed by the completion of the modified questionnaire of aptitude to physical activity (QAA-P) and the modifiable activity questionnaire (MAQ) [26]. Only sedentary adults, whose frequency of physical activity was less than twice per week, were enrolled.

Exclusion criteria included a history of neurological disease or major surgery in the year preceding the study, auditory or visual impairments that had not been corrected, cardiovascular disease or vascular peripheral attacks, and/or moderate to severe hypertension. In order to exclude participants with dementia or depression, a score lower than 26/30 on the Mini-Mental State Examination (MMSE) [27] and higher than 11 on the Geriatric Depression Scale (GDS) [28] resulted in exclusion. Ten participants did not meet inclusion criteria.

Assignment of the remaining 67 participants was based on the order of recruitment and on participants' willingness to engage in a 3-month fitness training program. Therefore, 32 participants were assigned to the experimental group, and the remaining 35 were assigned to the control group who did not receive any training. After completing the screening, seven participants in the training group and ten in the control group decided not to pursue the study for personal reasons. In the training group, there were no differences in baseline characteristics between the individuals who decided not to pursue and those who remained in the study. In the control group, those who discontinued were older ($P < 0.05$) and had lower scores ($P < 0.05$) on the similarities subtest of the WAIS-III.

The remaining participants in both the aerobic exercise group (F/M = 21/4; age (years) = 67.80 ± 6.60; education (years) = 14.36 ± 4.17) and the control group (F/M = 21/4; age (years) = 67.72 ± 6.01; education (years) = 12.92 ± 2.61) completed the study. Within these 50 participants, one participant in each group was excluded from statistical analyses due to missing Stroop test data. On a five-point health-rating scale (5 = excellent), the experimental (M = 4.21, SD = 0.74) and control groups (M = 4.17, SD = 0.72) average ratings were equivalent. Table 1 presents baseline characteristics of both groups.

Table 1: Participant's baseline characteristics.

	Control M (SD)	Training M (SD)
General characteristics		
Age	68.08 (5.85)	67.83 (6.74)
Education	12.96 (2.66)	14.42 (4.25)
General mental ability		
MMSE	29.20 (1.14)	28.62 (1.10)
Verbal intelligence		
Similarities	22.87 (4.41)	22.58 (4.89)
Mood assessment		
GDS	5.37 (4.36)	4.50 (2.83)
Fitness assessment		
MAQ	3.44 (2.62)	4.50 (4.45)

2.2. Procedure. During the pre-test session, the consent form was signed, and all screening tests and questionnaires were completed, along with the modified Stroop task (see description below). In the second session, a test of cardiorespiratory fitness (Rockport one-mile test, [29]) was completed. Then the training group participated in a 12-week aerobic fitness program (see below). In a post-test session, both groups were reevaluated with the same neuropsychological battery (including the Stroop task) and the Rockport one-mile fitness test. The study was completed within a 14-week period (1 week of pre-testing, 12 weeks of training, and 1 week of post-testing).

2.3. Aerobic Fitness Program. The 3-month (3 × 1 hour/week) physical exercise program was composed of stretching and cardiorespiratory exercises (fast walking and aerobic dancing). Adequate warm-up and cool-down periods and progressive and gradual increments in exercise duration and energy expenditure were implemented according to recommendations [30]. Duration of cardiorespiratory exercise was also gradually increased during the training program, beginning at 15 min per session and increasing until participants were exercising for 40 min per session. The training sessions were continuously supervised by two professional kinesiologists. Training session attendance was high, with participants attending 86.58% of sessions.

2.4. Pre- and Post-Test Measures: Cardiorespiratory Fitness Assessment. The Rockport one-mile test [29] was employed to evaluate cardiorespiratory fitness. This walking test provides an accurate estimation of the maximum level of oxygen consumption ($V_{O_2\,max}$; [29]). A strong correlation coefficient ($r = 0.88$) has been reported between the Rockport estimated $V_{O_2\,max}$ and a direct measure of $V_{O_2\,max}$ during an incremented test on a treadmill [29]. Participants wearing Polar S120 heart rate monitor (Polar Electro, Lake Success, NY, USA) were instructed to walk one mile without stopping, as fast as possible. The time required to complete the distance was manually recorded on a stopwatch. Heart rate frequency was recorded 1 min after the end of the walking test. $V_{O_2\,max}$ was estimated using the equation provided by [29] that takes into account participants' weight, age, sex, cardiac frequency post-exercise, and time to walk the one-mile distance.

2.5. Pre- and Post-Test Measures: Stroop Tasks. The present study utilized a Stroop test [23] that has four different conditions. Each condition included 100 stimuli (10 items per line) printed on a 21.5 × 28 cm sheet of paper. In the first (reading) condition, the participant had to read the words printed in black (i.e., red, green, blue, and yellow). In the second condition (naming), the participant needed to name the color of the rectangles. In the third condition (interference), the participant had to name the color of the ink in which the words are written. The meaning of each word had to be ignored, since it was incongruent with the color to name (e.g., the word "green" written in red). This condition is the inhibition only condition. The last condition (Inhibition/Switching) was similar to the third condition, except that 20 color words out of the 100 items were surrounded by a small box to indicate to the participant to read the word instead of naming its color. Therefore, the participant must alternate (or switch) in the inhibition/switching condition between naming the ink color of the words and reading the words. This is considered the most complex condition as it requires two executive processes (inhibition and switching). For all conditions, participants were to respond as quickly as possible, while making the least amount of errors. Reaction times (RTs) and the number of errors (corrected and uncorrected) were the main variables of interest.

3. Results

3.1. Participant's Baseline Characteristics. An ANOVA revealed no significant difference between groups on their level of formal education, $F(1,46) = 2,03$, $P < 0.16$, MMSE, $F(1,46) = 3,26$, $P < 0.08$, general verbal ability (score on the similarities subtest of the WAIS-III), $F(1,46) < 1$, GDS, $F(1,46) < 1$, and MAQ score, $F(1,46) = 1,01$, $P < 0.32$. Training and control groups were also comparable for age, $F(1,46) < 1$.

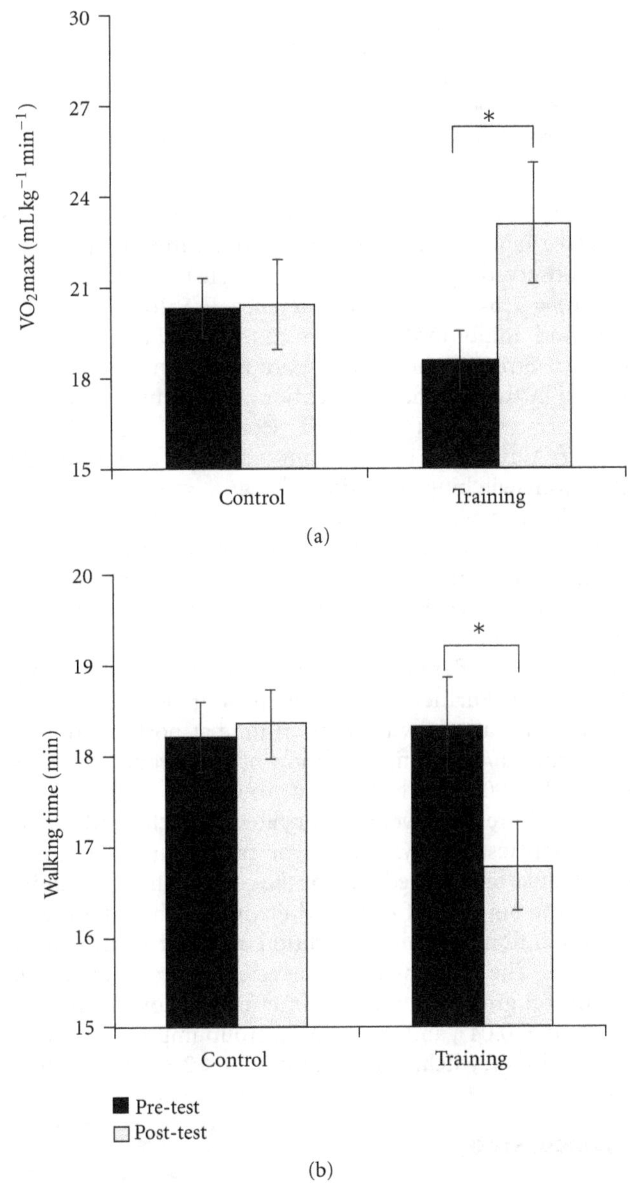

FIGURE 1: Mean and SE for $V_{O_2\,max}$ estimate (a) and walking time (b) in the Rockport one-mile test. $^*P < .001$.

3.2. Cardiorespiratory Fitness Assessment. A significant group × time interaction was found, $F(1,44) = 24.99$, $P < 0.001$, which confirmed that the participants in the training group showed significant improvement in the $V_{O_2\,max}$ estimate (see Figure 1(a)) after 3 months of physical fitness training, $F(1,23) = 39.00$, $P < 0.001$, while the $V_{O_2\,max}$ estimate of control participants remained unchanged, $F(1,23) < 1$. The analysis of walking time (see Figure 1(b)) also confirmed the benefits of the aerobic fitness intervention, as evidenced by a significant group × time interaction, $F(1,44) = 33.69$, $P < 0.001$. Participants in the training group walked the mile faster after the 12-week training program, $F(1,23) = 44.44$, $P < 0.001$, whereas the walk time of participants in the control group did not change significantly, $F(1,23) < 1$.

3.3. Stroop Task. At baseline, group performance on Stroop tasks (see Table 2) was equivalent as no significant differences were observed on the reading, $F(1, 46) < 1$, naming, $F(1,46) = 2,54$, $P < 0.19$, interference, $F(1,46) = 2.37$, $P < 0.13$, and inhibition/switching condition, $F(1,23) < 1$. For each Stroop condition, a score measuring the amount of change due to the intervention was computed as follows: pre-test minus post-test score (see Figure 2). An MANOVA revealed a significant effect of group for the inhibition/switching condition, $F(1,46) = 5.03$, $P < 0.03$. No difference was found for the reading, $F(1,46) < 1$, naming, $F(1,46) < 1$, and interference condition, $F(1,46) < 1$. Follow-up univariate analyses on the change score in the inhibition/switching condition confirm the effect of the intervention on the training group, $F(1,23) = 5.05$, $P < 0.03$, and no difference was found for the control group, $F(1,23) < 1$. Furthermore, the increase in aerobic capacity correlates negatively with reaction time at post-test only in the inhibition/switching condition of the Stroop task ($r = -0.54$; $P = .007$) for the training group.

Table 2 presents overall error rates for each condition of the Stroop test. Analyses on error rates using a Wilcoxon signed ranks test showed that for the control and the training group, the amount of corrected errors for the interference and inhibition/switching condition remains equivalent at month 3. The amount of uncorrected errors improved in the control group only for the interference condition ($Z = -2.10$, $P = 0.04$), and the training group improved only for the inhibition/switching condition ($Z = -2.86$, $P = 0.004$).

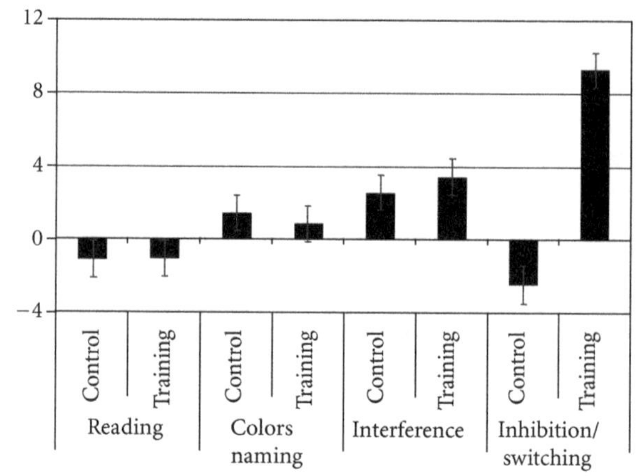

FIGURE 2: Mean (s) and SE for the change score on the Stroop test. $^*P < .05$.

4. Discussion

The results of the present study suggest that, in the elderly, the benefits of an aerobic training program occur primarily on executive functions and that these benefits can be seen after only three months of physical training. As a first step, we confirm based on the Rockport walk test that our trained group demonstrates improved cardiorespiratory fitness when compared to the control group after 12 weeks of physical training. In addition, the training group showed a performance improvement on the Stroop task requiring multiple executive processes, the inhibition/switching condition. As inhibition alone was not improved, we explain this in terms of improvement in the switching domain. One explanation could be the type of exercise done during the training. As previously mentioned, aerobic dance exercise was part of the training our participants received. Research [31] has already supported improved cardiorespiratory endurance after 12 weeks of low-impact aerobic dance in a group of elderly women. In addition, similar to our findings, Coubard et al. [32] evaluated executive functions after contemporary dance training and demonstrated an executive function improvement after 5.7 months of contemporary dance that was seen only in a switching condition (rule shift cards sorting test) but not in an inhibition condition (Stroop task). Together with our results, this suggests that some types of exercise might selectively improve complex tasks involving switching and/or multiple executive processes.

The absence of a specific training effect on the Interference condition is at odds with some studies, including the review of Barenberg et al. [15]. For example, in a 4-month (3 × 1 hours/week) trial, Dustman et al. [33] demonstrated that the Stroop interference condition performance only improved for those aerobically trained. Interestingly, Blumenthal et al. [34] employing an aerobic training of the same duration and intensity did not replicate this finding. The choice of control group activities does not explain these divergent findings as both studies included a group who did not exercise. A possible confounding factor is that both studies computed the Stroop effect differently. In Dustman's study, RTs in the reading condition were subtracted from the "interference" condition, as a way to account for improved motor ability. It has been proposed [22] that these proportional interference scores minimize the effects of general slowing, which is often highlighted as a potential explanation of the magnitude of the Stroop effect in the elderly [35–37]. Therefore, the absence of an aerobic benefit in inhibition in Blumenthal's study and our study could have been hindered by other factors that are not task specific.

Blumenthal et al. [34] acknowledged two factors that could account for the difference in the findings between their study and that of Dustman et al. [33]: (1) different sample characteristics (age and male/female ratio) and (2) differences in aerobic fitness improvement levels. In fact, Blumenthal et al. [34] reported that their participants experienced less than 50% (11.6% versus 27%) of the improvement in $V_{O_2\,max}$ reported in Dustman study. In the current study, there were no differences in our two groups based on age or male/female ratio, and we demonstrate a significant improvement in $V_{O_2\,max}$ in our training group, as such our findings are not confounded by these factors.

TABLE 2: Participant's baseline and follow-up results (Mean (SD)) for the Stroop test.

	Control		Training	
	Before	After	Before	After
Reaction time (s)				
Reading	44.26 (6.87)	45.40 (6.84)	43.82 (6.29)	44.90 (6.45)
Colors naming	71.39 (16.69)	69.97 (15.83)	64.81 (11.40)	63.97 (9.06)
Interference	126.03 (30.39)	123.48 (35.81)	113.57 (25.49)	110.16 (27.41)
Inhibition/switching	132.55 (21.21)	135.04 (29.48)	135.56 (38.94)	126.24 (27.29)
Error				
Reading	0.17 (0.38)	0.08 (0.28)	0.08 (0.28)	0.13 (0.34)
Colors naming	0.92 (1.21)	0.92 (0.88)	1.38 (1.28)	0.75 (0.68)
Interference	2.17 (2.73)	1.71 (1.49)	2.08 (2.21)	1.75 (1.39)
Inhibition/switching	2.50 (2.36)	2.17 (1.83)	4.79 (4.03)	3.00 (3.11)

Finally, it is important to note that our results show that the improvement in cardiovascular fitness and in executive performance in our training group is correlated. The increase in cardiorespiratory fitness correlates negatively with reaction time in the inhibition/switching condition of the Stroop at post-test, suggesting that there is indeed a relationship between improved cardiorespiratory fitness and improvements in a Stroop condition requiring two executive processes. We did not find a significant correlation between cardiorespiratory fitness and the inhibition-only performance which is in line with a recent finding that suggests that an improvement in cardiorespiratory fitness is not prerequisite to an enhanced Stroop performance [38]. Smiley-Oyen et al. [38] had equivalent V_{O_2} peak improvements in both their aerobic (18%) and strength/flexibility exercise training groups (13%) after completing 10 months (3×1 hours/week) of training, and yet Stroop performance as measured by RTs and accuracy improved only in the aerobic group. This outcome highlights the possibility that the impact of aerobic exercise on the Stroop performance might not be directly mediated by changes in cardiorespiratory fitness per se. In light of this possibility, other mechanisms have been proposed such as enhancement of brain vascularization, an increased plasticity though neurogenesis, neurotrophic factors (e.g., brain-derived neurotrophic factor (BDNF)) [39], or other factors that improve neuronal viability [40, 41].

Two limitations affect the generalizability of our results. First, the method of assignment was done by self-selection, potentially placing more motivated individuals in our training group; a future study should involve a more systematic and randomized method of assignment. Second, our waiting-list control group was only assessed at pre and post time points, and as such, we cannot control for any effect of socialization that may have occurred in the training group since they came repeatedly over the 12-week period. A better approach would have been to propose a control intervention with the same training regime that includes physical activity but that does not increase cardiorespiratory fitness.

Future research is needed to clarify why in the present study participants in the training group did not improve on the Inhibition condition and why other published studies have reported improvement (Liu-Ambrose et al. [14], for instance). One promising avenue would be the use of imaging techniques as they have shown an age-related brain activation difference when performing a Stroop task [42]. Of particular interest, a recent study [43] has found distinct patterns of prefrontal activation between the inhibition condition and the inhibition/switching condition using functional near infrared spectroscopy (fNIRS). Therefore, brain imaging studies could contribute to the comprehension of the condition-related effect of aerobic training in aging that is observed with the Stroop paradigm, particularly in the inhibition/switching condition, known to be sensitive to cognitive decline in the elderly [44–47].

Conflict of Interests

The authors have no conflict of interests to disclose.

Acknowledgment

This study was supported by Canada Research Chair Program.

References

[1] O. A. Coubard, L. Ferrufino, M. Boura, A. Gripon, M. Renaud, and L. Bherer, "Attentional control in normal aging and Alzheimer's disease," *Neuropsychology*, vol. 25, no. 3, pp. 353–367, 2011.

[2] L. Bherer and S. Belleville, "Age-related differences in response preparation: the role of time uncertainty," *Journals of Gerontology. Series B*, vol. 59, no. 2, pp. P66–P74, 2004.

[3] A. Hampshire, A. Gruszka, S. J. Fallon, and A. M. Owen, "Inefficiency in self-organized attentional switching in the normal aging population is associated with decreased activity in the ventrolateral prefrontal cortex," *Journal of Cognitive Neuroscience*, vol. 20, no. 9, pp. 1670–1686, 2008.

[4] A. Miyake, N. P. Friedman, M. J. Emerson, A. H. Witzki, A. Howerter, and T. D. Wager, "The unity and diversity of executive functions and their contributions to complex "Frontal Lobe" tasks: a latent variable analysis," *Cognitive Psychology*, vol. 41, no. 1, pp. 49–100, 2000.

[5] R. L. Buckner, "Memory and executive function in aging and ad: multiple factors that cause decline and reserve factors that compensate," *Neuron*, vol. 44, no. 1, pp. 195–208, 2004.
[6] R. Cabeza, N. D. Anderson, J. K. Locantore, and A. R. McIntosh, "Aging gracefully: compensatory brain activity in high-performing older adults," *NeuroImage*, vol. 17, no. 3, pp. 1394–1402, 2002.
[7] A. M. Tucker and Y. Stern, "Cognitive reserve in aging," *Current Alzheimer Research*, vol. 8, no. 4, pp. 354–360, 2011.
[8] F. Sofi, D. Valecchi, D. Bacci et al., "Physical activity and risk of cognitive decline: a meta-analysis of prospective studies," *Journal of Internal Medicine*, vol. 269, no. 1, pp. 107–117, 2011.
[9] M. W. Voss, L. S. Nagamatsu, T. Liu-Ambrose, and A. F. Kramer, "Exercise, brain, and cognition across the life span," *Journal of Applied Physiology*, vol. 111, no. 5, pp. 1505–1513, 2011.
[10] C. J. Caspersen, K. E. Powell, and G. Christenson, "Physical activity, exercise and physical fitness: definitions and distinctions for health-related research," *Public Health Reports*, vol. 100, no. 2, pp. 126–131, 1985.
[11] A. F. Kramer, S. Hahn, N. J. Cohen et al., "Ageing, fitness and neurocognitive function," *Nature*, vol. 400, no. 6743, pp. 418–419, 1999.
[12] S. Colcombe and A. F. Kramer, "Fitness effects on the cognitive function of older adults: a meta-analytic study," *Psychological Science*, vol. 14, no. 2, pp. 125–130, 2003.
[13] M. Renaud, F. Maquestiaux, S. Joncas, M.-J. Kergoat, and L. Bherer, "The effect of three months of aerobic training on response preparation in older adults," *Frontiers in Aging Neuroscience*, vol. 2, 148, 2010.
[14] T. Liu-Ambrose, L. S. Nagamatsu, M. W. Voss, K. M. Khan, and T. C. Handy, "Resistance training and functional plasticity of the aging brain: a 12-month randomized controlled trial," *Neurobiology of Aging*, vol. 33, no. 8, pp. 1690–1698, 2012.
[15] J. Barenberg, T. Berse, and S. Dutke, "Executive functions in learning processes: do they benefit from physical activity?" *Educational Research Review*, vol. 6, no. 3, pp. 208–222, 2011.
[16] T. Harada, S. Okagawa, and K. Kubota, "Jogging improved performance of a behavioral branching task: implications for prefrontal activation," *Neuroscience Research*, vol. 49, no. 3, pp. 325–337, 2004.
[17] H. L. Hawkins, A. F. Kramer, and D. Capaldi, "Aging, exercise, and attention," *Psychology and aging*, vol. 7, no. 4, pp. 643–653, 1992.
[18] C. M. MacLeod, "Half a century of reseach on the stroop effect: an integrative review," *Psychological Bulletin*, vol. 109, no. 2, pp. 163–203, 1991.
[19] N. B. Cohn, R. E. Dustman, and D. C. Bradford, "Age-related decrements in stroop color test performance," *Journal of Clinical Psychology*, vol. 40, no. 5, pp. 1244–1250, 1984.
[20] A. K. Troyer, L. Leach, and E. Strauss, "Aging and response inhibition: normative data for the Victoria Stroop Test," *Aging, Neuropsychology, and Cognition B*, vol. 13, no. 1, pp. 20–35, 2006.
[21] R. West, "The effects of aging on controlled attention and conflict processing in the stroop task," *Journal of Cognitive Neuroscience*, vol. 16, no. 1, pp. 103–113, 2004.
[22] J. M. Bugg, E. L. DeLosh, D. B. Davalos, and H. P. Davis, "Age differences in stroop interference: contributions of general slowing and task-specific deficits," *Aging, Neuropsychology, and Cognition*, vol. 14, no. 2, pp. 155–167, 2007.
[23] N. Bohnen, J. Jolles, and A. Twijnstra, "Modification of the Stroop Color Word Test improves differentiation between patients with mild head injury and matched controls," *Clinical Neuropsychologist*, vol. 6, no. 2, pp. 178–184, 1992.
[24] P. Verhaeghen, "Aging and executive control: reports of a demise greatly exaggerated," *Current Directions in Psychological Science*, vol. 20, no. 3, pp. 174–180, 2011.
[25] L. Vaughan and K. Giovanello, "Executive function in daily life: age-related influences of executive processes on instrumental activities of daily living," *Psychology and Aging*, vol. 25, no. 2, pp. 343–355, 2010.
[26] A. Vuillemin, J. M. Oppert, F. Guillemin et al., "Self-administered questionnaire compared with interview to assess past-year physical activity," *Medicine and Science in Sports and Exercise*, vol. 32, no. 6, pp. 1119–1124, 2000.
[27] M. F. Folstein, S. E. Folstein, and P. R. McHugh, "'Mini mental state'. A practical method for grading the cognitive state of patients for the clinician," *Journal of Psychiatric Research*, vol. 12, no. 3, pp. 189–198, 1975.
[28] J. A. Yesavage, T. L. Brink, and T. L. Rose, "Development and validation of a geriatric depression screening scale: a preliminary report," *Journal of Psychiatric Research*, vol. 17, no. 1, pp. 37–49, 1982.
[29] G. M. Kline, J. P. Porcari, and R. Hintermeister, "Estimation of VO2max from a one-mile track walk, gender, age, and body weight," *Medicine and Science in Sports and Exercise*, vol. 19, no. 3, pp. 253–259, 1987.
[30] M. E. Nelson, W. J. Rejeski, S. N. Blair et al., "Physical activity and public health in older adults: recommendation from the American College of Sports Medicine and the American Heart Association," *Circulation*, vol. 116, no. 9, pp. 1094–1105, 2007.
[31] D. R. Hopkins, B. Murrah, W. W. K. Hoeger, and R. C. Rhodes, "Effect of low-impact aerobic dance on the functional fitness of elderly women," *Gerontologist*, vol. 30, no. 2, pp. 189–192, 1990.
[32] O. A. Coubard, S. Duretz, V. Lefebvre, P. Lapalus, and L. Ferrufino, "Practice of contemporary dance improves cognitive flexibility in aging," *Frontiers in Aging Neuroscience*, vol. 3, no. SEP, pp. 1–12, 2011.
[33] R. E. Dustman, R. O. Ruhling, and E. M. Russell, "Aerobic exercise training and improved neuropsychological function of older individuals," *Neurobiology of Aging*, vol. 5, no. 1, pp. 35–42, 1984.
[34] J. A. Blumenthal, C. F. Emery, D. J. Madden et al., "Cardiovascular and behavioral effects of aerobic exercise training in healthy older men and women," *Journals of Gerontology*, vol. 44, no. 5, pp. M147–M157, 1989.
[35] P. Verhaeghen and L. De Meersman, "Aging and the Stroop effect: a meta-analysis," *Psychology and Aging*, vol. 13, no. 1, pp. 120–126, 1998.
[36] P. Verhaeghen and J. Cerella, "Aging, executive control, and attention: a review of meta-analyses," *Neuroscience and Biobehavioral Reviews*, vol. 26, no. 7, pp. 849–857, 2002.
[37] T. A. Salthouse, "The Processing-speed theory of adult age differences in cognition," *Psychological Review*, vol. 103, no. 3, pp. 403–428, 1996.
[38] A. L. Smiley-Oyen, K. A. Lowry, S. J. Francois, M. L. Kohut, and P. Ekkekakis, "Exercise, fitness, and neurocognitive function in older adults: the "selective improvement" and "cardiovascular fitness" hypotheses," *Annals of Behavioral Medicine*, vol. 36, no. 3, pp. 280–291, 2008.
[39] I. Lista and G. Sorrentino, "Biological mechanisms of physical activity in preventing cognitive decline," *Cellular and Molecular Neurobiology*, vol. 30, no. 4, pp. 493–503, 2010.

[40] A. F. Kramer and K. I. Erickson, "Capitalizing on cortical plasticity: influence of physical activity on cognition and brain function," *Trends in Cognitive Sciences*, vol. 11, no. 8, pp. 342–348, 2007.

[41] K. I. Erickson, A. M. Weinstein, B. P. Sutton et al., "Beyond vascularization: aerobic fitness is associated with N-acetylaspartate and working memory," *Brain and Behavior*, vol. 2, no. 1, pp. 32–41, 2012.

[42] S. A. Langenecker, K. A. Nielson, and S. M. Rao, "fMRI of healthy older adults during Stroop interference," *NeuroImage*, vol. 21, no. 1, pp. 192–200, 2004.

[43] M. Laguë-Beauvais, J. Brunet, L. Gagnon, F. Lesage, and L. Bherer, "A fNIRS investigation of switching and inhibition during the modified Stroop task in younger and older adults," *NeuroImage*, vol. 64, pp. 485–495, 2013.

[44] E. M. Fine, D. C. Delis, S. R. Wetter et al., "Cognitive discrepancies versus apoe genotype as predictors of cognitive decline in normal-functioning elderly individuals: a longitudinal study," *American Journal of Geriatric Psychiatry*, vol. 16, no. 5, pp. 366–374, 2008.

[45] L. R. Clark, D. M. Schiehser, G. H. Weissberger, D. P. Salmon, D. C. Delis, and M. W. Bondi, "Specific measures of executive function predict cognitive decline in older adults," *Journal of the International Neuropsychological Society*, vol. 18, no. 1, pp. 118–127, 2012.

[46] S. R. Wetter, D. C. Delis, W. S. Houston et al., "Deficits in inhibition and flexibility are associated with the APOE-E4 allele in nondemented older adults," *Journal of Clinical and Experimental Neuropsychology*, vol. 27, no. 8, pp. 943–952, 2005.

[47] K. A. Hutchison, D. A. Balota, and J. M. Ducheck, "The utility of stroop task switching as a marker for early-stage alzheimer's disease," *Psychology and Aging*, vol. 25, no. 3, pp. 545–559, 2010.

11

Accelerometer Derived Activity Counts and Oxygen Consumption between Young and Older Individuals

Lucas Whitcher[1] and Charilaos Papadopoulos[2]

[1] *Department of Applied Arts and Sciences, University of Montana-Missoula College, Missoula, MT 95812, USA*
[2] *Department of Kinesiology, Pacific Lutheran University, Tacoma, WA 98447, USA*

Correspondence should be addressed to Charilaos Papadopoulos; papadoha@plu.edu

Academic Editor: F. R. Ferraro

The purpose of this investigation was to compare accelerometer activity counts and oxygen consumption between young and elderly individuals. Sixteen young (21.3 ± 2.5 yrs) and sixteen elderly (66.6 ± 2.9 yrs) participants completed 30 minutes of resting oxygen consumption to determine resting metabolic rate and four 6 min walking intensities ranging from 27 to 94 $m \cdot min^{-1}$. Resting oxygen uptake was significantly lower for the older participants. Exercise oxygen consumption was significantly higher for the elderly group. There were no significant differences in activity counts between groups at each of the exercise intensities. When using measured resting metabolic rate, activity counts of 824 and 2207 $counts \cdot min^{-1}$ were associated with moderate (3 METs) physical activity intensity for the older and young participants, respectively. However, using standard resting metabolic rate ($3.5\ mL \cdot kg^{-1} \cdot min^{-1}$), activity counts of 784 and 2009 $counts \cdot min^{-1}$ were associated with moderate physical activity intensity for the elderly and young participants, respectively. These findings indicate that activity counts are similar across age groups even though the oxygen consumption of exercise is greater among elderly individuals.

1. Introduction

Despite the importance of physical activity in maintaining and improving health and quality of life in those individuals over the age of 65, research suggests that less than 3% of elderly Americans [1] comply with the American College of Sports Medicine's physical activity recommendations [2, 3]. Given the correlation between physical activity and increased health, it is of interest to accurately measure physical activity levels within a population. However, the ability to quantify physical activity in individuals can be a problematic task. In addition, because the current recommendations for physical activity include both intensity and duration, there is a compulsory need that measurement tools do the same. Criterion methods, such as doubly labeled water and open-circuit spirometry, may not be plausible when examining large populations due to cost and/or an inability to obtain frequency and intensity of physical activity. Furthermore, the commonly used self-report instruments are subjective and rely on recall information, which may be limited when applied to an older population [4].

Accelerometers offer detailed information over extended periods pertaining to physical activity behavior. This information can be used to provide estimates of time spent in different levels of physical activity intensities and overall patterns of physical activity. Unfortunately, few applications to the elderly population have been made [5] and the raw output data can be difficult to interpret [1]. Moreover, accelerometer activity count cut-points used to determine physical activity intensity levels have been established from studies testing young participants [6–9]. To date, there are only very few studies that have sought to determine an activity count cut-point for determination of moderate physical activity intensity for elderly adults [8, 10, 11] and only one study has evaluated the relationship between oxygen consumption and activity counts of younger and older adults [8]. Furthermore, since investigations have shown that elderly individuals require a greater metabolic cost for walking at the same absolute intensity as young individuals [12, 13], it seems necessary to make such a comparison. Lastly, evidence suggests that the standard 3.5 $mL{\cdot}kg^{-1}{\cdot}min^{-1}$ may not represent the resting metabolic rate of the general population [14, 15] and that older adults may have a lower resting metabolic rate compared to younger individuals [14, 16]. Due to those differences at rest and during exercise between younger and older adults, the researchers hypothesized that a lower resting metabolic rate and higher oxygen consumption during exercise with similar accelerometer derived activity counts may result in a lower activity count threshold associated with moderate exercise intensity for older adults.

Therefore, the first purpose of this investigation was to compare accelerometer derived activity counts and oxygen consumption, measured during treadmill walking, between young and elderly participants. Secondly, we sought to determine the relationship between metabolic equivalent (MET) and accelerometer derived activity counts for each group of participants by using estimated and measured MET levels.

2. Methods

2.1. Participants. Thirty-two individuals, 16 elderly (age 66.6 ± 2.9 yrs) and 16 young (age 21.3 ± 2.5 yrs), recruited from the local community agreed to participate in this study. Participants were recruited from flyers posted at recreational facilities (e.g., senior centers) and bulletin boards at various locations (e.g., university, grocery stores). The primary inclusion criterion was the ability to walk unassisted on a treadmill. However, secondary inclusion criteria were used to further screen participants. Only participants that were healthy, free of injury within the past six months, and not taking medication (e.g., antidepressants, beta-blockers) or stimulants (e.g., caffeine, smoking) known to influence energy expenditure or exercise capacity were tested. All participants provided written informed consent and approval was obtained by the Central Washington University Human Subjects Review Committee.

2.2. Procedures. Participants attended a familiarization session prior to testing. During the familiarization session, participants rested for 10 minutes in a seated position while breathing through a mouthpiece and then walked at the various intensities to familiarize them with the walking speeds and grade on the treadmill. At least two days and no more than seven days after the familiarization session, a testing session was scheduled. Even though the majority (27 out of 32) of the tests were performed in the morning (before 9 a.m.), there were some tests that were performed at a later time mainly due to participant availability. Participants were instructed to refrain from caffeine and exercise on the day of testing. Also, participants were asked to withhold food consumption 3-4 hours prior to testing. Participants reported to the laboratory and after 10 min of rest to determine compliance with pretest instructions and answer last minute questions; height was recorded to the nearest centimeter (MED ART, St. Louis, MO) and weight was measured to the nearest 0.5 kg (Detecto-Medic, Brooklyn, NY). Body density and percent body fat were determined from skinfold measurements (Lange Skinfold Calipers, Cambridge Scientific Instruments Inc., Cambridge, MD) as described by Pollack et al. [17].

2.3. Resting Metabolic Rate. Indirect calorimetry (True Max 2400, Parvo Medics Inc., Sandy, Utah) was used for the measurement of resting metabolic rate. Gas analyzers were calibrated before each test with a gas tank of known concentration (16% O_2, 4% CO_2). Respiratory flows were measured with a pneumotachometer calibrated before each test with a syringe of known volume (3.0 L). Participants were then fitted with a mouthpiece that incorporates a two-way breathing valve apparatus (Hans Rudolph Inc., Kansas City, MO.). Initially participants were in a supine position but during pilot testing older participants indicated that they were uncomfortable and therefore all participants remained awake in a seated position for 30 min while expired gases were collected. Expired gases were sampled in 30 s intervals and averaged oxygen uptake values ($\dot{V}O_2$), both relative ($mL{\cdot}kg^{-1}{\cdot}min^{-1}$) and absolute ($L{\cdot}min^{-1}$), obtained from minutes 15 to 25 were used to calculate an individual's resting metabolic rate. In addition, heart rate (Polar Electro, USA) was monitored throughout the entire resting period and averaged during minutes 15–25 and this value was considered as the individual's resting heart rate.

2.4. Treadmill Exercise. Similar to the procedures of Copeland and Esliger [10], the treadmill bout consisted of 6 min stages with 5 min seated rest periods between stages. The four treadmill stages included walking at speeds of 27, 54, and 80 $m{\cdot}min^{-1}$ (1.0, 2.0, and 3.0 mph, resp.) and 0% grade, performed in random order, and a final stage of 94 $m{\cdot}min^{-1}$ (3.5 mph) and 2% grade. These intensities were selected to induce light, moderate, and vigorous physical activity. Based on pilot testing, the 94 $m{\cdot}min^{-1}$ and 2% grade stage was excluded from the random selection because this intensity was too difficult for some individuals to begin with, particularly in the absence of a warm-up and could have resulted in higher oxygen consumption on subsequent stages. All trials were performed on the same Quinton Q65 treadmill (Quinton Instruments Company, Seattle, WA). The speed and the grade were checked before each trial. Oxygen consumption during the treadmill bout was calculated by averaging the 30 s sampling rate values obtained in the final 3 min of each treadmill stage completed. In order to determine measured MET value per stage, averaged oxygen consumption per stage was divided by the individual's resting metabolic rate (measured $\dot{V}O_2$/measured resting metabolic rate) and by the standard (3.5 $mL{\cdot}kg^{-1}{\cdot}min^{-1}$) metabolic rate (measured $\dot{V}O_2/3.5$).

2.5. Accelerometers. Prior to the treadmill bout, participants were fitted with two Actigraph (Pensacola, Florida) accelerometers (one GT1M model and one GT3X model). The GT1M (mass, 27 g; width, 38 mm; height, 37 mm; thickness,

18 mm) is a newer smaller version of the discontinued Actigraph model 7164. This updated model has demonstrated similar activity counts per minute, when compared with the Actigraph 7164, at treadmill speeds of 54, 80, and 107 m·min^{-1} [18]. Unlike the GT1M model, which senses vertical accelerations, the GT3X detects accelerations along three planes of motion. According to the manufacturer, the GT1M and the GT3X models utilize the exact same activity filtering algorithm. Both activity monitors were initialized before each trial using the same laptop computer and using the ActiLife low frequency extension. In addition, the activity monitors were marked so that the same units were used for each participant. Accelerometers were securely mounted side by side along the anterior-axillary line of the right hip with an adjustable nylon belt. The activity counts recorded by the GT1M and the vertical axis activity counts from the GT3X were summed using 1 min sampling intervals (epochs) and averaged for the final 3 min of each treadmill stage. For the purposes of this investigation, the average activity counts from the GT1M and GT3X were used in the statistical analysis.

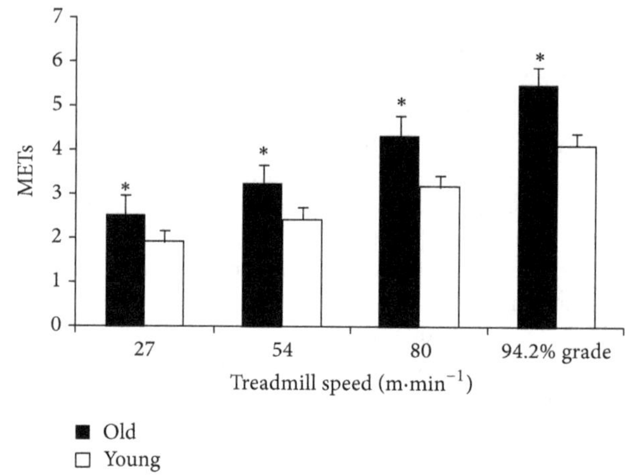

FIGURE 1: Treadmill speed and corresponding measured MET values among young and elderly participants. *Significantly greater than the younger group, $P < 0.05$.

2.6. Statistical Analysis. Body weight, height, and body composition were evaluated for significant differences between groups using a two-tailed independent t-test. Likewise, two-tailed independent t-tests were used to determine differences in heart rate and oxygen consumption between groups at rest. A two-way repeated measures (RM) analysis of variance (ANOVA) with one within factor (exercise intensity) and one between factor (elderly versus young) was used to evaluate differences between groups in averaged activity counts, oxygen consumption, and MET values for each of the intensities. To examine for differences between activity counts derived from the GT1M and GT3X Actigraph models, a two-way ANOVA was used as well. If statistical significance was found, Bonferroni *post hoc* test was used. A linear regression analysis was used to determine the relationship between measured METs and averaged vertical axis activity counts and between estimated METs and averaged vertical axis activity counts for each group (young and elderly). The prediction equation was determined from the entire data set for each group. Finally, activity counts corresponding to moderate intensity (3 METs) exercise were calculated from the developed regression equations. All data were analyzed using SPSS version 16.0. Data are expressed as means ± SD, and statistical significance was set at $P < 0.05$.

3. Results

Thirty-two individuals participated in the investigation (16 elderly and 16 young; Table 1). The young and elderly groups were similarly matched for gender (9 males and 7 females; 8 males and 8 females, resp.).

All participants completed the first three stages of treadmill walking. However, two of the elderly participants were unable to perform at the 94 m·min^{-1} and 2% grade. In one case, the participant declined to begin the final stage due to fatigue. In the other case, the participant began the final stage but requested to stop because of difficulty maintaining pace. Activity counts measured by the GT1M and GT3X Actigraph models are presented in Table 2.

There were no differences in activity counts between accelerometers for any of the exercise intensities, although the two-way RM ANOVA revealed significant difference for activity counts among the different intensities (Table 2). At rest, oxygen uptake relative to body mass among the elderly was significantly lower than the young group (3.49 ± 0.50 and 3.89 ± 0.28 mL·kg^{-1}·min^{-1}, resp.). There were no differences between groups in relative oxygen uptake (mL·kg^{-1}·min^{-1}) and heart rate at rest (Table 3). However, the two-way RM ANOVA showed a significant interaction between groups and exercise intensities. Bonferroni *post hoc* analysis indicated that oxygen uptake, measured MET, and heart rate values were significantly greater for the elderly participants at each of the intensities performed (Table 3).

Measured MET values were significantly greater among the elderly participants for each of the treadmill intensities (Figure 1).

A strong correlation (r = 0.89) between averaged activity counts and measured MET values existed among the young group (Figure 2(a)). Activity counts and estimated MET values were also strongly correlated (r = 0.91) for the young group (Figure 2(b)).

The relationships between activity counts and measured METs (Figure 3(a)) were moderate (r = 0.72) as it was the relationship (r = 0.76) between averaged activity counts and estimated METs (Figure 3(b)) for the older participants.

Based on the linear regression equations accelerometer activity counts of 824 (95% CI: 226–1719) and 2207 (95% CI: 1730–3008) counts·min^{-1} were associated with moderate (3 METs) physical activity intensity for the elderly and young participants, respectively, when using measured resting metabolic rate. Using the standard 3.5 mL·kg^{-1}·min^{-1}, linear regression equations indicated that moderate (3 METs) intensity physical activity was associated with 784 (95%

TABLE 1: Participants characteristics.

	n	Age (yrs)	Weight (kg)	Height (cm)	Percent body fat
Young	16	21.3 ± 2.5	72.8 ± 12.3	173.1 ± 8.4	18.9 ± 11.4
Elderly	16	66.6 ± 2.9*	77.7 ± 18.5	166.5 ± 9.2*	24.4 ± 9.1

*Significantly different from the young group, $P < 0.05$.

TABLE 2: Activity counts (counts·min^{-1}) during treadmill walking from uniaxial (GT1M) and triaxial (GT3X) accelerometers (n = 32).

	Treadmill speed (m·min^{-1})			
	27	54	80	94, 2% grade
Activity counts (GT1M)	302 ± 264#	1286 ± 481#	3000 ± 789#	3711 ± 881#
Activity counts (GT3X)	307 ± 276#	1184 ± 491#	2903 ± 817#	3651 ± 884#
Average activity counts	304 ± 271	1226 ± 483	2955 ± 809	3686 ± 882

#Significantly different among speeds, $P < 0.05$.

TABLE 3: Relative oxygen uptake (mL·kg·min^{-1}), heart rate, averaged activity counts, and measured MET values at rest and during treadmill walking in young (n = 16) and elderly subjects (n = 14).

		Rest	Treadmill speed (m·min^{-1})			
			27	54	80	94, 2% grade
Young	$\dot{V}O_2$	3.9 ± 0.3	7.6 ± 0.6#	9.4 ± 0.6#	12.4 ± 0.9#	16.0 ± 1.3#
	HR	67.3 ± 6.9	78.9 ± 7.7#	84.6 ± 6.7#	93.3 ± 8.3#	107.4 ± 13.9#
	MET		1.9 ± 0.2#	2.4 ± 0.3#	3.2 ± 0.3#	4.14 ± 0.4#
	AC		209 ± 130#	1188 ± 444#	2998 ± 739#	3689 ± 803#
Elderly	$\dot{V}O_2$	3.5 ± 0.5*	8.6 ± 1.4*#	11.0 ± 1.7*#	14.7 ± 2.0*#	18.5 ± 2.2*#
	HR	69.8 ± 9.8	86.7 ± 10.9*#	93.8 ± 10.5*#	109.2 ± 15.4*#	119.9 ± 14.6*#
	MET		2.5 ± 0.4*#	3.3 ± 0.6*#	4.3 ± 0.7*#	5.5 ± 0.9#
	AC		412 ± 352#	1267 ± 532#	2805 ± 891#	3506 ± 1032#

$\dot{V}O_2$: relative oxygen consumption (mL·kg·min^{-1}); HR: heart rate (bts·min^{-1}); AC: averaged activity counts (counts·min^{-1}).
*Significantly different from young group, $P < 0.05$.
#Significantly different among speeds, $P < 0.05$.

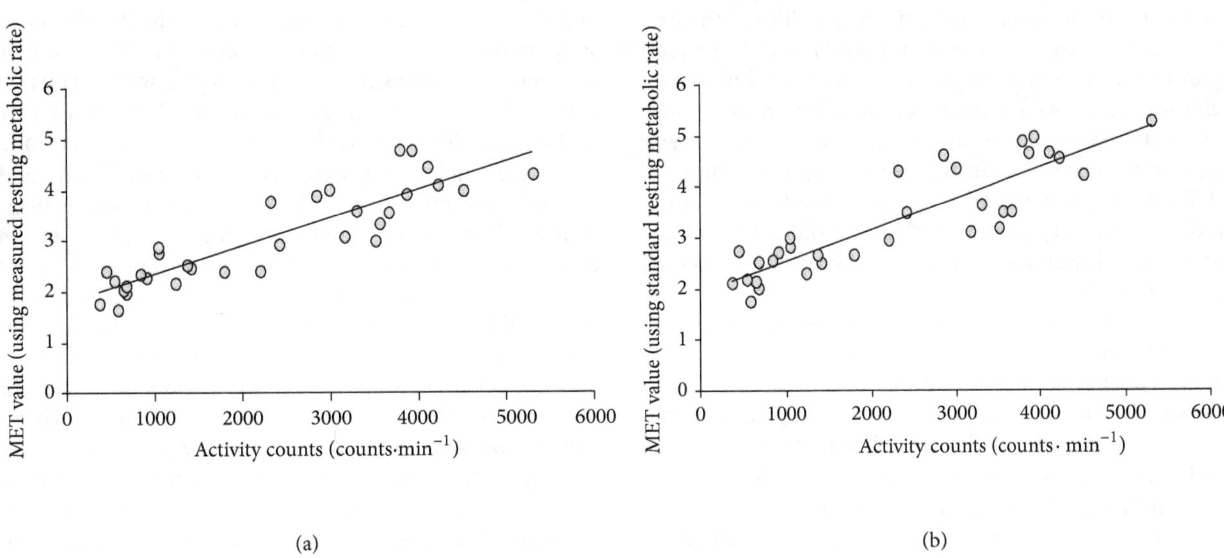

FIGURE 2: (a) Relationship between MET values and activity counts for young group using measured metabolic rate (R^2 = 0.80, standard error of estimate = 0.40). (b) Relationship between MET values and activity counts for young group using standard (3.5 mL·kg·min^{-1}) metabolic rate (R^2 = 0.82, standard error of estimate = 0.41).

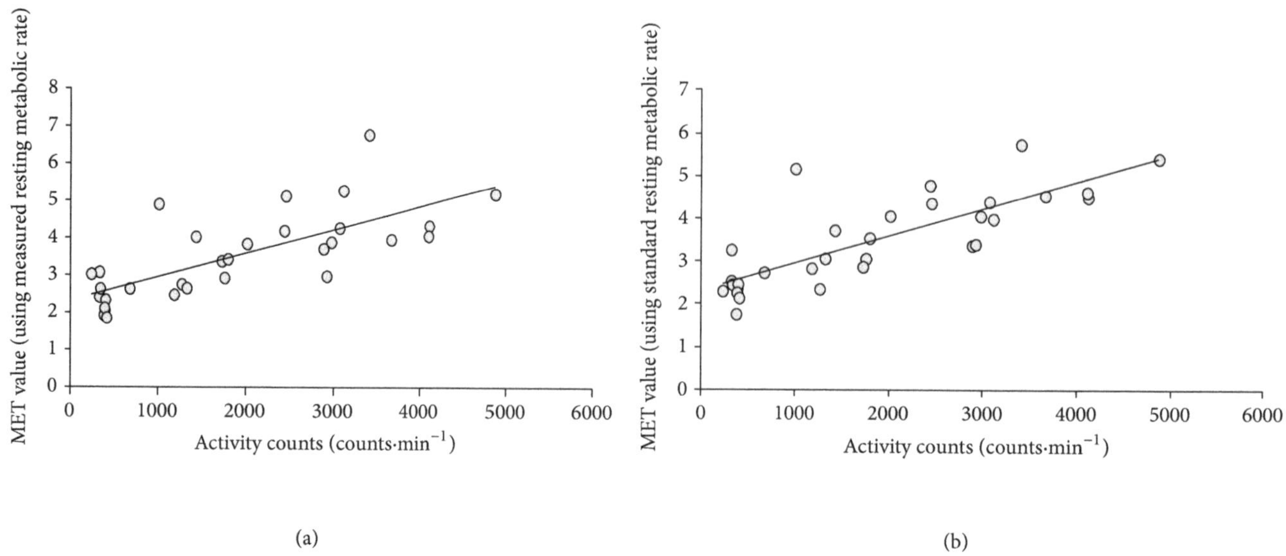

FIGURE 3: (a) Relationship between MET values and activity counts for elderly group using measured metabolic rate ($R^2 = 0.57$, standard error of estimate = 0.83). (b) Relationship between MET values and activity counts for elderly group using standard ($3.5\,mL{\cdot}kg{\cdot}min^{-1}$) metabolic rate ($R^2 = 0.52$, standard error of estimate = 0.85).

CI: 104–1859) and 2009 (95% CI: 1267–2320) counts·min^{-1} for the elderly and young participants, respectively.

4. Discussion

The purpose of this investigation was to compare treadmill derived activity counts, oxygen consumption, and MET values between young and elderly participants. Despite the widespread use of accelerometers for obtaining objective measures of physical activity, few applications to older populations have been made. Consequently, this study provides valuable information pertaining to the plausibility of the use of accelerometers within an elderly population. The main finding of the study is that despite no significant differences in accelerometer derived activity counts between older and younger participants at various walking intensities, there were significant differences in relative oxygen consumption and MET values at rest and all exercise intensities indicating that moderate intensity physical activity for older adults may be determined at lower accelerometer derived activity counts than younger adults.

Oxygen uptake values obtained during treadmill exercise from the younger individuals in this study are in agreement with data reported in the literature. Leenders et al. [19] reported oxygen uptake values in a group of young adults (age 23.7 ± 4), who performed treadmill walking exercises at speeds of 54, 80, and 94 m·min^{-1}, respectively. These values closely parallel those measured from the younger participants in our study (Table 3). Furthermore, oxygen consumption values associated with walking at the respective speeds in elderly individuals in this study are consistent with findings from previous investigations [10, 13].

In this investigation, elderly participants had significantly higher oxygen uptake values than the younger participants during treadmill walking across the range of intensities. Similar findings have demonstrated a 12% and 22% increase, among 65- and 80-year-old participants, respectively, in the energy cost of walking at speeds of 80 and 94 m·min^{-1}, compared with 25-year-olds [13]. Energy expenditure per mile walked, among elderly, has been shown to be 21% greater than younger individuals [12]. Others have found 31% greater energy cost of walking in older (age 74 ± 3) compared to younger adults (age 27 ± 3) [20]. The average oxygen consumption demonstrated by the elderly participants in this investigation ranged from 14 to 19% greater than the younger participants across the selected speeds. The data in our study support the idea of a greater energy cost in the elderly when compared to a younger cohort for varying walking intensities. Nonetheless, the underlying reasons for the increased energy cost among elderly individuals are not fully understood.

Interestingly, activity counts (counts·min^{-1}) did not differ between groups at any of the treadmill intensities performed. This is in agreement with the results by Miller et al. [8]. Several other studies have reported Actigraph activity counts per minute similar to ours for equivalent treadmill walking speeds [19, 21–23], although these studies have been specific to younger populations. Unfortunately, data concerning Actigraph activity counts produced during treadmill walking in older populations is limited. Therefore, few comparisons to this study can be made. However, an investigation similar to ours reported mean activity counts of 515, 1041, and 2504 counts·min^{-1} at speeds of 33.5, 54, and 80 m·min^{-1}, respectively, in a group of elderly participants (age 69.7 ± 3.5) [10]. Although these values closely resemble ours, the activity counts obtained from our sample of elderly individuals tend to be slightly higher. This difference can be attributed to different models of Actigraph accelerometer used to determine activity counts. Copeland and Esliger [10] used the 7164 model whereas in the present study we used the GT1M and GT3X models. A study by Kozey et al. [15] has shown that activity counts from the GT1M model are slightly but significantly higher than the 7164 model.

Research has indicated that the standard 3.5 mL·kg^{-1}·min^{-1} may not represent the resting metabolic rate of the general population and that resting metabolic rate may be lower in older individuals. Since previous studies by Copeland and Esliger [10] and Miller et al. [8] have not measured resting metabolic rate in older adults, this study aimed to determine measured MET values for each of the exercise intensities. To our knowledge, this attempt to identify the relationship between measured MET values and activity counts for a sample of elderly participants had not previously been performed. In agreement with previous research [14, 16], resting metabolic rate in our group of elderly individuals was significantly less than the younger participants. However, the average resting metabolic rate for the older participants was similar to the standard MET value of 3.5 mL·kg^{-1}·min^{-1} whereas the average resting metabolic rate for the younger adults was significantly higher than the standard MET value of 3.5 mL·kg^{-1}·min^{-1}. The average resting metabolic rates for both older and younger participants in this study are higher than other studies [14–16]. Some research indicates that casual seated resting metabolic rate approximates 3.6 mL·kg^{-1}·min^{-1} [24]. It is possible that the differences between the present study and previous studies are due to different positions during resting periods. While the mean measured MET value among the older individuals approached but was not equivalent to 6 METs at a walking speed of 94 m·min^{-1} 2% grade, five of them obtained values greater than 6 METs. At the intermediate treadmill speeds of 54 and 80 m·min^{-1}, all of the elderly participants were exercising at or above a moderate intensity. In contrast, the younger participants did not reach a level of moderate physical activity intensity until a treadmill speed of 80 m·min^{-1}. Furthermore, even at the fastest speeds, younger individuals were exercising well below a vigorous intensity.

Translating accelerometer activity counts to determine intensity of physical activity has proven to be a difficult task and has been questioned by some studies [25, 26]. The aim of the present study was not to develop any new regression equation. However, based on the data, we were able to determine an activity count threshold that is associated with moderate (3 METs) physical activity for this group of younger and older adults and compare this activity count threshold with current literature. The commonly used Actigraph activity count threshold for moderate physical activity intensity (≥1952 counts·min^{-1}), developed by Freedson et al. [6], was derived from exercise tests involving young adults. Similarly, Actigraph activity count cut-points for moderate physical activity intensity ranging from 1810 to 2260 counts·min^{-1} have been shown in other studies testing adults aged 20–45. In agreement with previous studies of younger adults, the present study found activity count cut-points for moderate physical activity intensity to be 2207 and 2009 counts·min^{-1} depending on either measured or standard resting metabolic rate. In contrast to those studies, Copeland and Esliger [10] and Miller et al. [8] have indicated a moderate intensity threshold value of 1041 and 1566 counts·min^{-1}, respectively, for their group of elderly individuals. In this investigation, the threshold value, equivalent to 3 METs, was 824 counts·min^{-1} when using measured resting metabolic rate and 784 counts·min^{-1} when using the standard resting metabolic rate. The activity count threshold associated with moderate intensity activity reported in this study is lower than the ones reported by previous research. Copeland and Esliger [10] did not attempt to determine cut-points of various intensities. The researchers simply used the activity counts that corresponded to a mean oxygen consumption of 13 mL·kg^{-1}·min^{-1}. In addition, Miller et al. [8] used a different methodology than previous research. Previous studies, including the present study, have used a discontinuous protocol. Participants exercised at various intensities for five minutes and rested between intensities for five or six minutes. Miller et al. [8] used a continuous walking and/or running protocol. It is therefore difficult to compare the activity counts reported in the present study and the one by Miller et al. [8].

The results of the present study, along with the results of previous research, may represent the need to establish agreeable metabolic equivalents for respective age groups to effectively determine physical activity intensity level activity count cut-points. These findings are of significant importance because recent epidemiological investigation pertaining to physical activity behaviors among elderly United States citizens reported a substantially low amount of time spent in moderate intensity activity. However, the activity count threshold employed for identifying moderate physical activity in adults aged 18–60$^+$ was 2020 counts·min^{-1} [1]. It is possible that previous epidemiological reports may be greatly underestimating the amount of time elderly populations spend performing moderate physical activity.

There are some limitations in this study. This sample size of younger and older adults is small and therefore the activity count threshold that is associated with moderate (3 METs) physical activity for this group of participants might not be generalizable to all older and younger adults. In addition, there were no participants between the ages of 30 and 55. Troiano et al. [1] have shown that accelerometry counts per minute do not change between ages of 18 and 59. In addition, the activity count thresholds established by Freedson et al. [6] were based on similar age group as ours. Therefore, the purpose of this study was to examine the differences in oxygen consumption and activity counts between a group of younger individuals (similar to the one by Freedson et al. [6]) and a group of older individuals above 60 years. The majority of the participants exercised below vigorous intensity (<6 METs). This limits the study from determining an activity count threshold associated with vigorous intensity. The intensity of 94 m·min^{-1} and 2% grade was used to elicit vigorous intensity. Two of the older participants were unable to complete this stage. It is difficult to elicit vigorous intensity for older adults due to either their lack of fitness, fear, or functional limitations.

5. Conclusions

Despite similarity in accelerometer activity counts produced during treadmill walking across a range of treadmill speeds among elderly and young participants, an increased oxygen uptake among elderly participants was evident. Therefore, accelerometers appear to be valid in their detection of exercise intensity across age groups. Moreover, translating activity counts into categorical levels of physical activity intensity cannot be done in the same manner for young and elderly individuals. Measurement of resting metabolic rate may offer the most effective way for determining the relationship between activity counts and the intensity level of physical activity performed. Further research is necessary in order to better understand the relationship between accelerometer activity counts and physical activity intensity levels for an elderly population.

Conflict of Interests

The authors declare that there is no conflict of interests regarding the publication of this paper.

Acknowledgments

The authors would like to thank all the participants in this study. This study was funded by the CWU Office of Graduate Studies and Research.

References

[1] R. P. Troiano, D. Berrigan, K. W. Dodd, L. C. Mâsse, T. Tilert, and M. Mcdowell, "Physical activity in the United States measured by accelerometer," *Medicine and Science in Sports and Exercise*, vol. 40, no. 1, pp. 181–188, 2008.

[2] R. R. Pate, M. Pratt, S. N. Blair et al., "Physical activity and public health: a recommendation from the Centers for Disease Control and Prevention and the American College of Sports Medicine," *Journal of the American Medical Association*, vol. 273, no. 5, pp. 402–407, 1995.

[3] W. L. Haskell, I.-M. Lee, R. R. Pate et al., "Physical activity and public health: updated recommendation for adults from the American College of Sports Medicine and the American Heart Association," *Circulation*, vol. 116, no. 9, pp. 1081–1093, 2007.

[4] R. J. Shephard, "Limits to the measurement of habitual physical activity by questionnaires," *British Journal of Sports Medicine*, vol. 37, no. 3, pp. 197–206, 2003.

[5] M. G. Davis and K. R. Fox, "Physical activity patterns assessed by accelerometry in older people," *European Journal of Applied Physiology*, vol. 100, no. 5, pp. 581–589, 2007.

[6] P. S. Freedson, E. Melanson, and J. Sirard, "Calibration of the computer science and applications, Inc. accelerometer," *Medicine and Science in Sports and Exercise*, vol. 30, no. 5, pp. 777–781, 1998.

[7] D. Hendelman, K. Miller, C. Baggett, E. Debold, and P. Freedson, "Validity of accelerometry for the assessment of moderate intensity physical activity in the field," *Medicine and Science in Sports and Exercise*, vol. 32, supplement 9, pp. S442–S449, 2000.

[8] N. E. Miller, S. J. Strath, A. M. Swartz, and S. E. Cashin, "Estimating absolute and relative physical activity intensity across age via accelerometry in adults," *Journal of Aging and Physical Activity*, vol. 18, no. 2, pp. 158–170, 2010.

[9] A. Yngve, A. Nilsson, M. Sjöström, and U. Ekelund, "Effect of monitor placement and of activity setting on the MTI accelerometer output," *Medicine and Science in Sports and Exercise*, vol. 35, no. 2, pp. 320–326, 2003.

[10] J. L. Copeland and D. W. Esliger, "Accelerometer assessment of physical activity in active, healthy older adults," *Journal of Aging and Physical Activity*, vol. 17, no. 1, pp. 17–30, 2009.

[11] K. S. Hall, C. A. Howe, S. R. Rana, C. L. Martin, and M. C. Morey, "METs and accelerometry of walking in older adults: standard versus measured energy cost," *Medicine and Science in Sports and Exercise*, vol. 45, no. 3, pp. 574–582, 2013.

[12] A. M. Harris, L. M. Lanningham-Foster, S. K. McCrady, and J. A. Levine, "Nonexercise movement in elderly compared with young people," *The American Journal of Physiology—Endocrinology and Metabolism*, vol. 292, no. 4, pp. E1207–E1212, 2007.

[13] D. Malatesta, D. Simar, Y. Dauvilliers et al., "Energy cost of walking and gait instability in healthy 65- and 80-yr-olds," *Journal of Applied Physiology*, vol. 95, no. 6, pp. 2248–2256, 2003.

[14] N. M. Byrne, A. P. Hills, G. R. Hunter, R. L. Weinsier, and Y. Schutz, "Metabolic equivalent: one size does not fit all," *Journal of Applied Physiology*, vol. 99, no. 3, pp. 1112–1119, 2005.

[15] S. L. Kozey, J. W. Staudenmayer, R. P. Troiano, and P. S. Freedson, "Comparison of the actigraph 7164 and the actigraph GT1M during self-paced locomotion," *Medicine and Science in Sports and Exercise*, vol. 42, no. 5, pp. 971–976, 2010.

[16] M. Kwan, J. Woo, and T. Kwok, "The standard oxygen consumption value equivalent to one metabolic equivalent (3.5 mL/min/kg) is not appropriate for elderly people," *International Journal of Food Sciences and Nutrition*, vol. 55, no. 3, pp. 179–182, 2004.

[17] M. L. Pollack, D. H. Schmidt, and A. S. Jackson, "Measurement of cardiorespiratory fitness and body composition in the clinical setting," *Comprehensive Therapy*, vol. 6, no. 9, pp. 12–27, 1980.

[18] M. G. Abel, J. C. Hannon, K. Sell, T. Lillie, G. Conlin, and D. Anderson, "Validation of the Kenz lifecorder EX and actigraph GT1M accelerometers for walking and running in adults," *Applied Physiology, Nutrition and Metabolism*, vol. 33, no. 6, pp. 1155–1164, 2008.

[19] N. Y. J. M. Leenders, T. E. Nelson, and W. M. Sherman, "Ability of different physical activity monitors to detect movement during treadmill walking," *International Journal of Sports Medicine*, vol. 24, no. 1, pp. 43–50, 2003.

[20] O. S. Mian, J. M. Thom, L. P. Ardigò, M. V. Narici, and A. E. Minetti, "Metabolic cost, mechanical work, and efficiency during walking in young and older men," *Acta Physiologica*, vol. 186, no. 2, pp. 127–139, 2006.

[21] G. A. King, N. Torres, C. Potter, T. J. Brooks, and K. J. Coleman, "Comparison of activity monitors to estimate energy cost of treadmill exercise," *Medicine and Science in Sports and Exercise*, vol. 36, no. 7, pp. 1244–1251, 2004.

[22] G. J. Welk, S. N. Blair, K. Wood, S. Jones, and R. W. Thompson, "A comparative evaluation of three accelerometry-based physical activity monitors," *Medicine and Science in Sports and Exercise*, vol. 32, no. 9, pp. S489–S497, 2000.

[23] G. J. Welk, J. A. Schaben, and J. R. Morrow Jr., "Reliability of accelerometry-based activity monitors: a generalizability study," *Medicine and Science in Sports and Exercise*, vol. 36, no. 9, pp. 1637–1645, 2004.

[24] D. P. Swain, B. C. Leutholtz, M. E. King, L. A. Haas, and J. David Branch, "Relationship between % heart rate reserve and % VO2 reserve in treadmill exercise," *Medicine and Science in Sports and Exercise*, vol. 30, no. 2, pp. 318–321, 1998.

[25] J. Staudenmayer, D. Pober, S. Crouter, D. Bassett, and P. Freedson, "An artificial neural network to estimate physical activity energy expenditure and identify physical activity type from an accelerometer," *Journal of Applied Physiology*, vol. 107, no. 4, pp. 1300–1307, 2009.

[26] K. Lyden, S. L. Kozey, J. W. Staudenmeyer, and P. S. Freedson, "A comprehensive evaluation of commonly used accelerometer energy expenditure and MET prediction equations," *European Journal of Applied Physiology*, vol. 111, no. 2, pp. 187–201, 2011.

12

Following Up on Clinical Recommendations in Transitions from Hospital to Nursing Home

Lisa B. Caruso,[1] Soe Soe Thwin,[1,2] and Gary H. Brandeis[1]

[1] *Boston University Geriatric Services, Boston University School of Medicine, Boston Medical Center, 88 East Newton Street, Robinson 2, Boston, MA 02118, USA*

[2] *Massachusetts Veterans Epidemiology Research and Information Center (MAVERIC), New England VA Healthcare System, 150 South Huntington Avenue, Boston, MA 02130, USA*

Correspondence should be addressed to Gary H. Brandeis; garyhb@bu.edu

Academic Editor: Marja J. Aartsen

Following up on recommendations made at the time of a hospital discharge is important to patient safety. While data is lacking, specifically around the transition of patient to nursing home, it has been postulated that missed items such as laboratory tests may result in adverse patient outcomes. To determine the extent of this problem, a retrospective cohort study of subjects discharged from an academic medical center and admitted to nursing homes (NH) was followed to determine the type of discharge recommendations and the rate of completion. In addition, for the purpose of generalizability, the 30-day hospital readmission rate was calculated. 152 recommendations were made on 51 subjects. Almost a quarter of the recommendations made by the hospital discharging team were not acted upon. Furthermore, for the majority of those recommendations that were not acted upon, a reason could not be determined. In concert with national data, 20% of the subjects returned to the hospital within 30 days. Further investigation is warranted to determine if an association exists between missed recommendations and hospital readmission from the nursing home setting.

1. Introduction

Transitional care is "a set of actions designed to ensure the coordination and continuity of healthcare as patients transfer between different locations or different levels of care in the same location [1]." Errors in transitional care can occur in several ways. Medication errors are made when a patient either receives the wrong medication at the destination site or an indicated medication is omitted from the discharge instructions. Another error that commonly occurs in transitional care is test follow-up error, that is, if a test is pending but not acknowledged in the discharge. In a study performed at a major teaching hospital in New York with a diverse patient population, 41% of the study participants with tests pending at the time of discharge had at least one test follow-up error [2]. A follow-up study found that, of recommended workups, 35.9% were not completed within six months of discharge [3]. Recently, Weiner and colleagues reported that half of the medical specialty referrals among an ambulatory population aged ≥65 were not completed by 180 days [4]. Another study found that physicians, including both inpatient and outpatient physicians, were unaware of 61% of abnormal test results that were considered "actionable." Yet, they were unable to determine if these "missed results" were associated with adverse patient outcomes. These investigators noted that failure to follow-up test results may account for one-quarter of diagnosis-related malpractice cases [5]. These investigators and others recommend further work to design better follow-up systems [6]. The American Medical Directors Association (AMDA) has responded by formulating an 80-page online document entitled "Transitions of Care in the Long-Term Care Continuum" that includes a universal transfer form. This form includes a page for tests and appointments. All these initiatives are designed to improve patient care as the patient moves in and out of various healthcare settings [7].

As the patient moves from site to site, the opportunities for neglecting communication or to follow up on unresolved medical problems rise dramatically [8]. While the standard of care is for a discharge summary to accompany the patient when leaving the hospital and transitioning to NH, this document has been known to be missing or incomplete on arrival [9]. Were and colleagues reviewed hospital discharge summaries from two Midwestern hospitals with computerized electronic health records (EHR) and found that the discharge summaries were inadequate at documenting tests with pending results and the appropriate follow-up [10]. Several authors have suggested returning to handwritten forms or checklists to aid in communication when a patient is transferred from one site of care to another [1].

When a person is discharged from the hospital, a discharge summary is prepared. Today it is universally typed. It may be dictated or entered into the computer by the hospital discharging team. Generally, the discharging team is composed of a physician (attending or resident) and may also include a nonphysician practitioner (nurse practitioner or physician assistant) and/or nurse. It is their responsibility to list recommendations for future care of the patient to the provider in the next site of care.

For this study, the next site of care was the nursing home, where the physician and/or the nonphysician practitioner reviewed the recommendations to determine future actions. Studies examining specific items that are missed from transition from acute care hospital to nursing home are lacking. To our knowledge, the only research examining this transition was published by Gandara and colleagues who found that 47.2% of discharge packets from one healthcare system were missing the mention of pending test results. Gandara examined only the discharge documentation that was generated by the acute care hospitals [11]. To date, there are no studies which assess the completion of follow-up items through the entire episode of the transition of care in the NH.

The purpose of this study was to determine the number and types of follow-up recommendations generated during an acute care admission documented in the EHR that were completed within 180 days of hospital discharge to a NH and while the subjects were in the NH. Reasons for not completing the recommendations were also investigated. A secondary purpose was to determine the hospital readmission rate. Even though our study was too small to make any association between missed follow-up recommendations and hospital readmissions, reporting the 30-day hospital readmission rate adds to the generalizability of the study.

2. Design and Methods

2.1. Subjects. A medical record review was performed retrospectively on a cohort of patients discharged to nursing homes. Subjects were eligible if they were ≥65 years old and had been discharged from any medical or surgical inpatient service at Boston Medical Center, Boston, MA (BMC), between January 1, 2007, and June 30, 2007, and admitted to one of ten nursing homes (skilled nursing facilities/nursing facilities) in the greater Boston, MA area, serviced by Boston University Geriatric Services. Subjects were excluded if they were admitted to the nursing home for hospice care or if their records or charts were not available at the NH at the time of record review (i.e., charts had already been sent to off-site storage). All patients that met enrollment criteria were entered into the database. Using SAS 9.1, ten subjects from each month of the six-month study period were randomly selected to establish a convenience sample of sixty patients. Subjects were followed for 180 days after hospital discharge or until they were discharged from the NH, died, or returned to the acute hospital and did not return to the NH.

2.2. Data Collection. A data collection form was adapted from Moore et al. [3]. The original Moore form was tested for interrater reliability and found to have high reliability (κ, 0.89). The inpatient record, the discharge summary, and nursing home records were reviewed by study investigators (LBC, GHB) and four geriatric nurse practitioners. All clinicians extracting data were trained on completion of the data collection form. Inpatient medical records were either available electronically via Sunrise Clinical Manager system or available online as part of BMC's archival medical record system, GRID (Synergize-Streamlined Document Management). The medical provider notes from NH visits were hand-written in the nursing home record or available electronically as part of GE Centricity EHR. The data were collected electronically via a Microsoft 2003 ACCESS based software programmed with range and logic checks to ensure efficient and accurate electronic data entry. Once the data were entered into the database, all subjects were given a deidentifying number to ensure anonymity.

2.3. Analytic Variables. Data collection included demographic characteristics of the subject (age, race, ethnicity, and insurance), length of stay in the NH, and recommendations made during the inpatient stay including the category of recommendation (diagnostic procedures, subspecialty referrals, laboratory tests, physical exam reviews, and medication changes or monitoring), completion status of the recommendations, and reasons documented in the medical record describing why recommendations were not completed. Subspecialty referrals included appointments that were recommended to be made for neurology, endocrine, cardiology, psychiatry, gastroenterology, and general and surgical subspecialties. Laboratory tests included recommendations for basic metabolic panels, complete blood counts, PET scans, pending pathology reports, and urine culture results. Medication changes or monitoring included duration of antibiotic treatment, monitoring levels of medications, deep vein thrombosis prophylaxis, and titration of medications.

2.4. Data Analysis. The data were analyzed using SAS 9.1. Summary statistics describing the pattern of recommendation completeness were generated. The protocol was approved by the Boston University Medical Campus Institutional Review Board.

Table 1: Baseline characteristics of the study sample ($N = 51$).

Characteristic	Frequency (%)
Age in yrs (mean ± SD)	80.6 ± 9.3
Race	
White	25 (49)
Black	23 (45)
Hispanic	3 (6)
Gender	
Female	42 (82)
Male	9 (18)
Language	
English	34 (67)
Non-English	17 (33)
Insurance	
Medicare	42 (82)
Medicaid	2 (4)
Medicare managed care	3 (6)
Medicare advantage (i.e., senior care options)	3 (6)
Other	1 (2)
Hospital length of stay in days (mean ± SD)	6.1 ± 3.4

Table 2: Categories of recommendations made by the hospital discharging team.

Type of procedure	Frequency (%)
Diagnostic procedures	7 (4.6)
Subspecialty referrals	46 (30.3)
Laboratory tests	36 (23.7)
Physical exam reviews	15 (9.9)
Medication changes/monitor	27 (17.8)
Other	21 (13.9)
Total number of recommendations	152

Table 3: Types of recommendations not pursued by 6 months following hospital discharge.

Recommendations	Total number of recommendations not completed (%)
Diagnostic procedures (%)	3 (8)
Subspecialty referrals (%)	13 (35)
Laboratory tests (%)	9 (24)
Physical exam (%)	2 (5)
Med changes (%)	6 (16)
Other (%)	4 (11)
Total	37

3. Results

There were 222 subjects ≥65 years old at the time of discharge from Boston Medical Center, Boston, MA, between January 1, 2007, and June 30, 2007, who were admitted to one of ten nursing homes serviced by Boston University Geriatric Services. Sixty records were consecutively reviewed to obtain the analytic sample of 51 subjects. Four subjects were not admitted to the NH from BMC, four subjects had incomplete records, and one subject had a duplicate medical record number so could only be used once. No subjects were on hospice at the time of NH admission. Table 1 shows the baseline characteristics of the study sample. The average age was 80.6 ± 9.3 (range 65–106). The sample was mostly white women with Medicare as the primary payer source. The length of stay at the hospital was 6.1 ± 3.4 days (range 1 to 16 days) prior to NH admission. The majority of the subjects were discharged from the geriatrics (36%), general internal medicine (32%), and family medicine (4%) services. 16% were discharged from a surgical service. The remainder were discharged from other specialty services such as neurology or oncology.

Table 2 lists the categories of recommendations made for the 51 subjects. A total of 152 recommendations were made by inpatient providers. The most common type of recommendation was a subspecialty referral followed by laboratory tests and medication changes or monitoring. Of the 152 recommendations made, 37 (24%) had no documentation of follow-up within six months of the hospital discharge. 32 of these recommendations were identified from the discharge summary, and 5 were found on review of the inpatient hospital record (GRID and Centricity).

Table 3 lists the categories of recommendations that were not completed within 180 days of hospital discharge. Of those 37, the receiving NH provider team documented reasons for declining 13 (35%); no reason was documented for the remaining 24 (65%).

The number of follow-up recommendations for each subject varied (range 0–8) with the mode being 2. As the number of recommendations made increased, the number followed decreased. For those subjects with one, two, and three to eight follow-up recommendations, 88%, 53%, and 23% were completed, respectively. During the study period, 23 of 51 subjects (45%) had hospital readmissions during the study period. 10 of these 51 returned within 30 days (20%).

4. Discussion

We tracked recommendations made during acute care hospital inpatient stays for subjects discharged to a NH. Almost a quarter of recommendations made during the inpatient stay were not followed after the transition of care. The three most common recommendations not followed in our study were (1) subspecialty referrals, (2) laboratory tests, and (3) medication changes/monitoring.

While, to our knowledge, there are no studies similar to ours for comparison, it may be instructive to look at the findings of Moore and colleagues who examined discharges from hospital to community [3]. As expected, Moore's sample was younger (average age of 58) [3]. Our finding of 24% of recommendations not completed compares to Moore's finding of 35.9% of recommended workups not completed after hospital discharge. Our rate was likely lower because there was a dedicated team that saw the patient within a week of discharge and who were more attuned to following up outstanding items due to the higher vulnerability of patients being admitted to the nursing home.

Moore found that the three most common categories of recommendations not followed were (1) diagnostic procedures, (2) subspecialty referrals, and (3) laboratory tests. Diagnostic procedures were the least common type of recommendation needing follow-up in our study (4.6% of all recommendations). This difference may be due to the fact that our sample of older, more frail NH subjects may have been thought to need fewer diagnostic procedures as opposed to outpatients in the Moore study [3]. It is also possible that diagnostic procedures were easier to obtain at BMC, and so they were able to occur during the acute hospitalization.

It has been estimated that 20%–33% of older patients are rehospitalized within 30 days [12]. Our results are consistent with these figures. However, our sample represents a select, frail population. One may posit that the rate at which subjects were readmitted may have been higher if not for the EHR and the single medical practice within one medical center that cared for these NH residents. Strengths of the study include the use of an integrated EHR. Accepting providers at the NH had access to all documentation from the acute care hospitalization.

The current study has several limitations. First, the sample size was small. It is a single site study from a safety net hospital with an integrated geriatrics practice. Due to time and resource constraints, only 60 discharges were selected and 51 were reviewed. In addition, we were unable to compare the qualities of our small sample to the unselected population. However, our randomization method should mitigate any differences between the groups. Second, while the acute care portion of the record was electronic, all NHs used paper records. Third, while we were able to determine the readmission rate of the study population, because of the cross-sectional design of the study, we were limited in our ability to relate readmissions to noncompletion of recommendations. Lastly, tracking of pending lab tests for most subjects was dependent on what was documented in the discharge summary and the inpatient progress notes. From the recent study published by Walz and colleagues, 32% of the patients discharged from acute care to subacute care were discharged with pending lab tests alone, not including any other type of recommendation [13].

A question remains for future investigation: does a relationship exist between noncompletion of inpatient recommendations and hospital readmissions? While the present study was not able to determine an association, there does seem to be face validity to the premise that missed recommendations would lead to hospital readmissions especially in patients with multiple comorbidities and functional impairments.

As has been previously observed, many inpatient recommendations are not followed. Specifically, in our study, the rate of nonfollow-up is less than the others have found. We believe that the use of an EHR is a major reason. The receiving team at the NH had access to the inpatient record. In most cases, the receiving provider also had access to the entire outpatient record prior to the acute hospitalization. We would not expect that all recommendations by the inpatient care team would be followed by the NH admitting team. The NH team providers have expertise in NH care and likely determine that some acute care recommendations are not justified. Other potential reasons why some acute care recommendations were not followed could have been (1) the NH providers had a reason for not following the recommendation, such as a change in the goals of care, but did not document it, (2) the NH providers missed the recommendation, or (3) the patient was discharged from the NH before the recommendation could be acted upon.

Since this study was completed, several hospital wide initiatives have been instituted at BMC to decrease any missed recommendations. First, all future primary care and specialty care appointments are automatically entered into the discharge summary. Second, the names of the members of the discharging team, including the attending and house staff, are listed along with the outpatient primary care provider. Third, any medication that was added or changed during the hospitalization is documented on the discharge summary, thus reconciling the prehospital medication list with the discharge medication list. Fourth, a separate section titled "outstanding issues" has been added to prompt the house staff to enter items for follow-up. However, the electronic discharge summary does not automatically download any outstanding laboratory values at the time of discharge.

Nationally, other efforts are being made to improve transitional care, given the currently limited interoperability between EHRs in various sites of care. Interact II is an initiative to "improve care and reduce the frequency of potentially avoidable transfers to the acute hospital [14]." The Resident Transfer Form, found in the Interact II Tool Kit, provides a medical summary, a reason for transfer as well as cognitive and functional baselines, active behavioral and social issues, and important contact numbers. Adopting standardized approaches to transfers helps ensure that important issues needing follow up are communicated to receiving providers. There is early evidence that standardizing the transitional care process using Interact II leads to a decrease in avoidable hospitalizations from NH [15]. Perhaps the rate of unresolved medical recommendations would decrease as well.

Boockvar and Burack have found that management-level organizational relationships between nursing homes and hospitals are associated with more optimal transfers [16]. While the NHs in our study were not affiliated with BMC, they did provide Internet connections so that BMC providers could access BMC's EHR. Improved organizational relationships between NHs and hospitals will help to efficiently and cost-effectively provide transitional care. As NHs purchase EHRs, it will be important that they are compatible with those of the hospitals. As we leave the era of not having information because it was not written down or communicated, we risk entering the era of having the data but being unable to access it.

The majority of hospital discharge recommendations were followed in the NH, yet a quarter were not. The reasons why are only partially understood. While organizations such as AMDA have written guidelines to help with transitions, much work needs to be done to operationalize the discharge process [7]. An EHR that is accessible across key sites of care will be an important component.

5. Conclusions

Almost a quarter of the recommendations for subjects discharged from an acute care hospital to a nursing home are not followed after transitions of care. Noncompletion was associated with an increasing number of recommendations, lack of documentation in the discharge summary, and the type of recommendation. Establishing better processes of communication during transitions of care may help to reduce noncompletion of recommendations and enhance their appropriateness. One process that was instituted at BMC added a formal section "outstanding issues" to the discharge summary. Further work needs to be done to allow EHR to automatically add "outstanding issues" to the discharge transfer form.

Conflict of Interests

The authors declare that there is no conflict of interests regarding the publication of this paper.

Acknowledgments

The authors would like to thank Kimberly Claude, NP, Katherine Concilio, NP, Julie Miller, NP, and Debbie Sylvester, NP, for their assistance with data collection. Funding for this work was supported by Boston Medical Center, Department of Risk Management, Boston, MA.

References

[1] E. A. Coleman and C. Boult, "Improving the quality of transitional care for persons with complex care needs," *Journal of the American Geriatrics Society*, vol. 51, no. 4, pp. 556–557, 2003.

[2] C. Moore, J. Wisnivesky, S. Williams, and T. McGinn, "Medical errors related to discontinuity of care from an inpatient to an outpatient setting," *Journal of General Internal Medicine*, vol. 18, no. 8, pp. 646–651, 2003.

[3] C. Moore, T. McGinn, and E. Halm, "Tying up loose ends: discharging patients with unresolved medical issues," *Archives of Internal Medicine*, vol. 167, no. 12, pp. 1305–1311, 2007.

[4] M. Weiner, A. J. Perkins, and C. M. Callahan, "Errors in completion of referrals among older urban adults in ambulatory care," *Journal of Evaluation in Clinical Practice*, vol. 16, no. 1, pp. 76–81, 2010.

[5] C. L. Roy, E. C. Poon, A. S. Karson et al., "Patient safety concerns arising from test results that return after hospital discharge," *Annals of Internal Medicine*, vol. 143, no. 2, pp. 121–128, 2005.

[6] A. J. Forster, H. J. Murff, J. F. Peterson, T. K. Gandhi, and D. W. Bates, "The incidence and severity of adverse events affecting patients after discharge from the hospital," *Annals of Internal Medicine*, vol. 138, no. 3, pp. 161–167, 2003.

[7] AMDA, "Transitions of Care in the Long-Term Care Continuum," 2010, http://www.amda.com/tools/clinical/TOCCPG/index.html.

[8] J. E. Morley, "Transitions," *Journal of the American Medical Directors Association*, vol. 11, no. 9, pp. 607–611, 2010.

[9] V. K. Lee, C. J. Westley, and K. Fletcher, "If at first you don't succeed: efforts to improve collaboration between nursing homes and a health system," *Topics in Advanced Practice Nursing*, vol. 4, no. 3, pp. 1–8, 2004.

[10] M. C. Were, X. Li, J. Kesterson et al., "Adequacy of hospital discharge summaries in documenting tests with pending results and outpatient follow-up providers," *Journal of General Internal Medicine*, vol. 24, no. 9, pp. 1002–1006, 2009.

[11] E. Gandara, T. Moniz, J. Ungar et al., "Communication and information deficits in patients discharged to rehabilitation facilities: an evaluation of five acute care hospitals," *Journal of Hospital Medicine*, vol. 4, no. 8, pp. E28–E33, 2009.

[12] P. Wendling, "Readmission affects 1 in 3 elderly patients," *Caring for the Ages*, vol. 10, no. 9, pp. 4–5, 2009.

[13] S. E. Walz, M. Smith, E. Cox, J. Sattin, and A. J. H. Kind, "Pending laboratory tests and the hospital discharge summary in patients discharged to sub-acute care," *Journal of General Internal Medicine*, vol. 26, no. 4, pp. 393–398, 2011.

[14] I. I. Interact, 2011, http://interact2.net/index.aspx.

[15] J. G. Ouslander, G. Lamb, R. Tappen et al., "Interventions to reduce hospitalizations from nursing homes: evaluation of the INTERACT II collaborative quality improvement project," *Journal of the American Geriatrics Society*, vol. 59, no. 4, pp. 745–753, 2011.

[16] K. S. Boockvar and O. R. Burack, "Organizational relationships between nursing homes and hospitals and quality of care during hospital-nursing home patient transfers," *Journal of the American Geriatrics Society*, vol. 55, no. 7, pp. 1078–1084, 2007.

13

Picture your Nursing Home: Exploring the Sense of Home of Older Residents through Photography

J. van Hoof,[1,2] M. M. Verhagen,[1,3] E. J. M. Wouters,[1,2] H. R. Marston,[4] M. D. Rijnaard,[2] and B. M. Janssen[3]

[1]*Centre for Healthcare and Technology (Fontys EGT), Fontys University of Applied Sciences, Dominee Theodor Fliednerstraat 2, 5631 BN Eindhoven, Netherlands*
[2]*Institute of Allied Health Professions, Fontys University of Applied Sciences, Dominee Theodor Fliednerstraat 2, 5631 BN Eindhoven, Netherlands*
[3]*Section of Applied Gerontology, Institute of Nursing, Fontys University of Applied Sciences, Dominee Theodor Fliednerstraat 2, 5631 BN Eindhoven, Netherlands*
[4]*Centre for Research Computing, Faculty of Mathematics, Computing and Technology, Open University, Milton Keynes, Buckinghamshire, MK6 7AA, UK*

Correspondence should be addressed to J. van Hoof; joost.vanhoof@fontys.nl

Academic Editor: Maddalena Illario

The quality of the built environment can impact the quality of life and the sense of home of nursing home residents. This study investigated (1) which factors in the physical and social environment correlate with the sense of home of the residents and (2) which environmental factors are most meaningful. Twelve participants engaged in a qualitative study, in which photography was as a supportive tool for subsequent interviews. The data were analysed based on the six phases by Braun and Clarke. The four themes identified are (1) the physical view; (2) mobility and accessibility; (3) space, place, and personal belongings; and (4) the social environment and activities. A holistic understanding of which features of the built environment are appreciated by the residents can lead to the design and retrofitting of nursing homes that are more in line with personal wishes.

1. Introduction

For older people who can no longer age in place, nursing homes provide an alternative place of residence where care and assistance are offered by professionals. The needs and wishes of older residents in terms of the architectural quality of the nursing home environment should ideally be respected and implemented as much as possible. It is questionable whether the nursing home is a place where one feels at home which corresponds to how residents experience the environment in which they reside. Furthermore, such questions correspond to what is needed for residents to feel at home in the first instance, which, in turn, should be considered in the constant process of evaluation and action. Creating attractive nursing homes, from both setting and social perspective, in which residents can feel at home, is a core challenge of nursing home organisations, in particular, their care staff and facility managers [1–4]. Too often, existing nursing homes do not meet the needs of the current generations of residents, and this mismatch leads to suboptimal living conditions that are experienced 24 hours a day.

In order to create this form of environment, namely, a true nursing "home," it is essential to address the experiences and views of the residents in studies and empower the thoughts of these residents through a combination of inclusive design strategies [5, 6]. Despite the laudability of small-scale initiatives in healthcare [7, 8], (future) residents are often overlooked and not included in design and development processes.

In the second half of the 20th century, the design of nursing homes was conducted by experts in the field, and this isolated approach traditionally resulted in high-rise hospital-like buildings [2]. In such cases, the quality of the building

Table 1: Characteristics of the participants.

Participant	Sex [M/F]	Age	Marital status	Education	Limitations
1	M	84	Widowed	Primary education	Mobility
2	M	94	Widowed	Secondary education	Mobility, early dementia
3	F	85	Widowed	Secondary education	Mobility
4	F	88	Widowed	Primary education	Mobility
5	F	74	Widowed	Secondary education	Mobility, CVA
6	F	87	Widowed	Primary education	Mobility, hearing
7	M	95	Widowed	Higher education	Mobility, sight
8	F	64	Unmarried	Higher education	Mobility
9	M	78	Married	Higher education	Mobility, CVA
10	F	83	Widowed	Primary education	Mobility, psychiatric symptoms
11	F	62	Unmarried	Primary education	Mental/intellectual problems
12	F	67	Married	Secondary education	Mobility, psychiatric symptoms

was often expressed in terms of technological, functional, and economic requirements, and factors related to the residents were given less attention. A more holistic vision of healthcare is currently emerging which considers the consequences of the built environment on the well-being of the residents [2]. For instance, Van Steenwinkel et al. [2] conducted a study focusing on how the built environment contributes to a feeling of homeliness of older people living in different contexts in Belgium. Van Dijck-Heinen et al. [3] investigated the sense of home among permanent and temporary residents of nursing homes in the Netherlands. Both studies concluded that a sense of home is a multifactorial phenomenon which is highly influenced by environmental, social, and personal characteristics. When one experiences a positive sense of home, one might experience a feeling of familiarity [9]. Duyvendak [10] also uses the two metaphors "heaven" and "haven" to describe a sense of home in a better way. Heaven refers to a place where you can be yourself, feel connected with like-minded people, and perform your favourite activities. Haven is a safe, comfortable, predictable place. When referring to the characteristics of "haven," this is primarily associated with the physical environment [10]. On the one hand, there is an elaborate set of literatures related to heaven and how social interactions with significant others play an important role in experiencing a sense of home. The literature related to haven, on the other hand, which deals with the built environment and personal belongings, is less abundant [4]. Despite these research efforts, there is a gap in the literature with respect to what might "influence" a sense of home and the general well-being of, and according to, nursing home residents with physical limitations and gerontopsychiatric health problems.

Therefore, this study explores (1) which factors in the physical and social environment correlate with the sense of home of the residents and (2) which environmental factors are most meaningful. The goal of this study is to gain insight into the experiences and views of actual residents in order to understand their needs in relation to the design of nursing homes and in order to make these nursing homes more fitting and facilitating to the social context of residents. This study is part of a larger programme called "Nursing Home of the Future," which investigates the architectural, technological, and social aspects of future nursing homes and the sense of home of the residents [1, 11–13].

2. Methodology

A qualitative methodology was chosen for this study, comprising photography and in-depth interviews with nursing home residents, as a way to involve the least voiced people in our society through creativity and dialogue [5]. The Critical Appraisal Skills Programme's checklist for qualitative research [14] was used as a guide for this study. In the following sections we describe (1) the settings, ethics, and participants, (2) photography approach, (3) interviews, and (4) the data analysis.

2.1. Settings, Ethics, and Participants. In April and May 2014, interviews and the field study were conducted in two wards of the same nursing home in Eindhoven, the Netherlands, including 12 participants (Table 1). The study aimed to include both residents with physical limitations and gerontopsychiatric health problems in order to gain a more diverse set of results. The inclusion criteria for this research were as follows: participants had to be at least 55 years of age, had to reside in a nursing home for at least six months, had to be able to communicate in Dutch, had to be able to take pictures with a photo camera independently or with the help of (in)formal carers, had to be able to make a selection of important photos independently, and had to be able to participate in an interview of at least 30 minutes.

A total of nine residents with physical limitations (out of 25 who were asked to participate) and three additional gerontopsychiatric residents (who were selected by the care organisation) consented to their participation. Prospective participants and their relatives received an information letter from the principal care professional, which was approved by the hosting care organisation. Informed consent was obtained from the participants in conjunction with their initial family carers by signing the given consent forms. All documentation was treated anonymously. Moreover, no persons or images of persons were included in these photos in a recognisable way. Participants were asked not to take explicit pictures or photographs of people who did not want to be photographed.

The personal data from the participants were obtained with a checklist, which was based on the Tilburg Frailty Indicator (TFI) [15], an instrument used to quantify the frailty of older people from their own perspective. The study population consisted of 8 females and 4 males. The age of the participants ranged from 62 to 95 years. Eight of the participants were widowed, two respondents were married, and two were unmarried. All participants were born in the Netherlands. The level of education varied from primary education only (n = 5) to secondary (n = 4) and higher education (n = 3). Eight participants indicated, using the TFI, they felt healthy, three participants had no clear indication of their overall health, and one participant indicated not feeling healthy. The duration of residence in the nursing home ranged from 8 months to 8 years. Every participant had a single-person room, with private sanitary facilities. The participants had stated that they were satisfied with their living environment.

2.2. Photography. As pointed out by Annemans et al. [16], we experience the built environment through our senses. Therefore, a visual research method was chosen for this study [17], in which people are interviewed based on photographs they have taken themselves with cameras supplied to them by the researcher. Radley [17] concluded that what pictures portray and what stories narrate are better thought of as versions of our experience of the world than as constructions of the world that we experience.

Photography is a method that has been used in research for decades and which allows participants to create a record of an event, capture a complex phenomenon, or tell a story through images [18–21]. As taking photos does not rely on language alone, it can be used with vulnerable populations who might not normally be included in research [18, 22], for example, in researching frail older persons and nursing home residents. Previously, photography methods have been applied in the domains of housing, communities, and the built environment [16, 23–28].

Images provide a lasting record of an event or in the case of this study an architectural or social scene, required to study the relationship of humans and their living environments. A photo only serves as a conduit to enhanced, thoughtful, and deliberative narrative, instead of as a replacement of words. Photography allows complex environmental, health, and social issues to be captured and then shared with other people [16, 18]. There are numerous photography methodologies available for researchers, including photovoice, photo-elicitation, and photo-production methods. As this study tries to capture the real-life experiences of nursing home residents, the photo-production method was applied, which builds on the principles of photo-elicitation [17]. In line with Annemans et al. [16], this study wanted to gain a good understanding of what has been made visible on the photos, in addition to why and how. The photo-production method enables researchers to experience a phenomenon from another point of view, in this study, the nursing home as a living environment. The older residents, who serve as participants, are experts of their own situation and environment, and they can highlight the positive and negative features in the built environment.

Studies by other researchers, for instance, Yuan and Dong [28], suggest that asking older people to make pictures to document their experiences is not always straightforward. In this study, the selection procedure, the instructions, and manual were tools to tackle potential operational challenges.

At the beginning of this study, the participants received a short explanation of the goal of the study and how to use the camera, including a leaflet-sized written and visual manual on how to use the camera. The manual also contained the study's time plan, its goals, and contact details of the principal researcher (M. M. Verhagen). The participants were asked to share their experiences and views concerning their living environment and which of the factors of the living environment were most and least meaningful, through taking photographs of characteristic elements and situations.

The research team chose to provide the participants with disposable cameras instead of digital cameras for three reasons. First, traditional cameras may be more familiar to the participants, as is stated by Novek et al. [29], and can be operated as long as residents have sufficient strength and dexterity in their hands. Second, disposable cameras are cheaper than digital cameras and when dropped are not as easily damaged. Third, using disposable cameras limits the number of pictures participants could take, limiting the choice in the selection procedure. A disadvantage of disposable cameras is that pictures need to be developed, which is time consuming and costs money and one does not know the end results immediately. Digital cameras yield digital output, which is easier to process for data analysis. Moreover, participants may be less cautious with the disposable camera as they know it is of a lower value. With both methods, pictures can be supplied to the participants after the research as a token of appreciation of their contribution to the research.

In this study, participants were supplied with a camera for one week up to a week and a half (in late April and early May 2014) and were asked to take pictures of their living environment. The reel of the camera contained 27 photos, which should be sufficient for taking the most important pictures, but participants were free in the number of pictures they took. The participants did not keep a log of the things they photographed, although the researchers were aware that due to privacy restrictions not every situation could be photographed [30]. Even though notes from the logs could be used during the elicitation process, we assumed that the limited number of pictures would not require a log. Support, for instance, by family carers, could be provided to the participants for taking the photographs, but the decision to take a picture and the choice for scene that was to be photographed had to be that of the participant. After the time period, the cameras were collected by the principal investigator and sent off for development of the photos. Upon completion, the principal investigator returned to the participants and invited them to choose a top-5 ranking of their photographs. The top-5 ranking was used as a basis for the interviews held by the principal investigator in May 2014, as participants could use the selection as

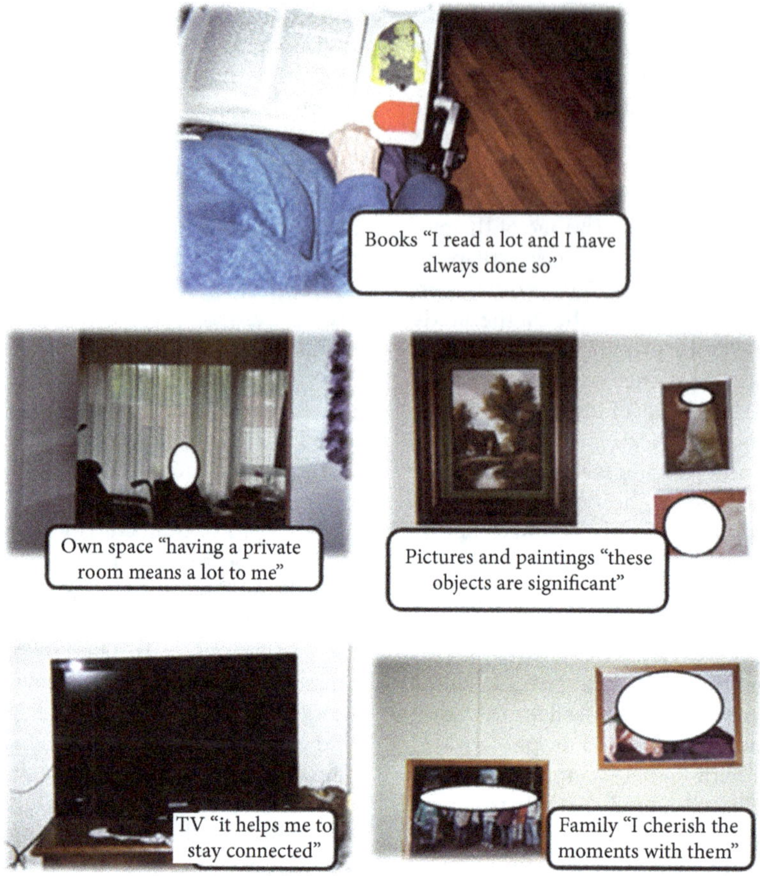
Books "I read a lot and I have always done so"
Own space "having a private room means a lot to me"
Pictures and paintings "these objects are significant"
TV "it helps me to stay connected"
Family "I cherish the moments with them"

FIGURE 1: Example of the top-5 pictures of one of the participants, showing personal belongings, a private room, and social relationships. The top-5 ranking does not necessarily show building-related photos only.

a foundation for what they wanted to discuss in the interview [31].

2.3. Interviews. During the subsequent photo-elicitation interviewing phase, participants talked about the photographs and how they attributed social and personal meanings and values to these photographs. All interviews were conducted within the private rooms of the residents. The interviews had the character of a conversation in which participants were asked about their experiences and views of their living environment and their sense of home. The interviews varied between 30 and 60 minutes each, depending on the richness of the conversation and the attention span of the participants.

Each interview commenced with an introduction and participants were asked about their personal background, the reasons for admission, and health status (Table 1). The opening question included whether participants could describe their experiences concerning their living environment in general. Thereafter, the top-5 photographs taken were discussed in terms of the contents of the photographic material. This resulted in participants being asked to describe why the particular pictures were selected and the meaning of the pictures to the individual. The top-5 ranking was supplemented by items from a topic list, which is an overview of research themes and accompanying questions. The list was based on the work of Van Steenwinkel et al. [2] and van Dijck-Heinen et al. [3]. The participants were free to add items to the topic list, as long as these were relevant to the study. The topic list contained items relating to the living environment, such as (1) appreciation (choice, most meaningful features), (2) the choice for the top 5 (choice, meaning, positive features, and improvements), (3) experiences, wishes, and expectations of the living environment, (4) experience of the sense of home (which experiences, positive experiences, and improvements), and (5) experiences in relation to the living environment (which experiences, positive experiences, and improvements).

2.4. Data Analysis. All interviews were recorded with a voice recorder and transcribed verbatim. The data were analysed based on the six phases by Braun and Clarke [32]. First, all transcripts were read in their entirety. Then, the top-5 photographs were compared to the transcripts (Figure 1), which were used in conjunction with the photographs, and were evaluated in terms of the values that are attributed to the statements made by the participants and the photographs they had taken.

For instance, were these statements either positive or negative? Then, the first set of codes was being generated through open coding. Thereafter, codes were added to the transcripts. The researchers, bearing the research questions in mind, systematically highlighted the relevant information (open coding). Open coding concerns the process of unravelling all of the collected data into fragments or codes. Similar codes and quotes were clustered and labelled, and themes emerged from this process. Together, the research team organised the codes and clustered them into smaller thematic groups. The final themes were grouped in amalgamation with the photographs that reflected aspects of these themes, which is a form of axial coding. Thereafter, these themes were reviewed and then defined and named. In order to guarantee the anonymity and privacy of participants, the photographs showing people were processed in order to white out faces. Names of people and institutions, appearing in quotes, were deleted from the written texts or were changed.

3. Results

There are numerous factors and subfactors which influence the sense of home. The thematic analysis led to the identification of four themes: (1) the physical view; (2) mobility and accessibility; (3) space, place, and personal belongings; and (4) the social environment and activities. These themes are further elaborated in the following sections.

3.1. The Physical View. The theme named the physical view encompasses the green environment in which the nursing home is located and the views from the building. Every participant stated that they appreciated the green environment of the nursing home, which is located in a park landscape. Living amongst nature is considered a positive perspective. A number of residents stated that the environment is beautiful, healthy, and green. This does not mean that all residents can appreciate the landscape by going outside, but in such cases the view of nature is considered to be attractive and pretty. To some, the green environment provides a sense of freedom. In total, the green environment was placed four times at the top 5 of photographs by the residents and the view from the nursing home five times. Three out of twelve participants mentioned the green environment. Words association with the green environment included "enjoying," "healthy air," "freedom," and "nice and green."

> *A green environment. Yes, it is healthy and beautiful, isn't it? [...] It is so nice, well, you need to enjoy it, I can really enjoy it. I always say that it is the small things that matter. That is the way it is, and you need to appreciate that. (Participant 5)*

Seven participants mentioned the view. Word association with the view included "beautiful," "nice," and "freedom." One of the participants talked about the photo she took staring out of the window, which she experienced as freedom.

> *I always look outside from the window over there. Freedom, aren't I allowed to say that? (Participant 1)*

Participants did not make a distinction between the types of view from the room. Any type of view was appreciated in this study, whether it was a park, traffic, a playground with children, or a building. The main reason for appreciating the view was that it gives them something to look at during daytime.

> *It is beautiful view, over this piece of art, the water tower. (Participant 9)*

A regular feature was the importance of birds. At one of the living rooms in the gerontopsychiatric ward there was a wild crow, eating from a net of peanuts hanging in front of the window. One of the respondents stated that this bird was the main source of distraction and a "resident of the ward" as if it were a pet animal.

3.2. Mobility. Several participants spoke of elements which can be classified within the theme of mobility, which relate to freedom, independence, and interior design. One of the residents spoke of the elevator, which is hard to operate when seated in a wheelchair. The hoist was mentioned as being an essential element in the room in order to be comfortable and to aid getting out of the chair. The bathroom can be a source of joy, if people can access it without difficulties, and they can wash and shower themselves. Another participant spoke of the washbasin in her room, which is hard to use, and therefore, it was photographed.

> *Yes, this one is about the sanitary equipment. You need to have a decent washbasin ... one of those washbasins for the disabled, so to say. So you can wash your hands without having to stretch to absurd proportions. (Participant 8)*

> *A little difficult, isn't it? It, of course, does not feel like living at home, but on the other side it is pleasant to have someone around the corner when you need to go to the bathroom, so to say. (Participant 6)*

Two participants indicated that the taxi service was important in order to travel to places such as the supermarket and to see relatives. One of the participants stated that the waiting times are often too long, although they should be around 30 minutes at the most.

> *I'm happy that there is a taxi service. It opens the way to somewhere else. But things don't go smoothly. (Participant 9)*

Participant 7 showed a picture of him being lifted out of the bed. The hoist was named "James," in analogy to a butler, but the respondent said there was nothing interesting about the technology itself. No special meaning was given to the hoist, other than that it supported the personal mobility of the participant.

In relation to mobility, being dependent and the lack of freedom were the least appreciated features in the lives of the residents. One of the participants mentioned their wish to be able to walk again, because it would improve their sense of being independent. One of the respondents mentioned the feeling of not being able to do things alone and thought that this aspect was the worst of living in a nursing home. One of the female residents took a picture of her diseased hands (arthritis) and described them as a source of "sadness." Another resident stated that having to sit all day makes one feel dependent on others, because one has to ask others to do things for them, and another one felt locked-up occasionally.

> *The nursing home, it is something you have to experience yourself for once. Having to sit here all day, being dependent, having to ask for everything. It is hard to cope. (Participant 4)*

> *Well, I cannot say that I always enjoy myself, but that is more a matter of my character than of the environment I think. [. . .] Yes, I do feel locked-up once in a while. (Participant 7)*

One participant stated that he had lost the sense of freedom because he was no longer allowed to drive around in a mobility scooter, which also emerged in the theme of mobility.

> *Yes, because of the mobility scooter that was taken away from me, I lost a great part of my freedom. (Participant 7)*

3.3. Space, Place, and Personal Belongings. Many photographs were taken by participants based on pieces of furniture or personal belongings that are present in their room. The theme also concerns being able to decorate their own room and deciding which personal items are important in this process. Three of the participants took photographs of their television set. These residents cannot think of having to abandon the television, as it helps them get through the day and to keep up to date with the world news. This is actually one of the few comments about technology by the residents.

A regular feature was the importance of flowers. Flowers contribute to a homely atmosphere, as was acknowledged by multiple participants. Drawings of grandchildren meant a lot to the participants, because they represented memories of loved ones. One of the residents explicitly stated personal belongings and having a nice chair are important to her.

> *Yes here, the fact that I have a comfortable chair and many of my personal things. That is something I like. (Participant 6)*

Having access to either a single-person room or an allocated space in the communal areas is subthemed as having a private place in this study. This theme emerged from the analysis of the photographs. Five participants took photographs of their own private place. This was either their own room (4 participants) or a place somewhere else in the nursing home. Additional pictures were taken of picture frames with smaller photos of the relatives, which were found in the private rooms. During meal times, the residents have their own place around the table. The private room means pleasure and joy in living. One of the participants wished that their own room would have a more attractive atmosphere but has the impression that personal belongings and furniture would not fit inside. She does not know what the possibilities are for bringing items, and she does not want to burden others with having to carry loads.

> *I wish the room were bit cozier, but there is nothing at home that would fit in here. I have large cabinets, and I have a large clock too. It would be nice if I could put it here, but I don't bother to carry heavy loads. And a small cabinet as well, and a large one, but I am not sure whether it will stand in the way. We need space for the patient hoist and it would not be enough [with the cabinet]. (Participant 3)*

Two participants stated that living in the nursing home will never be like living at home but that they have accepted the situation and are satisfied. Two other participants stated that they do not experience a sense of home at all. One of the residents stated it feels like being in a shared student dormitory.

> *Do I have to give a grade for it? Well, I don't have a sense of home. It feels like I live in a student house, we are going back to our teenage years, living in a room and getting pocket money. (Participant 5)*

For one of the participants, the common living room is the main source of a sense of home. Two of the participants stated that they would rather return to their old home. They did realise that this was no longer an option. Four of the participants stated that the way they are being cared for positively contributes to a sense of home. Two residents experienced a sense of home inside of their private rooms.

> *Because I am rather mobile, and have my own stuff around, I do feel at home in my room. (Participant 6)*

One participant mentioned the entrance as being important. She calls the entrance her private spot and forms a sense of mental freedom. Residents may have a sense of being locked.

> *The entrance is important. Because it is also the exit. (Participant 5)*

> *Without this little place, I don't make it through the day. There is a lot of buzz. (Participant 10)*

Finally, one of the participants mentioned the cleaning tools and products in her room. The meaning of these items was a sense that the room was kept clean and tidy. She was worried that the current cleaning regimen of cleaning twice a week was reduced to once a week, which she considered to be insufficient.

3.4. Social Environment and Activities. The theme named social environment and activities encompasses the contacts with care professional and relatives and being engaged in activities. The participants indicated a great appreciation for the care staff; in particular, the personal contact and the treatment were considered positive. A number of participants indicated that they valued their contact with relatives as most positive, in particular, having close contacts and being visited on a regular basis.

A number of times, participants spoke of their interaction with care professionals. Five out of twelve participants stated that these professionals contributed positively to their quality of life. One of the participants took a picture of herself with a care professional. It was perceived important to have a positive personal contact with the caregiver and being able to get along well with them.

> *Well, yes, the contact with the care professionals. Well, yes, you need to be on speaking terms, so we can get along well. (Participant 9)*

Five of the participants mentioned the importance of relatives during the interviews and included spouses, children, grandchildren, great grandchildren, parents, and siblings. One of the participants mentioned that he appreciated that his wife came to visit him every day at 18:00.

> *The fact that my wife comes visit me every day is the thing I appreciate most. (Participant 9)*

A number of participants spoke about the activities that were being organised, such as the cooking club, arts, and crafts such as paint workshops, and reminiscence activities conducted in the activity space. One of the residents spoke of the small shop on the ground floor which keeps her occupied and allows her to buy clothes. Two others indicated missing a large store in the direct neighbourhood for buying groceries.

> *Oh that is so nice. I had to go to the small store a while ago. If I cannot buy the things I want, they will actually buy it for me. (Participant 10)*

Having dinner is an ingredient for employing a nice atmosphere to multiple participants. One of the participants took a photograph of a Chinese meal, which he found illustrative of the atmosphere and the memory he had of the dinner. Another participant took a photo of a quality restaurant and the quality food that was served there. She said she missed good quality food in the nursing home. In the two wards of the nursing home, food and drinks were experienced differently. Food, to the participants, is related to appreciation of the living environment which is a positive or negative sense.

> *Sometimes, the food is alright, and at other times it is very bad. I have the choice between two meals, and I guess I always chose the wrong meal. (Participant 7)*

> *I appreciate the food the most. It looks so tasty and it actually tastes good. People told me I was getting served wartime meals; well these meals were definitely not served during the war. It is all rubbish what they said. (Participant 10)*

A number of residents valued the dining atmosphere, especially in relation to being seated around a table together.

> *Particularly going to the dining room is nice. We all sit together around a table with certain people. The table is nicely set. You sit around the table like you used to do at home. (Participant 2)*

4. Discussion and Conclusion

4.1. Reflections on the Results. The focus of this study was the sense of home. This is a complicated and multifactorial phenomenon, which contributes to a sense of identity and well-being of nursing home residents [3, 33–35]. The themes which seem to have a relationship with the experienced sense of home in this study seem consistent with the findings of Sixsmith [36]. In this study, 22 adults were questioned about which factors were associated with their experienced sense of home. 20 categories were formed which were categorised into three layers of perceiving a home, namely, physical, social, and personal.

Feeling at home is a layered emotion [10], and in order to experience a sense of home, one should feel familiar within the environment. A home can either be a country, a city, a neighbourhood, a house or a park bench [9], or, in the context of this study, a nursing home. This, however, does not mean that it is a naturalness that nursing home residents experience a sense of home by just the fact that they live in such a facility. Not all of the residents in this study felt at home, even though they could point out factors in the environment that were important to them. The feeling, that is, the sense of home, that we are talking about is a secondary emotion, and this is a conscious experience of the experienced "more reflexive" primary emotions [37]. Additional emotions play a role, which can differ per individual and one's circumstances. Our study showed that certain social events, including having meals together with fellow residents, contribute to positive emotions that, in turn, positively contribute to their personal sense of home.

A well-experienced balance between autonomy and safety/security also contributes to a positive sense of home [2, 38]. In this study, residents express concerns and limitations related to their sense of autonomy, for instance, when speaking of the need for assistance and help with mobility. At the same time, the sense of security is also hampered in the nursing home, as people are dependent on others for help. In the words of these residents, their sense of home is affected in a negative fashion. This can be explained through the nature of nursing homes, in which more emphasis is put on the provision of a safe and secure environment, whereas residents like to see an environment in which their personal autonomy is enhanced. If a person does not experience a good sense of home, he or she may feel anxious and uncertain [9], and this, in turn, may be aggravated by the fact that the sense of autonomy and security in a nursing home environment may be lower than that for people who still live in their own homes. Duyvendak [39] also reported that people can feel homesick and nostalgic when they experience a lack of sense of home. One's own home can be seen as a secure place from which they can explore the world around themselves [2]. By furnishing one's home with personal belongings, for instance, one enables reminiscence and positive memories [2, 34, 40, 41]. In this study, residents mentioned the importance of personal belongings as a way to connect with their past and as a source of familiarity.

4.2. There Is More to It Than Just the Built Environment. When architects design buildings, it is often thought that the built environment and the architectural design dictate how people experience the space and the interactions that will take place. To residents, the built environment may be of a different level of importance compared to the more basic needs and a well-functioning and stimulating social environment. This does not rule out the need for age-friendly solutions and accessibility. Primarily, residents value good communication with care professionals and relatives the most, as well as having a sense of autonomy, independence, and freedom. These are all human values. This is in line with findings from a review by Xu et al. [42] on the quality of life in relation to nursing home features. The researchers concluded that there were serious questions about whether any elements of the nursing home's structure can improve residents' quality of life. Rural facilities (green environments) and facilities with a higher percentage of private rooms had better residents' self-reported quality of life. This is in line with the statements by the residents that they valued a green environment. Moreover, it suggests that the built environment has a role to play in the quality of life of older people but that the social environment should also be considered when planning and designing a new facility.

According to Brown et al. [24], place attachments are the positive bonds that people form with places and which arise from affective, behavioural, and cognitive ties between individuals or groups and their sociophysical settings. The built environment cannot be seen on its own without regarding the social context. Moreover, place attachments can also change, as old attachments evolve or are disrupted and new attachments form [24]. Admission to a nursing home is a major life-event, as most individuals do not wish to leave the home they have been living in for a long time in order to move to a nursing home [43]. Nevertheless, "*there seem to be good reasons to assert that living in an institution and being 'at home' is not a contradiction in terms*" [44, page 221]. In this study, residents spoke of (social) activities that took place in a certain room or part of the nursing home, for instance, eating in the communal living room. These activities and spaces were mentioned at the same time, as if they were linked together. The activities were the main contributor to the development of a sense of home and may be a starting point to improve living conditions for people who have been admitted to a nursing home.

Still, features of the built environment have a role to play. Features of the built environment that matter are the green environment, the view from the rooms, and having personal belongings in a private room where residents can withdraw. When these important features of a nursing home are present, residents have a basis to develop a sense of home. Moreover, these features are within reach of architects designing nursing home facilities. It is, therefore, an important task for architects to create environments which meet the needs of future residents and may even contribute to social interaction, for example, by designing rooms where one can meet up and interact with others and where visitors are invited and feel welcome. The need for having both social and architectural components which have to be fulfilled in order to get a sense of home matches the findings by Van Steenwinkel et al. [2] of people who resided in the community. In our study, participants indicated that having flower arrangements and having a positive and homely atmosphere and habits, like eating together, are important for experiencing a sense of home. These statements are in line with earlier findings by Cooney [45].

What this study has shown once more is that nursing home residents are independent and unique in their needs and wishes. It is important not to offer standardised arrangements for nursing homes. Instead, residents should have the freedom to live the lives they want to lead and make changes to their room (by adding personal belongings) without hampering the provision of care. People in general express their sense of identity through their personal belongings [10, 46], and these belongings can "move" the sense of home to the nursing home environment [47]. Relatives can play a role in the development of a sense of home in the nursing home, for instance, in eating together, decorating their room, saying goodbye to their former home, and the creation of a new home together with other residents. The photographs and outcomes of the interviews may actually act as the stimulus for social action and change [48]. In line with such actions, it should be interesting to explore the degree of freedom a nursing home resident has in relation to making modifications to the home environment or private room.

4.3. Reflections on the Methodology. The methodology applied in this study can be utilised across a wide range of settings, including older people with dementia, with autism, and with cognitive impairments. People have a strong visual tool to express wishes and needs, when words are often too limited to describe how people think or feel about something. In fact, the methodology could also be expanded to indoor environmental research and studies concerning building services engineering at home and in office buildings. The photographs allow for a direct and complete expression of thoughts and expressions and provide a qualitative methodology which is not entirely new to the field [16, 28, 49] but is not applied on a large scale in nursing homes. There are some things that can be improved in future studies concerning nursing home residents.

First of all, the researcher could undertake the photography in conjunction with the participants and conduct the interviews directly afterwards or even during the photography sessions. The participants will be able to remember why a certain picture was taken in the first instance and provide a better description. This is particularly true when it takes some weeks to have the photographs developed (as traditional photography is getting out of fashion and is no longer optimally supported by the market chain). Using a digital camera is more costly but solves the challenge of having to wait. In addition, using disposable cameras resulted in half of the photographs being blurred and, therefore, not useful for the study. When dealing with poorly taken photographs, one could ask for making top 5 without the photographs but by describing what has been photographed in order to find answers to the research question. When taking photographs together with the participants, one can do a secondary check with the participants by again showing the photographs and the transcripts in a later stage as a form of member check. Given the small sample size of the current study, it would be recommended to work with larger groups. This would also allow for the application of the so-called photovoice methodology [17] in which themes can be found through interactions in a group.

4.4. Conclusions. The major challenge for practice is how to incorporate the factors identified in this study in the design and planning of the built environment and how to stimulate social interactions in order to improve the sense of home of residents. The residents' sense of home is not similar to the design of housing alone. The implications thereof are that improving a sense of home is a multifactorial assignment in which many factors need to be addressed and that it encompasses more than just a good design of the built environment. This is also reflected by the statements of the residents included in this study, as a sense of home was not experienced by all of them. The treatment by others, including relatives and care professionals, is another important factor that is valued and has an impact on the sense of home.

The improvement of the experienced sense of home can be achieved through the residents themselves on the one hand and the care professionals on the other hand, for instance, by making changes to the built environment and social interactions. An inclusive approach to the design of nursing homes can combine creative and interviewing techniques which help create an ideal home situation. It can provide a way of participation for the least voiced. In the future, nursing home organisations and family carers could engage in similar creative methods in order to find out which aspects of the built environment are appreciated most and how rooms should be designed and decorated. This would be a method to stimulate social change which is inclusive.

Conflict of Interests

There is no conflict of interests.

Acknowledgments

All participants of the sessions and interviews are thanked for their willingness to share their views. The hosting care organisation (*Vitalis Woonzorg Groep* in Eindhoven) and the coordinators are thanked for facilitating the research. The Province of Noord-Brabant (*Algemene Subsidieverordening Noord-Brabant, grant "Samen Slim in Zorg," as part of the Activiteitenplan Brabant Medical School (BMS) 2013*) and Stichting Promotie Installatietechniek (PIT) are thanked for their financial support. The paper processing charges were funded by the "Fontys Denk Groter Prijs." Being a preliminary study for the Nursing Home of the Future Programme, the writing of this paper was partly supported by the RAAK (Regional Attention and Action for Knowledge circulation) scheme [01-05P]. This scheme is managed by the Foundation Innovation Alliance (SIA: Stichting Innovatie Alliantie), with funding from the Dutch Ministry of Education, Culture and Science (OCW).

References

[1] J. van Hoof, M. H. Wetzels, A. M. C. Dooremalen et al., "Technological and architectural solutions for Dutch nursing homes: results of a multidisciplinary mind mapping session with professional stakeholders," *Technology in Society*, vol. 36, no. 1, pp. 1–12, 2014.

[2] I. Van Steenwinkel, S. Baumers, and A. Heylighen, "Home in later life: a framework for the architecture of home environments," *Home Cultures*, vol. 9, no. 2, pp. 195–217, 2012.

[3] C. J. M. L. van Dijck-Heinen, E. J. M. Wouters, B. M. Janssen, and J. van Hoof, "The environmental design of residential care facilities: a sense of home through the eyes of nursing home residents," *International Journal for Innovative Research in Science & Technology*, vol. 1, no. 4, pp. 57–69, 2014.

[4] J. van Hoof, M. L. Janssen, C. M. C. Heesakkers et al., "The importance of personal possessions for the development of a sense of home of nursing home residents," *Journal of Housing for the Elderly*. In press.

[5] G. Munten, M. Legius, T. Niessen et al., *Practice Development. Naar duurzame veranderingen van zorg- en onderwijspraktijken*, Boom Lemma, The Hague, The Netherlands, 2012, (Dutch).

[6] B. McCormack, K. Manley, and A. Titchen, *Practice Development in Nursing and Healthcare*, Wiley-Blackwell, Oxford, UK, 2nd edition, 2013.

[7] J. van Hoof, H. S. M. Kort, and H. van Waarde, "Housing and care for older adults with dementia: a European perspective," *Journal of Housing and the Built Environment*, vol. 24, no. 3, pp. 369–390, 2009.

[8] E. van Zadelhoff and H. Verbeek, *Morgen mag ik naar het verpleeghuis! Toekomstvisie op zorg voor mensen met dementie*, Boom-Lemma, The Hague, The Netherlands, 2012, (Dutch).

[9] J. W. Duyvendak and P. van der Graaf, *Thuisvoelen in de Buurt: Een Opgave voor Stedelijke Vernieuwing*, NICIS, The Hague, The Netherlands, 2008, (Dutch).

[10] J. W. Duyvendak, "Thuisvoelen. Een korte introductie op drie artikelen," *Sociologie*, vol. 5, no. 2, pp. 257–260, 2009, (Dutch).

[11] J. van Hoof, M. H. Wetzels, A. M. Dooremalen et al., "The Essential Elements for a Nursing Home According to Stakeholders from Healthcare and Technology. Perspectives from multiple simultaneous monodisciplinary workshops," *Journal of Housing For the Elderly*, vol. 28, no. 4, pp. 329–356, 2014.

[12] J. van Hoof, A. M. C. Dooremalen, M. H. Wetzels et al., "Exploring technological and architectural solutions for nursing home residents, care professionals and technical staff: focus groups with professional stakeholders," *International Journal for Innovative Research in Science & Technology*, vol. 1, no. 3, pp. 90–105, 2014.

[13] J. van Hoof and E. J. M. Wouters, Eds., *Het verpleeghuis van de toekomst is (een) thuis*, Bohn Stafleu van Loghum, Houten, The Netherlands, 2014 (Dutch).

[14] Critical Appraisal Skills Programme (CASP), *Qualitative Research Checklist 31.05.13*, Critical Appraisal Skills Programme (CASP), Oxford, UK, 2011, http://www.casp-uk.net/wp-content/uploads/2011/11/CASP-Qualitative-Research-Checklist-31.05.13.pdf.

[15] R. J. J. Gobbens, M. A. L. M. van Assen, K. G. Luijkx, M. T. Wijnen-Sponselee, and J. M. G. A. Schols, "The tilburg frailty indicator: psychometric properties," *Journal of the American Medical Directors Association*, vol. 11, no. 5, pp. 344–355, 2010.

[16] M. Annemans, C. Van Audenhove, H. Vermolen, and A. Heylighen, "Hospital reality from a lying perspective: exploring a sensory research approach," in *Designing Inclusive Systems*, P. Langdon, P. Clarkson, and P. Robinson, Eds., pp. 3–12, Springer, London, UK, 2012.

[17] A. Radley, "What people do with pictures," *Visual Studies*, vol. 25, no. 3, pp. 268–279, 2010.

[18] D. Evans, J. Robertson, and A. Candy, "Use of photovoice with people with younger onset dementia," *Dementia*, 2014.

[19] S. Warren, "'Show me how it feels to work here': using photography to research organizational aesthetics," *Ephemera*, vol. 2, no. 3, pp. 224–245, 2002.

[20] J. Collier, *Visual Anthropology: Photography as a Research Method*, Holt Rinehart and Winston, New York, NY, USA, 1967.

[21] C. Mills and L. Hoeber, "Using photo-elicitation to examine artefacts in a sport club: logistical considerations and strategies throughout the research process," *Qualitiative Research in Sport, Exercise and Health*, vol. 5, no. 1, pp. 1–20, 2013.

[22] K. C. Hergenrather, S. D. Rhodes, C. A. Cowan, G. Bardhoshi, and S. Pula, "Photovoice as community-based participatory research: a qualitative review," *The American Journal of Health Behavior*, vol. 33, no. 6, pp. 686–698, 2009.

[23] S. M. D. Grieb, R. M. Joseph, A. Pridget, H. Smith, R. Harris, and J. Ellen, "Understanding housing and health through the lens of transitional housing members in a high-incarceration Baltimore City neighborhood: the GROUP Ministries Photovoice Project to promote community redevelopment," *Health & Place*, vol. 21, pp. 20–28, 2013.

[24] B. B. Brown, I. Altman, and C. M. Werner, "Place attachment," in *International Encyclopedia of Housing and Home*, S. J. Smith, Ed., pp. 183–188, Elsevier, Amsterdam, The Netherlands, 2012.

[25] A. P. Belon, L. M. Nieuwendyk, H. Vallianatos, and C. I. Nykiforuk, "How community environment shapes physical activity: perceptions revealed through the PhotoVoice method," *Social Science & Medicine*, vol. 116, pp. 10–21, 2014.

[26] C. Fusco, F. Moola, G. Faulkner, R. Buliung, and V. Richichi, "Toward an understanding of children's perceptions of their transport geographies: (non)active school travel and visual representations of the built environment," *Journal of Transport Geography*, vol. 20, no. 1, pp. 62–70, 2012.

[27] G. Nelson, A. Stefancic, J. Rae et al., "Early implementation evaluation of a multi-site housing first intervention for homeless people with mental illness: a mixed methods approach," *Evaluation and Program Planning*, vol. 43, pp. 16–26, 2014.

[28] S. Yuan and H. Dong, "Adapting data collection methods for different participants of the user study," in *Proceedings of the DRS 2014: Design's Big Debates*, Y.-K. Lim, K. Niedderer, J. Redström et al., Eds., pp. 1519–1525, Umeå Institute of Design, Umeå University, Umeå, Sweden, 2014.

[29] S. Novek, T. Morris-Oswald, and V. Menec, "Using photovoice with older adults: some methodological strengths and issues," *Ageing and Society*, vol. 32, no. 3, pp. 451–470, 2012.

[30] A. Radley and D. Taylor, "Images of recovery: a photo-elicitation study on the hospital ward," *Qualitative Health Research*, vol. 13, no. 1, pp. 77–99, 2003.

[31] J. L. Oliffe and J. L. Bottorff, "Further than the eye can see? Photo elicitation and research with men," *Qualitative Health Research*, vol. 17, no. 6, pp. 850–858, 2007.

[32] V. Braun and V. Clarke, "Using thematic analysis in psychology," *Qualitative Research in Psychology*, vol. 3, no. 2, pp. 77–101, 2006.

[33] L. Groger, "A nursing home can be a home," *Journal of Aging Studies*, vol. 9, no. 2, pp. 137–153, 1995.

[34] G. D. Rowles, F. Oswald, and E. G. Hunter, "Interior living environments in old age," in *Annual Review of Gerontology and Geriatrics. Volume 23*, H.-W. Wahl, R. J. Scheidt, and P. G. Windley, Eds., pp. 167–194, Springer, New York, NY, USA, 2003.

[35] H. Chaudhury and G. D. Rowles, "Between the shores of recollection and imagination: self, aging and home," in *Home and Identity in Late Life. International Perspectives*, G. D. Rowles and H. Chaudhury, Eds., pp. 3–18, Springer, New York, NY, USA, 2005.

[36] J. Sixsmith, "The meaning of home: an exploratory study of environmental experience," *Journal of Environmental Psychology*, vol. 6, no. 4, pp. 281–298, 1986.

[37] A. R. Damasio, "Emotions and feelings," in *Feelings and Emotions: The Amsterdam Symposium*, A. S. R. Manstead, N. Frijda, and A. Fisher, Eds., pp. 49–57, Cambridge University Press, Cambridge, UK, 2004.

[38] P. A. Parmelee and M. P. Lawton, "The design of special environments for the aged," in *Handbook of the Psychology of Aging*, J. E. Birren and K. W. Schaie, Eds., pp. 465–489, Academic Press, San Diego, Calif, USA, 3rd edition, 1990.

[39] J. W. Duyvendak, *The Politics of Home: Belonging and Nostalgia in Western Europe and the United States*, Palgrave Macmillan, Basingstoke, UK, 2011.

[40] G. D. Rowles and J. F. Watkins, "History, habit, heart and hearth. On making spaces into places," in *Aging Independently: Living Arrangements and Mobility*, K. W. Schaie, H.-W. Wahl, H. Mollenkopf, and F. Oswald, Eds., pp. 77–96, Springer, New York, NY, USA, 2003.

[41] S. Wapner, J. Demick, and J. P. Redondo, "Cherished posessions and adaptation of older people to nursing homes," *The International Journal of Aging and Human Development*, vol. 31, no. 3, pp. 219–235, 1990.

[42] D. Xu, R. L. Kane, and T. A. Shamliyan, "Effect of nursing home characteristics on residents' quality of life: a systematic review," *Archives of Gerontology and Geriatrics*, vol. 57, no. 2, pp. 127–142, 2013.

[43] C. Gillsjö, D. Schwartz-Barcott, and I. Von Post, "Home: the place the older adult can not imagine living without," *BMC Geriatrics*, vol. 11, article 10, 2011.

[44] H. W. Wahl, "Environmental influences on aging and behavior," in *Handbook of the Psychology of Aging*, J. E. Birren and K. W. Schaie, Eds., pp. 215–237, Elsevier, San Diego, Calif, USA, 5th edition, 2011.

[45] A. Cooney, "'Finding home': a grounded theory on how older people 'find home' in long-term care settings," *International Journal of Older People Nursing*, vol. 7, no. 3, pp. 188–199, 2012.

[46] D. L. Kahn, "Making the best of it: adapting to the ambivalence of a nursing home environment," *Qualitative Health Research*, vol. 9, no. 1, pp. 119–132, 1999.

[47] D. Shenk, K. Kuwahara, and D. Zablotsky, "Older women's attachments to their home and possessions," *Journal of Aging Studies*, vol. 18, no. 2, pp. 157–169, 2004.

[48] C. Wang and M. A. Burris, "Photovoice: concept, methodology and use for participatory needs assessment," *Health Education and Behavior*, vol. 24, no. 3, pp. 369–387, 1997.

[49] M. Annemans, C. Van Audenhove, H. Vermolen, and A. Heylighen, "Being transported into the unknown: how patients experience the route to the operation room," in *Inclusive Designing: Joining Usability, Accessibility and Inclusion*, P. M. Langdon, J. Lazar, A. Heylighen, and H. Dong, Eds., pp. 189–200, Springer, London, UK, 2014.

14

Older Adults with Hoarding Behaviour Aging in Place: Looking to a Collaborative Community-Based Planning Approach for Solutions

Kyle Y. Whitfield,[1] Jason S. Daniels,[1] Keri Flesaker,[2] and Doneka Simmons[3]

[1] *Faculty of Extension, University of Alberta, Enterprise Square, Room 2-215, 10230 Jasper Avenue, Edmonton, Alberta, Canada T5J 4P6*
[2] *Department of Educational Psychology, University of Alberta, 6-102 Education North, Edmonton, Alberta, Canada T6G 2G5*
[3] *Senior Association of Greater Edmonton, 15 Sir Winston Churchill Square, Edmonton, Alberta, Canada T5J 2E5*

Correspondence should be addressed to Kyle Y. Whitfield, kyle.whitfield@ualberta.ca

Academic Editor: Frank Oswald

This paper reports on and synthesizes new research that examines how a collaborative community response can promote successful aging in place for older adults with hoarding behaviour. Through interviews with older adults with hoarding behaviour, who used a particular community support and a focus group interview with members of the community collaborative that directed supports for this population, our findings suggest that there were valuable outcomes for both groups. These older adults with hoarding behaviour were able to remain in their own homes, their safety was enhanced, their sense of isolation was minimized, empowerment was fostered, and they gained valuable insight into their behaviour. The members of the community collaborative were able to access the expertise of other professionals, maximize their own expertise, and they generated an enhanced understanding of the experience of older adults living with hoarding behaviour in Edmonton. This study is a significant addition to the much too sparse literature about the community planning needs of older adults with hoarding behaviour. It offers knowledge that is integral to theories and principles of better aging in place but attempts to translate this into practice.

1. Introduction

Older adults with hoarding behaviour are often at a high risk of being homeless making aging in place extremely complex. This paper reports on a study that examines the value of a community-based planning approach that responds to the needs of this population, a population that is both increasing in number and that is very seldom studied [1]. It synthesizes new research about the complexities associated with remaining in one's own home when he/she is over 55 and has compulsive hoarding behaviour. And it examines how a collaborative community response promotes successful aging in place for this population. Not only are community-based services necessary to better understand because they are central to all health sectors [2], but also current research surrounding those with hoarding behaviour is mostly focussed on methods addressing individual-level behavioural characteristics of hoarding through cognitive behavioural therapy (cf., the extensive work of Frost and Steketee). Missing are descriptions of community-based planning approaches for health and social service sectors working hard to make aging in place a possibility.

For older individuals with hoarding behaviour, aging in place is complex because hoarding behaviour is multifaceted; it touches on social, environmental, familial, and personal issues [3]. Aging in place is also not simple for those with hoarding behavior because they want to remain living in their own homes, neighbourhoods and communities which seem to require that a collection of agencies, often representing different sectors, understand their needs in order to help them stay in the community and age in place. In this paper, aging in place refers to an ideal where people can age in the familiarity of their homes, neighbourhoods, and communities where their quality of life is maximized by the availability and accessibility of supports and services that respond to their needs and capacities [4, 5]. Aging in place, in addition, is about belonging to a community that supports one's many needs, for example, physically, socially, mentally, environmentally, and so forth [6]. To understand the varying aspects of aging in place in late life, older individuals with hoarding behaviour need to be further understood so their aging journey is successful; collaborative approaches by community support agencies can help to make that possible.

In our case, social and health related organizations from different sectors, that in some way supported people with hoarding behaviour in Edmonton, AB, Canada, were brought together in 2007 through the leadership of the social worker of a seniors support agency called SAGE (Seniors Association of Greater Edmonton). After having visited a number of individuals with hoarding behaviour (age 55+) in her professional role, she noticed, as did those members of the imminent community collaborative, that those with hoarding behaviour were at a high risk for being evicted from their homes, and they experienced shame associated with their hoarding resulting in isolation, as well as depression; they were at risk of falling in their own homes, and generally, they were living in unsanitary conditions. To approach this highly vulnerable population, to respond to some of their needs, especially to prevent their potential eviction, a concerted effort by a broad representation of social, health, and other agencies was necessary. The collaborative met together regularly (e.g., once every 2 months over the years and as of June 2011, it continues to meet) to continually plan for and improve the support of older adults with hoarding behaviour in the Edmonton area.

Although little is still known about the effects of one's neighbourhood on the mental health of older adults, positive mental health in later life may be influenced by the way in which older people feel about their neighbourhood [7]. It is fair to conclude, therefore, that for older adults with hoarding behaviour, place matters and the role of place as locality is key when making meaning at both the individual and the collective levels. In particular, local place is an important factor in identity, in ones sense of community, and attachment; this is crucial to the determinants of attachment, satisfaction, and behaviour [8]. Also important is place and the person-place relationship are very much grounded in a context of fear over loss of place [9] and the obliteration of locality [10]. Aging and compulsive hoarding behaviour need to be examined in concert with one another.

As our aging population rapidly increases, the number of older adults with hoarding behaviour will also quickly increase. Although hoarding behaviour usually begins in early adolescents, its severity increases with age [11]. Results from the Hopkins Epidemiology of Personality Disorder Study found that the odds of hoarding were over two times as great in the oldest compared with the youngest age group [12], and in a study of hoarding-related complaints to public health departments in Massachusetts, 40% of individuals that hoarded were involved with elder service agencies [13].

Referring to Frost and Hartl [14] when defining hoarding behaviour, there are key characteristics: the acquisition of and failure to discard a large number of possessions that seem to be of little use or limited value; cluttered living spaces that cannot be used as intended; significant distress and/or impairment associated with the clutter. Hoarded possessions clutter living spaces until rooms are difficult or impossible to use for their designed purpose, causing significant stress to the individuals themselves. Possessions may be purchased through compulsive buying [15] and/or through acquiring things like newspapers or discarded items from dumpsters [16]. Some individuals may even steal new possessions. After acquiring possessions, discarding these items is extremely difficult [17]. In serious instances, household clutter may interfere with and prevent daily activities, like food preparation, moving freely in one's home, and using the bathroom [11, 17]. And as clutter increases, falling, fire, sanitation issues, depression, and isolation are possible, creating significant risk for a number of outcomes but especially eviction and thus homelessness [18].

Community collaboration is one way to respond to social and health needs of a population. In fact, genuine collaborate is say to be the very thing that successfully reforms health systems [14]. Although there are many ways to define collaboration, most definitions emphasize the importance of shared responsibility and a team approach [20], and using a collaborative approach can significantly increase the available pool of resources from which team members can draw [21]. A response to the multiple challenges of older adults with hoarding behaviour requires a comprehensive and far-reaching approach, more than one single agency can provide alone [22, 23]. Philosophically, collaboration is rooted in systems theory which says that entities in a system are dependent on one another [24] and ecological theory in particular proposes that causes and solutions of health and/or social problems are beyond the individual and are associated with such determinants as the health and social services that we receive [25]. Service recipients can benefit from a collaborative approach to the provision of community health services as can the agencies participating in the collaborative [26–28]. Using a collective made up of representative agencies to support this vulnerable population creates potential for an approach that builds on the strengths of all those involved.

2. Methods

Between January 2007 and January 2010, approximately 75 older adults (ages 55+) with hoarding behaviour in Edmonton, AB, Canada, were provided with community supports to prevent them from being evicted from their homes [29]. The Seniors Association of Greater Edmonton (SAGE) offers support through a program referred to as *This Full House*. And *This Full House* is a direct outcome of the work of the community collaborative. The aim of *This Full House* for older individuals with hoarding behaviour is to prevent eviction from their home, improve their health and well-being, maintain positive social contacts, and contribute to the building of a healthy community [29]. As the population of potential participants with hoarding behaviour in Edmonton is not particularly large, a small-n approach was used in an attempt to create heuristic generalizations which Tsoukas [30] defines as opportunities to refine analytic understanding and to make more incisive distinctions than were previously possible. Small-n studies are not designed to support or refute a theory, but rather, to further refine it. As such, the purpose of this study is to further examine the role of a collaborative planning approach in a community setting when seeking to help those over 55 years with issues relevant to having compulsive hoarding behaviour and wanting to age well in one's community.

To further understand the value of collaboration and, in particular, its role and value in this community support, interviews and a focus group were conducted with seniors with hoarding issues involved with *This Full House* and with the community collaborative. All interviews were semistructured and conducted by a third party researcher (i.e., Research Assistant). Ethics approval for this research was received from the University of Alberta, Research Ethics Board.

2.1. Interviews with Individuals with Hoarding Behaviour. Individual interviews were conducted with five ($N = 5$) individuals with hoarding behaviour involved with *This Full House*, all of whom were over the age of 55. The semistructured, face to face interviews took place at a location expressed as being most comfortable to the interviewee, for example, at their homes, at a university office, at a nearby coffee shop. These study participants were first contacted by the social worker from SAGE who directs *This Full House*. The individuals with hoarding behaviour had either referred themselves to *This Full House* or had been referred to it by one of their health care practitioners or family members. At an appointment with the individuals, the social worker informed them about the study asking if they might be interested in being interviewed by a researcher about their experience with *This Full House*. If they agreed (which all five did), she gave them a one-page written description of the study. She then went through the summary of the study ensuring they understood what was being requested from them. With their agreement, their telephone numbers were provided to the researcher (i.e., Research Assistant) who contacted them and established a location and time to meet for the interview. The aim of the one-hour interviews was to gather information regarding their experience with *This Full House*. In particular, the interview was used to understand their perceptions of the impact of or value of their association with *This Full House*, that is, the aspects of the program they benefitted from most.

2.2. Focus Group with the Community Collaborative Members. A community collaborative made up of social and health related agency representatives providing insights into the ongoing development of *This Full House* was formed. The focus group interview included ten members ($N = 10$) (of the possible 11 members in total) and was conducted in a face-to-face manner for approximately 1.5 hours. Members of this collaborative represented a number of expert groups: social workers, home care nurses, geriatric neuropsychologists, geriatric nurses, fire and safety investigators, public health practitioners, and environmental health and safety officers. The focus group questions centered on the nature of the working relationship between and amongst the members and their observations about the value and impact their work may have had on the service users, that is, those with hoarding behaviour. The questions guiding the semistructured interview were generated from key themes highlighted in the literature (i.e., health services, collaboration, community support, etc.) that aligned with the purpose of the study.

3. Results

Use of a grounded theory framework was quite valuable for our data analysis. Grounded theory means that the data analysis essentially, is "grounded" in the data [31]. Therefore, the concepts and themes we describe in our results have evolved from and are embedded in the data collected and have been mined through a process of conceptual ordering. Grounded theories are said to provide further insight, to enhance understanding, and to be used as a guide to inform action (i.e., acting on the results). As Strauss and Corbin [31] describe in more detail, our interview data, in the form of pages of the exact words from the interview, was organized into categories that were not predetermined but that evolved after reading and rereading this data many times. And that, mainly described ideas and offered explanations from interviewees that had commonalities to each other. The themes described here are those that were mentioned frequently and carried the same meaning.

Because our aim in this study was to further our understanding of how older adults with hoarding behaviour were supported by a particular community-based planning approach, grounded theory provided the most effective means of organizing, reducing, and understanding the data. Suggested below is a picture that describes how the work of the community collaborative, because of its high level of collaboration, resulted in many important benefits for older people with hoarding behaviour that align well with and facilitate the goals and ideals associated with an aging in place model. The picture also describes how the community collaborative members valued their experience on the team.

3.1. The Work of the Community Collaborative Benefitted People with Hoarding Behaviour. As a result of this group working together to respond to the needs of older adults with hoarding behaviour, several themes evolved from the data demonstrating direct benefits for these individuals: being able to remain in their own homes; reducing their potential for harm, and minimizing their isolation all which allowed them to experience a feeling of empowerment which also helped them to generate insight into issues surrounding their hoarding behaviour.

3.1.1. Remaining in Own Home. There are considerable challenges associated with aging in one place for older individuals with hoarding behaviour. They can be at significant risk of being evicted from their homes and their behaviour can be a major public health concern leading to eviction as a result of violating building, fire, or property maintenance codes. It may not be until a particular emergency occurs (i.e., water leakage, fire, and pest infestation) that a landlord is notified [32]. One focus group member describes their role, as a member of the community collaborative, in minimizing evictions for this population:

> *"Our legislation says that we do have the right to go into any public or private place if we believe there may be a public health nuisance... and if that means we have to order their suite cleaned out, we'll do it. Um, because you can't get control of bedbugs and cockroaches unless you treat all the suites and if somebody's hoarding, you can't get rid of them... so, so they have to clean up."*

The five interviewees in this study were all in a situation where eviction from their homes was a potential, but they were able to remain at home as a result of a community-based approach that addressed some of their needs. Prior to the existence of this community collective, one focus group member describes how the health inspector had to play all roles and visit clients once a week and "nag people into cleaning up, which was mostly unsuccessful." For example, when there is a potential home eviction for individuals with hoarding behaviour, the social worker and a public health worker, together with the client and other members of the collaborative, that is, where necessary such as a fire and safety representative, provide input into the problem-solving process. A professional organizer usually assists with the practical aspects associated with cleaning up including heavy lifting, removing garbage, and reorganizing resulting in "[these clients being able to] stay living at home without being on the street and [being] homeless." Being able to age in one's own home, one's neighbourhood, and community fosters independence significantly impacts a more positive relationship in the person-place relationship [33].

The five people with hoarding behaviour that we interviewed spoke about the value of being able to remain living in their own homes. One person found it motivating to have someone help him/her to clean up his/her apartment, "it's the motivation of having someone there plus... the helper doing the heavy lifting and heavy carrying... making... 76 thousand trips to the garbage bin... its stressful but helpful [and] I certainly would not have been able to hire a company on my own [...] if the program had not been in effect [and] I would be in deep do-do with Capital Health." For another individual, what helped him remain in his own home was having the home care worker put him in touch with the social worker and the cleaning person who helped him find ways to deal with issues of parting with his stuff. And for this gentleman, the social worker supported him by suggesting options: "she made life more convenient for me by offering me options." And for another person, the social worker and the cleaner reminded her that the condition of her house, the bugs, the mouse droppings, the make up from years ago, the shiny covered magazines all over, and the infestation that she had, was not her fault and she could probably face organizing and cleaning it with encouragement and the help of a plan.

3.1.2. Reducing Harm and Promoting Safety. Hoarding behaviour creates a significant safety risk for the individual him/her self and for the community [32]. Harm reduction is a core principle that is essential to address the needs of those with compulsive hoarding behaviour because promoting safety is foremost [13]. In this case, focusing on harm reduction by the community collective ensured that safety was embedded within all the actions, initiatives, and supports they provided. One focus group member talks about the value of taking on this strategic focus: "We subsequently learned the value of focusing on a harm reduction approach wherein we address issues of harm first so that the person [with hoarding behaviour], at least, will be safe. Even though they may be living with a significant amount of stuff every day of their lives, but at least they are safe." A harm reduction philosophy considers behaviour change to be incremental and assumes that people will maintain their behaviour change when they have decision-making power to influence their goals and put them into action [34].

This focus on safety and reducing harm or the potential for harm helped the individuals with hoarding behaviour buy into the larger process at hand, that is, to contribute to the building of healthy neighbourhoods, supporting their well-being, and helping them stay in their homes as long as possible. Instead of suddenly or immediately removing the person from a potentially unsafe environment or situation, the aim instead is first to reduce the potential for harm and create a safe place to live. In the case of these five individuals, it meant such things as: hiring a person to help them remove and reorganize their excessive items, getting help to fumigate their apartments, openly talking about their hoarding situation to help them reflect upon it, receiving nonjudgemental support, and establishing a plan to minimize household items. One interviewee describes the value of setting goals and generating a plan, "we set a plan and the social worker would come back and generally we would accomplish that goal whatever it was." It also meant helping the person at risk of potential eviction, for example, to respond to requests made by the Public Health Inspector. One person with hoarding behaviour describes the role of this service (i.e., *This Full House*): "they sort of mediate [between varying agencies] and rub off the sharp corners." Reducing harm by promoting safety enables an aging in place philosophy and model as both can facilitate positive and long-term aging in one location.

3.1.3. Minimizing Loneliness. The community collaborative, used in this study as a planning approach helped to address the problem of isolation for these older adults. Several of the representative organizations of the community collaborative, that is, a social worker, public health nurse, geriatric nurse, and so forth, offer home visitation to many of their clients and observe their living environment. As observed by one community collaborative member, "a lot of these seniors are very lonely, very isolated, and so the fact that they have someone that's coming to their home often, helps." Another member talked about the impact of the support group (which is provided for people with hoarding behaviour on a monthly basis as part of *This Full House* services) on minimizing their sense of loneliness and connecting with people that have similar experiences: "[there is] value of that coming together, meeting with other people and seeing and hearing that you're not alone." Two interviewees with hoarding behaviour confirmed this same sentiment, about the importance of feeling connected to a group: "the group has helped me" and "[I realized] you are not the odd one out." As a result of not feeling alone and part of a group, interviewees with hoarding behaviour said that they felt empowered.

3.1.4. Fostering Empowerment. Empowerment can be an outcome of collaborative relationships; it offers a catalyst for new community programs and other supports, changes in policies, and advancing health practices [35, 36]. The members of the community collaborative intentionally aimed to facilitate empowerment using it as a principle to guide their work that addressed the needs of older individuals with hoarding behaviour in the greater Edmonton area. During the focus group interview, one member describes how empowerment as a guiding principle was translated into action benefitting a particular individual with hoarding behaviour:

> *"We [the community collaborative] have entertained some really creative approaches in terms of dealing with management [i.e., housing manager] and having the client lead those interventions [...] as opposed to, we [the service providers] meet[ing] with management, then... meet[ing] with the client... we really include the client in those interventions, so that the client really is aware of everyone that's involved, what's being discussed and then they are really empowered to be part of the action plan."*

When individuals with hoarding behaviour are more involved in directing their own support, they may experience greater control in such decision making which can lead to empowerment [13]. As observed by another community collaborative member, "[empowerment provides] a sense of control in a situation that they may feel a lack of control."

3.1.5. Communicating Insight into Their Hoarding Behaviour. The most successful reported treatment for those with compulsive hoarding behaviour is the use of behavioural treatment, in other words, a cognitive behavioural model [37]. To be motivated to discard their possessions, insight into their hoarding behaviour is significant [14, 38]. Members of the community collaborative said that individuals with hoarding behaviour seemed to gain insight into their behaviour as a result of the support provided by this collaborative. This observation was expressed during the focus group interview by the social worker:

> *"... the insights that come out as a part of the intervention, as you go along, then they [clients with hoarding behaviour] start to reveal some insight as to "how did I ever get to this place? and, "I can't believe this happened to me" and "I can't believe that I'm actually, I'm making some decisions now that I was not able to before"."*

During an individual interview, one individual with hoarding behaviour reflected on the changes in her own behaviour of accumulating things: "I would still be walking down one little path between the bathroom, bedroom and one side of the kitchen and that would have been it." Another interviewee with hoarding behavior expresses insight into her hoarding behavior: "they [the social worker] finally were able to get me to accept... this condition... that it probably was not my fault and that I could probably face it... it's been a great support... eye opening." And another person said something similar: "when I think how far I came from the first day.... it [my behavior] improved." She also said "I need to continue both thinking about and maybe following up [...] with counseling [...] is there an answer why I have become a person who allows clutter around myself [...]?". In the one-on-one interviews, individuals reported an improved feeling of independence and a sense of empowerment. This occurred because the collaborative team joined forces, they were united by a common goal of supporting, to the best of their ability, the needs of this population who they noticed to be struggling more and more and who they were being called upon more frequently to try to assist.

3.2. Participating in the Community Collaborative Benefitted the Group Members, Individually and Collectively. On individual and collective levels, the members of the community collaborative experienced three significant benefits as a consequence of participating in this group. For example, members of the collaborative were able to access the expertise of other professionals, they maximized the use of their own skills and knowledge and significantly enhanced their understanding of hoarding behaviour.

3.2.1. Accessing Expertise from the Other Group Members. Working on the collaborative team allowed the individual members an opportunity to access a broader range of skills and knowledge than those who were found solely in their own area of expertise or their own organization. In one instance, a professional social worker described how she could now present the risks associated with hoarding behaviour more objectively to a client with greater confidence as she could make reference to and more easily call on the authoritative role of the local fire department. Because the firefighter and social worker were both members of the collaborative, a close working partnership was facilitated. This benefit was expressed in this way: "when I mention to her [the client with compulsive hoarding behavior] the possibility of having someone from [the fire department] come and just do an assessment to let her know what her risk level is [i.e., of eviction from her home], she was suddenly open to that." As a result of working collaboratively, members also got to know more about the professional resources available to them in the community through their ongoing communication together. As one health professional of the community collaborative said: "it is a professional benefit to see and use the expertise around this table for the benefit of the individual clients."

Evaluating collaborative planning practices must consider not just the purpose of the collaboration but the value of its relational interactions [28]. For example, asking how social relations are changed can reveal how certain conditions are impacted for the group. Access to new areas of expertise is one descriptor of the quality of social relations. The sharing of expertise between and amongst the members was said to directly benefit the older people with hoarding behaviour using the services of *This Full House*. In the words of one member of the community collaborative, "a benefit of the collaborative process was working with everybody, to partner, to ensure that we're getting our clients the best support."

3.2.2. Maximizing their Own Expertise. Participating in this group allowed team members to maximize the use of their own expertise. One member, a public health inspector, recounted a time when such a collaborative approach was not used to support older adults with hoarding behaviour illustrating the tremendous limitations of working in isolation:

> *"Before... [the community collaborative existed] it was [up to]... the health inspector to try and play all roles and just sort of go and visit once a week and try and nag people into cleaning up. Which was mostly unsuccessful and wasn't really our job. I mean we are not social workers, we're not mental health workers, we are public health inspectors."*

Functioning alone, the health inspector had to operate as the only contact for this client group. Working in isolation took away time from the job he/she was actually trained and hired to do forcing them to work beyond their professional scope of practice. As further evidence of the value of being able to maximize one's own expertise, the professional organizer, who provides hands-on assistance with the cleanup of client homes, can now maximize her cleaning and organizational skills while directing clients' emotional issues to a trained professional. As described by the social worker during the focus group interview: "A big portion of her [the professional organizer's] time was addressing the [clients] emotional issues. So we've now learned that when those issues come up, it's a direct link back to me."

3.2.3. Enhancing Their Knowledge of Hoarding Behaviour. Members of the community collaborative described how their partnering with one another as professionals helped to enhance their knowledge and understanding of compulsive hoarding behaviour. Gaining new knowledge and a more "enlightened understanding" of compulsive hoarding behaviour was said to be the result of participating in this ongoing process. One member of the collaborative described the value of the increase of his knowledge stating "another professional benefit [of being a member of the community collaborative] is deepening my personal understanding of what hoarding is and what the dynamics are. Certainly, it's helped me in recognizing that it's multi-faceted." Group members said they were then able to take their learning back to their representative organizations: "I think working with [the collaborative] has really helped to educate me and hopefully the rest of [name of organization]." Successful aging in place requires that support by community-based organizations exists that it is available and accessible and responsive to a variety of their needs; therefore, knowledge about aging and its long list of associated issues, such as compulsive hoarding behaviour, is imperative.

4. Discussion

The aim of our discussion is to explain several matters that underpin the major themes of our results. Explaining why such themes evolved and their relationship to the broader phenomenon being studied is what Strauss and Corbin refer to as the process of theorizing [31]. At the heart of this study is community-based planning as a phenomenon of which a number of related concepts are embedded: aging in place, social support, collaboration, vulnerable populations, and community services. Overall, our research attempted to discover how a collaborative approach to planning for and addressing the needs of older adults with hoarding behaviour, living in the community, provided value. For these vulnerable adults living in Edmonton, Alberta, Canada, a collaborative planning approach that involved multiple agencies (representing varying sectors) that worked continuously to improve their quality of life made a difference. And, the members of this community collaborative also benefitted. From this approach they were able to access the professional expertise of the other group members, maximize the use of their own skills and knowledge, overall, giving them an opportunity to generate new insights into hoarding behaviour which they described as helping them provide the best possible care and support to this population. It is feasible; therefore, to use such results to inform the many ways to age in place more successfully in late life.

Currently there is no systemic, long-term process to support older people living in the community that have compulsive hoarding behavior. Nor in Canada, is there an overall strategy to plan for our aging population, therefore aging in place, at a national, political scale, is not yet a priority. But, because people with this behavior will increase in numbers, and the complexities associated with their need to live safely in their own communities, a national strategy must also address their specific and unique needs. As emphasized by The Canadian Health Services Research Foundation [39], our study also finds a need for enhanced integration, cooperation, and coordination at the system and at the service delivery levels. That is, integration and collaboration between health and social services, between ranges of sectors, between disciplines of front line workers, and between government ministries. Collaboration and integration need to be part of the foundation upon which aging in one's own home and community can be realized. In addition, our study supports the findings of Keonig et al. [3] who found that when having to facilitate ethical dilemmas for this population, older adults with hoarding behavior benefit from the use of teams whose members have a variety of disciplines.

Well evidenced in the health services planning literature, applied to an aging population, is the need for improved collaboration, both at a principle and a practice-based level [35]. Our study also confirms and emphasizes this important need. Not only do our findings align with the literature but it provides further insight into the challenges associated with older individuals that want and deserve to remain in their own homes. Our particular case is specific to older individuals that have hoarding behaviour that were supported through the efforts of a community collaborative planning approach. Our study adds to the current aging in place literature and extends it. The current literature supports collaboration and integration at varying levels of the health and social support system. But studies that examine community planning approaches grounded in collaboration are uncommon. This population will increase in numbers over time and they deserve to remain in their own communities with the support of surrounding agencies and organizations that work togather to best support older individuals with hoarding behaviour to age well in their own homes.

5. Conclusions

At the heart of several concepts and themes arising from interviews with older people with compulsive hoarding behavior and members of a community collaborative working to support this population is an approach founded on collaboration between and amongst service providers. Results demonstrated that when a highly collaborative approach to planning is used, there were quite direct benefits for older adults with hoarding behavior and, at the same time, there were benefits for the members of the community collaborative. This approach to planning for the health and social needs of this population resulted in people with hoarding behavior being able to remain in their own homes when eviction was a potential, enhancing their safety, helping to minimize their isolation, and creating opportunities to increase control in their own decision making. The members of the community collaborative could now access the expertise of other professionals, maximize their own expertise, and they generated new insight and understanding of the experience of older adults living with hoarding behaviour in Edmonton. Our study needs to be viewed within certain boundaries. Although our data conveys that this approach to planning has quite positive outcomes, our data is short term and situational. Our use of a single, one-time only interview method only allows us to draw insights and observations about that moment in time and not over an extended trajectory. As well, our study is grounded in five interviews with older adults with compulsive hoarding behavior. And although a collaborative approach to addressing the needs of older people with hoarding behaviour conveyed comprehensive benefits, collaboration as a planning approach is rarely the complete answer or solution to people's social and health needs. Health Integrated Delivery systems, for example, are far more comprehensive but do view collaborative planning as a core principle [2]. Viewed in this light, aging in place may not always be possible, but it must be realized that community-level social and health related supports maximize the quality of later life while aging at home [5]. And further building on that is the need for a well-coordinated model of care [5, 35] where supports are comprehensive, easily accessible, and well connected [5].

Acknowledgments

The authors are grateful to the Seniors Association for Greater Edmonton for helping to facilitate this study. As well, they very much appreciate the individuals with hoarding behaviour and professionals that agreed to participate in an interview. This research was made possible through a University of Alberta, Faculty of Extension Research Grant.

References

[1] S. A. Luchian, R. J. McNally, and J. M. Hooley, "Cognitive aspects of nonclinical obsessive-compulsive hoarding," *Behaviour Research and Therapy*, vol. 45, no. 7, pp. 1657–1662, 2007.

[2] F. Lega, "Organisational design for health integrated delivery systems: theory and practice," *Health Policy*, vol. 81, no. 2-3, pp. 258–279, 2007.

[3] T. Koenig, R. Chapin, and R. Spano, "Using multi-disciplinary teams to address ethical dilemmas with older adults who hoard," *Journal of Gerontological Social Work*, vol. 53, no. 2, pp. 137–147, 2010.

[4] C. Dye, D. Willoughby, and D. Battisto, "Advice from rural elders: what it takes to age in place," *Educational Gerontology*, vol. 37, no. 1, pp. 74–93, 2011.

[5] Institute for Life Course and Aging, *Mapping Aging in Place in a Changing Neighborhood*, University of Toronto, Toronto, Canada, 2008.

[6] A. Bookman, "Innovative models of aging in place: transforming our communities for an aging population," *Community Work and Family*, vol. 11, no. 4, pp. 419–438, 2008.

[7] C. Gale, E Dennison, C. Cooper, and A. Sayer, "Neighbourhood environment and positive mental health in older people: the Hertfordshire Cohort Study," *Health and Place*, vol. 17, no. 4, pp. 867–874, 2011.

[8] R. Stedman, "Toward a social psychology of place: predicting behavior from place-based cognitions, attitude, and identity," *Environment and Behavior*, vol. 34, no. 5, pp. 561–581, 2002.

[9] E. Relph, "Geographical experiences and being-in-the-world: the phenomenological origins of geography," in *Dwelling, Place and Environment*, D. Seamon and R. Mugerauer, Eds., pp. 15–32, Columbia University, New York, NY, USA, 1985.

[10] D. Massey, "The conceptualization of place," in *A Place in the World?* D. Massey and P. Jess, Eds., pp. 45–86, Open University Press, Milton Keynes, UK, 1995.

[11] J. Grisham, R. O. Frost, G. Steketee, H. J. Kim, and S. Hood, "Age of onset of compulsive hoarding," *Journal of Anxiety Disorders*, vol. 20, no. 5, pp. 675–686, 2006.

[12] J. F. Samuels, O. J. Bienvenu, M. A. Grados et al., "Prevalence and correlates of hoarding behaviour in a community-based sample," *Behaviour Research and Therapy*, vol. 46, no. 7, pp. 836–844, 2008.

[13] R. O. Frost, G. Steketee, and L. Williams, "Hoarding: a community health problem," *Health and Social Care in the Community*, vol. 8, no. 4, pp. 229–234, 2000.

[14] R. O. Frost and T. L. Hartl, "A cognitive-behavioral model of compulsive hoarding," *Behaviour Research and Therapy*, vol. 34, no. 4, pp. 341–350, 1996.

[15] R. O. Frost and G. Steketee, *Stuff: Compulsive Hoarding and the Meaning of Things*, Houghton Mifflin Harcourt, Boston, Mass, USA, 2009.

[16] R. O. Frost, H. J. Kim, C. Morris, C. Bloss, M. Murray-Close, and G. Steketee, "Hoarding, compulsive buying and reasons for saving," *Behaviour Research and Therapy*, vol. 36, no. 7-8, pp. 657–664, 1998.

[17] G. Steketee and R. O. Frost, *Compulsive Hoarding and Acquiring: Therapist Guide*, Oxford University Press, New York, NY, USA, 2006.

[18] C. L. Damecour and M. Charron, "Hoarding: a symptom, not a syndrome," *Journal of Clinical Psychiatry*, vol. 59, no. 5, pp. 267–272, 1998.

[19] R. Lindstrom, S. M. MacLeod, and A. Levy, "Twisting the lion's tail: collaborative health policy making in British Columbia," *Healthcare Papers*, vol. 11, no. 2, 2011.

[20] E. A. Henneman, J. L. Lee, and J. I. Cohen, "Collaboration: a concept analysis," *Journal of Advanced Nursing*, vol. 21, no. 1, pp. 103–109, 1995.

[21] M. M. Friend and L. Cook, *Interactions: Collaboration Skills for School Professionals*, Allyn and Bacon, Boston, Mass, USA, 5th edition, 2007.

[22] J. G. Emshoff, A. J. Darnell, D. A. Darnell, S. W. Erickson, S. Schneider, and R. Hudgins, "Systems change as an outcome and a process in the work of community collaboratives for health," *American Journal of Community Psychology*, vol. 39, no. 3-4, pp. 255–267, 2007.

[23] C. A. McAiney, L. M. Hillier, M. Ringland, and N. Cooper, "Getting a bigger bang for your buck: a collaborative approach to enhancing dementia education planning in long-term care homes," *Healthcare Policy*, vol. 5, no. 2, pp. e125–e140, 2009.

[24] F. Capra, *The Web of Life: A New Understanding of Living Systems*, Anchor Books, New York, NY, USA, 1996.

[25] J. Mikkonen and D. Raphael, *Social Determinants of Health: The Canadian Facts*, York University School of Health Policy and Management, Toronto, Canada, 2010.

[26] S. Dieleman, K. Farris, D. Feeny, J. A. Johnson, R. T. Tsuyuki, and S. Brilliant, "Primary health care teams: team members' perceptions of the collaborative process," *Journal of Interprofessional Care*, vol. 18, no. 1, pp. 75–78, 2004.

[27] P. Drew, B. Jones, and D. Norton, "Team effectiveness in primary care networks in Alberta," *Healthcare Quarterly*, vol. 13, no. 3, pp. 33–38, 2010.

[28] P. Healey, "Collaborative planning in perspective," *Planning Theory*, vol. 2, no. 2, pp. 101–123, 2003.

[29] D. Simmons, "This full house: an intervention program to assist elderly compulsive hoarders," 2009, http://www.seniorscouncil.net/uploads/files/This%20Full%20House.pdf.

[30] H. Tsoukas, "Craving for generality and small-N studies: a Wittgensteinian approach towards the epistemology of the particular in organization and management studies," in *The Sage Handbook of Organizational Research Methods*, D. A. Buchanan and A. Bryman, Eds., pp. 285–301, Sage, London, UK, 2009.

[31] A. Strauss and J. Corbin, *Basics of Qualitative Research*, Sage, London, UK, 1998.

[32] C. Rodriguez, L. Panero, and A. Tannen, "Personalized intervention for hoarders at risk of eviction," *Frontline Reports*, vol. 61, no. 2, p. 205, 2010.

[33] K. Johansson, S. Josephsson, and M. Lilja, "Creating possibilities for action in the presence of environmental barriers in the process of 'ageing in place'," *Ageing & Society*, vol. 29, no. 1, pp. 49–70, 2009.

[34] S. J. Rogers and T. Ruefli, "Does harm reduction programming make a difference in the lives of highly marginalized, at-risk drug users?" *Harm Reduction Journal*, vol. 1, pp. 1–7, 2004.

[35] R. Hebert, P. Durand, A. Tournigy, and PRISMA Group, "PRISMA: a new model of integrated service delivery for the frail older people in Canada," *International Journal of Integrated Care*, vol. 3, 2003, http://www.ijic.org/.

[36] S. Fawcett, A. Paine-Andrews, V. T. Francisco et al., "Using empowerment theory in collaborative partnerships for community health and development," *American Journal of Community Psychology*, vol. 23, no. 5, pp. 677–697, 1995.

[37] J. A. Cermele, L. Melendez-Pallitto, and G. J. Pandina, "Intervention in compulsive hoarding: a case study," *Behavior Modification*, vol. 25, no. 2, pp. 214–232, 2001.

[38] T. L. Hartl and R. O. Frost, "Cognitive-behavioral treatment of compulsive hoarding: a multiple baseline experimental case study," *Behaviour Research and Therapy*, vol. 37, no. 5, pp. 451–461, 1999.

[39] Canadian Health Services Research Foundation, "Better with age: health systems planning for the aging population," 2011, http://www.chsrf.ca/.

15

Effects of Gait and Cognitive Task Difficulty on Cognitive-Motor Interference in Aging

Prudence Plummer-D'Amato, Briana Brancato, Mallory Dantowitz, Stephanie Birken, Christina Bonke, and Erin Furey

Department of Physical Therapy, Northeastern University, 360 Huntington Avenue, 6 Robinson Hall, Boston, MA 02115-5000, USA

Correspondence should be addressed to Prudence Plummer-D'Amato, pplummer@neu.edu

Academic Editor: Kirk Erickson

Although gait-related dual-task interference in aging is well established, the effect of gait and cognitive task difficulty on dual-task interference is poorly understood. The purpose of this study was to examine the effect of gait and cognitive task difficulty on cognitive-motor interference in aging. Fifteen older adults (72.1 years, SD 5.2) and 20 young adults (21.7 years, SD 1.6) performed three walking tasks of varying difficulty (self-selected speed, fast speed, and fast speed with obstacle crossing) under single- and dual-task conditions. The cognitive tasks were the auditory Stroop task and the clock task. There was a significant Group × Gait Task × Cognitive Task interaction for the dual-task effect on gait speed. After adjusting for education, there were no significant effects of gait or cognitive task difficulty on the dual-task effects on cognitive task performance. The results of this study provide evidence that gait task difficulty influences dual-task effects on gait speed, especially in older adults. Moreover, the effects of gait task difficulty on dual-task interference appear to be influenced by the difficulty of the cognitive task. Education is an important factor influencing cognitive-motor interference effects on cognition, but not gait.

1. Introduction

Functional community ambulation requires an ability to perform cognitive tasks while walking and an ability to adapt to extrinsic environmental factors that increase the complexity of mobility, such as obstacle avoidance (e.g., curbs) and time-critical tasks (e.g., crossing the street within the time constraints imposed by traffic signals) [1]. A reduced capacity for dual-task walking may limit community mobility. Research has shown that healthy older adults experience significant decrements in gait speed when cognitive tasks are performed while walking [2], a phenomenon referred to as dual-task interference or cognitive-motor interference.

A limitation of the existing research on dual-task interference in aging is that it has focused predominantly on dual-task performance during unobstructed walking at preferred gait speed. Therefore, the effect of dual-task interference on gait and cognitive performance during more attention-demanding gait tasks remains largely unknown. Furthermore, because slowing down during unobstructed walking in the gait laboratory is inconsequential for successful completion of the motor task, individuals may place more importance on performing the cognitive task [3]. Indeed, healthy young and older adults appear to place greater priority on the secondary (nongait) task in many dual-task situations [4, 5]. It seems reasonable to assume that when gait task complexity increases and there is a greater potential threat to stability, individuals would place more importance on completing the gait task safely. The current study explores how gait task difficulty affects cognitive-motor interference.

Bock et al. [4] examined the dual-task costs of performing cognitive and gait tasks of varying difficulty in both young and older adults. The authors concluded that in dual-task conditions, older adults were at greater risk for falls than young adults. However, the effect of task difficulty on dual-task interference was not explicitly analyzed and remains unclear. Numerous studies have examined dual-task effects on gait during obstacle avoidance in older adults [6–15], but none have directly compared the dual-task effects during obstacle negotiation to those during unobstructed walking.

Kelly et al. [16] recently examined the effects of walking task difficulty (usual walking versus narrow-based walking) on dual-task performance in young adults. They found that walking task difficulty affected walking performance but not cognitive performance. Because this study included only dual-task conditions with specific instructions to focus primarily on either the cognitive task or the gait task, it is not known what effect task difficulty has on a person's default prioritization; that is, the way in which the person chooses to allocate his attention in the absence of explicit instruction. Moreover, the study included only young adults, so age-related differences in the effects of task difficulty on dual-task interference are not currently known.

The purpose of this study was to determine the effect of gait and cognitive task difficulty on dual-task interference in healthy young adults and older adults. We specifically compare obstructed and unobstructed gait because of the relevance to community ambulation. We hypothesized that as the difficulty of the gait task increased, attention to gait would increase, resulting in smaller dual-task effects relative to simple walking (unobstructed at self-selected speed). We focus on gait speed as the measure of gait performance in dual-task conditions, since meta-analysis results show that cognitive-motor interference effects across a range of cognitive tasks are prominent in gait speed [2]. Furthermore, because research has shown that dual-task effects on gait vary according to the type of cognitive task [17], we explore our hypothesis in two different cognitive-motor dual-task combinations.

2. Methods

2.1. Participants. Twenty young adults (mean age 21.7 years, range 20–27) and 15 older adults (mean age 72.1 years, range 66–84) were recruited through advertisements at Northeastern University and local senior centers. To be included, participants had to be 18–30 years or older than 65 years, be able to walk independently in the community for at least 50 meters, have intact cognition according to the Mini-Mental State Exam (score > 23), and have normal or corrected-to-normal hearing and vision. Participants were excluded if they had a history of neurological disorders, any orthopedic conditions affecting gait, reported more than 2 falls in the past year, had an acute hospital stay within the last 3 months, or had a lower extremity amputation. Participants who met the selection criteria signed an informed consent form. The study was approved by the Institutional Review Board at Northeastern University.

Demographic information was collected for each participant, including age, gender, and education. Cognitive abilities of the participants were characterized using the Mini-Mental State Exam [18], Digit Substitution Test [19], Stroop Color-Word Interference Test [20], Comprehensive Trail Making Tests [21], and the Activities-specific Balance Confidence (ABC) Scale [22]. Functional mobility was assessed using the Timed Up and Go test (TUG) [23].

2.2. Procedures. Each participant performed three gait tasks and two different cognitive tasks in isolation (single-task conditions) and each gait task in combination with each of the cognitive tasks (dual-task conditions). The cognitive tasks were the auditory Stroop [24] and the "clock task" [25]. In the auditory Stroop task, participants heard the words "high" and "low" spoken in either a high pitch (360 Hz) or a low pitch (180 Hz). The participants were instructed to indicate the pitch of the word they heard (ignoring the actual word presented) by responding verbally "high" or "low" as accurately and as quickly as possible. In the clock task, the participants heard a time (e.g., one-twenty-five) and were required to determine whether the two hands of the clock at the given time were in the same half (left/right) or opposite halves. If the hands were the same half, participants were asked to respond "yes;" if the hands were in opposite halves, the participants were asked to respond "no." There were no clock-task stimuli in which one of the hands was exactly on the twelve or six (e.g., one-thirty). For each task, the participants completed at least two practice blocks of 30 trials while sitting. Single-task performance in each cognitive task was recorded in sitting and was always performed immediately before the dual-task conditions. Both the Stroop and clock tasks were produced using DirectRT (Empirisoft, New York, NY, USA). The stimuli were delivered through wireless headphones and participant responses were recorded through a wireless microphone (Logitech, Newark, CA). For both cognitive tasks, we measured reaction time (in milliseconds) and accuracy (percent of correct responses). Our assumption was that the clock task was more difficult because it required greater cognitive processing.

The three gait tasks were walking at self-selected speed (SS), walking at fastest comfortable speed (FC), and walking at fastest comfortable speed while stepping over an obstacle (OB). The three gait tasks were chosen to provide differing levels of task difficulty. A critical assumption was that walking at fastest comfortable speed was more attention-demanding than walking at preferred (self-selected) speed, and that walking fast and stepping over an obstacle further increased the demands of the task. All gait tasks involved participants walking across a 6.1-meter Platinum GAITRite walkway, which contains pressure activated sensors. The associated software computes spatio-temporal parameters of gait. The participants started and finished each pass 2 meters beyond the end of the walkway so that only steady state gait data were captured. Participants completed 6 passes of the walkway for each condition and the average of the 6 passes was used for analysis. In the OB condition, a 15 cm high hurdle was placed at the 4.5 m mark of the GAITRite walkway. The order of the three gait tasks was randomized, but was performed in the same order for the single-task and the two dual-task (Stroop, clock) blocks. Block order (single, Stroop, clock) was also randomized across participants.

2.3. Measures of Dual-Task Interference. To analyze the effect of task difficulty on dual-task interference, we calculated the dual-task effect (DTE) on both gait speed and cognitive task performance (reaction time and accuracy). Dual-task effects

Table 1: Characteristics (mean, SD) of sample.

Variable	Young adults (n = 20)	Older adults (n = 15)	$P^{\dagger}$
Age	21.7 (1.6)	72.1 (5.2)	<.001
Female gender (number, %)	18 (90%)	12 (80%)	.418
Education (years)	15.3 (0.7)	12.4 (2.0)	<.001
MMSE[a] (max. 30)	28.6 (1.1)	27.5 (2.2)	.080
Activities-specific balance confidence scale (max. 100)	95.8 (4.9)	85.9 (10.9)	.004
Digit symbol copy (time in seconds to complete)	57.4 (6.9)	84.1 (21.0)	.001
Digit symbol substitution (number correct in 90 seconds)	74.2 (9.1)	46.1 (13.2)	<.001
Stroop color-word interference[b]	24.1 (7.5)	35.8 (13.0)	.005
Comprehensive trail-making test interference[c] (seconds)	13.8 (9.7)	35.1 (24.8)	.006
TUG (seconds)	7.4 (0.7)	9.6 (2.4)	.003

† t-test for independent samples.
Abbreviations: MMSE: Mini Mental State Examination; TUG: Timed Up and Go test; P value is for t-test comparing young and older adults.
[a]MMSE measures global cognitive function; Digit symbol modalities test measures speed of processing and attention; Stroop and Trail Making Tests measure executive function; TUG measures balance during functional performance.
[b]Stroop interference score calculated as difference in number correct between baseline condition and interference condition.
[c]Trail-making test interference score calculated as difference in time (seconds) between time to complete Trail 5 and Trail 1.

on gait speed (DTEg) and clock and Stroop-task accuracy (DTEacc) were calculated as follows [16]:

$$\text{DTE} = \frac{(\text{dual task} - \text{single task})}{\text{single task}} \times 100\%. \quad (1)$$

Whereas a decrease in gait speed and accuracy represent performance decrement, an increase in reaction time (i.e., slower response) represents performance decline, therefore DTE on reaction time (DTErt) was calculated as follows [16]:

$$\text{DTE} = \frac{-(\text{dual task} - \text{single task})}{\text{single task}} \times 100\%. \quad (2)$$

Thus, for each variable, negative values for DTE indicate that performance deteriorated under dual-task conditions (i.e., dual-task cost), and positive values represent an improvement in the dual-task condition relative to single-task performance (i.e., dual-task benefit).

2.4. Statistical Analysis. The young and older adults were compared on profile measures using independent t-tests. To verify whether the clock task required greater cognitive processing than the Stroop task, we conducted paired t-tests on mean reaction times for the two tasks in the single-task (sitting) condition for each group. To determine whether participants increased their SS gait speed as instructed in the FC and OB conditions, we analyzed changes in gait speed across conditions with a 3 Gait Task (SS, FC, OB) × 3 Cognitive Task (single, Stroop, clock) ANOVA for each group. Tukey's post hoc tests were used as needed.

To analyze the effects of gait and cognitive task difficulty on dual-task interference, we applied a 3 Gait Task (SS, FC, OB) × 2 Cognitive Task (Stroop, clock) × 2 Group (young, older) repeated measures ANCOVA with education (years) as covariate to each dependent variable (DTEg, DTErt, DTEacc). Significant three-way interactions were followed up with two-way analyses and post hoc tests as needed. The partial eta squared (η_p^2) is presented as a measure of effect size for each repeated measures ANCOVA. By convention, 0.01 indicates a small effect size, 0.06 is moderate, and 0.14 represents a large effect [26]. Due to technical issues three older adults and one young adult were missing gait data from one or more of the gait tasks. Listwise deletion meant that these subjects were excluded from the analyses for gait variables, resulting in minor variations in degrees of freedom. All analyses were performed using SPSS 18.0 (SPSS Inc., Chicago, IL, USA).

3. Results

The young and older adults did not differ in global cognition assessed using the MMSE, but there were significant differences in specific cognitive domains, including executive function, inhibition of habitual response, and speed of processing (Table 1). The older adults also had significantly lower balance self-efficacy and took longer to complete the TUG. However, the differences between the groups on the cognitive and mobility measures were not considered clinically meaningful, since the older adults performed within normal limits for their age [21, 27, 28]. On average, the young adults had more years of education than the older adults (Table 1).

The mean reaction time while sitting (single-task) for the clock task (young adults M = 1403 ms, SD = 271; older adults M = 1889 ms, SD = 433) was significantly longer than that for the Stroop task (young adults M = 805 ms, SD = 109; older adults M = 956 ms, SD = 216) for both young adults, $t(19) = -10.5$, $P < .001$, $d = 2.9$, and older adults, $t(14) = -9.5$, $P < .001$, $d = 2.7$. Thus, consistent with our assumption, the clock task required greater cognitive processing than the Stroop task. In both tasks, mean reaction time of older adults was slower than young adults.

3.1. Task Difficulty and Dual-Task Interference on Gait Speed. The mean gait speeds for young and older adults in each condition and each gait task are shown in Table 2.

TABLE 2: Mean (SD) gait speeds (m/s) for each condition and each gait task. Values are only from the subjects with gait speed data for all conditions.

Gait task	Young adults (n = 19)								Older adults (n = 12)							
	Single-task		Dual-stroop		Dual-clock		Mean		Single-task		Dual-stroop		Dual-clock		Mean	
SS	1.50	(0.17)	1.49	(0.16)	1.46	(0.22)	**1.48**	(0.17)	1.31	(0.29)	1.24[a]	(0.26)	1.28	(0.31)	**1.28**	(0.29)
FC	1.97[b]	(0.21)	1.90	(0.17)	1.90[a,b]	(0.20)	**1.93**[b]	(0.19)	1.51[b]	(0.37)	1.44[b]	(0.39)	1.39[a,b]	(0.36)	**1.44**[b]	(0.37)
OB	1.96[c]	(0.21)	1.88[a,c]	(0.19)	1.87[a,c]	(0.21)	**1.90**[c]	(0.20)	1.42[c,d]	(0.40)	1.32[a,c,d]	(0.36)	1.30[a,d]	(0.36)	**1.35**[d]	(0.37)
Mean	**1.81**	(0.17)	**1.76**[a]	(0.15)	**1.75**[a]	(0.18)	**1.77**	(0.24)	**1.41**	(0.35)	**1.33**	(0.33)	**1.32**[a]	(0.34)	**1.36***	(0.24)

SS: walking at self-selected speed, FC: walking at fastest comfortable speed, OB: walking at fastest comfortable speed with obstacle crossing.
[a]Significant differences between single-task and dual-task (none of the differences between the two dual-tasks were significant), $P \leq .05$ (Tukey's HSD).
[b]Significant differences between self-selected and fast, $P \leq .05$ (Tukey's HSD).
[c]Significant differences between self-selected and fast obstacle, $P \leq .05$ (Tukey's HSD).
[d]Significant differences between fast and fast obstacle, $P \leq .05$ (Tukey's HSD).
*Significant difference between older adults and young adults, $P < .001$.

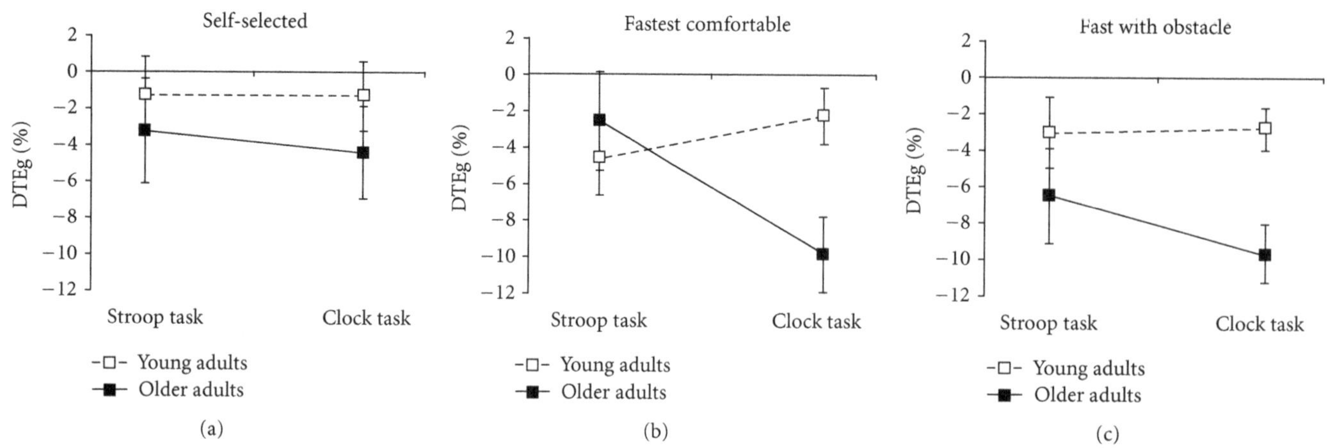

FIGURE 1: Dual-task effects on gait speed (DTEg) shown as a function of cognitive task and group for (a) walking at self-selected speed, (b) walking at fastest comfortable speed, and (c) walking at fastest comfortable speed and stepping over on obstacle. The interaction between cognitive task and group was significant for the fast comfortable walking condition (b), but not for the other two gait tasks. Error bars indicate standard error of the mean. DTEg are adjusted values for education in the Gait Task × Cognitive Task × Group ANCOVA; $n = 19$ young adults, $n = 12$ older adults.

Participants significantly increased their walking speed when instructed to walk at their fastest comfortable speed. Among young adults, there were no significant differences in average gait speed between FC and OB for single-task or dual-task walking (Table 2). However, for older adults, average gait speed in OB was significantly slower than FC (Table 2). Table 2 also illustrates that there were significant declines in gait speed during the Stroop and clock tasks relative to single-task walking in both groups during the obstacle condition. Both groups had a significant reduction in FC walking speed for the clock task but not the Stroop task. In the SS condition, the older adults reduced their gait speed during Stroop but not clock task. Young adults had no significant change in gait speed in either dual-task in SS.

These findings are corroborated by the significant Gait Task × Cognitive Task × Group interaction effect on DTEg, $F(2, 56) = 3.17$, $P = .050$, $\eta_p^2 = .10$. Although the statistical significance was marginal, the effect size was large. Follow up two-way ANCOVAs revealed that the three-way interaction occurred because the Cognitive Task × Group interaction was significant for the FC gait task ($P < .001$; $\eta_p^2 = .39$), but not for SS ($P = .794$; $\eta_p^2 < .01$) or OB ($P = .376$; $\eta_p^2 = .03$) (Figure 1). Specifically, in FC, the dual-task cost (negative DTE) on gait speed for the older adults during the clock task was significantly greater than that of young adults, and was also greater than DTEg during the Stroop task for either group (Figure 1). In SS and OB, there was no effect of cognitive task on DTEg for either group, although Figure 1 shows a tendency for a larger dual-task cost in the clock task in OB among older adults.

3.2. Task Difficulty and Dual-Task Interference on Cognition. Young adults had mean accuracy of 99% (SD 0.01) in the Stroop task and 97.2% (SD 0.1) in the clock task. Older adults, on average, were significantly less accurate than young adults ($P < .001$), with lower mean accuracy in the clock task ($M = 83.6\%$, SD = 0.2) than the Stroop task ($M = 93.1\%$, SD = 0.1) ($P = .045$). Mean values for DTErt and DTEacc for each gait task and cognitive task are presented in Table 3. After adjusting for education, there were no significant main effects or interaction effects in the Gait Task × Cognitive Task × Group ANCOVA on DTErt or DTEacc. As illustrated by the wide confidence intervals in Table 3, there was large variability in the dual-task effects on both reaction time and accuracy for the Stroop and clock tasks.

Education was significantly related to DTEacc in the OB condition ($r = .38$, $P = .026$); lower levels of education were weakly associated with larger dual-task costs in accuracy on the clock task during obstacle crossing. Before adjusting for education, the three-way interaction on DTEacc was significant due to a Gait Task × Cognitive Task interaction for older adults but not young adults: dual-task cost on accuracy was significantly greater in the clock task during OB than in any other task among older adults; the effect was not significant after adjusting for education.

4. Discussion

The purpose of this study was to determine the effect of gait and cognitive task difficulty on dual-task interference in aging. An important finding was that young adults were able to maintain fast walking speed in the obstructed condition with or without a simultaneous cognitive task, whereas older adults could not maintain fast walking speed in the obstructed condition even when no additional cognitive task was required. However, fast-obstacle walking speeds for older adults were still significantly faster than self-selected gait speed during single-task and Stroop task, but not in the clock task. In other words, although older adults reduced their gait speed in the fast-obstructed condition relative to fast-unobstructed walking, they were still able to walk faster than their preferred speed, except when they had to perform the clock task while stepping over the obstacle. This suggests that

Table 3: Adjusted means (95% confidence intervals) for dual-task effects on reaction time (DTErt) and accuracy (DTEacc) for each cognitive task as a function of gait task. Positive values indicate a dual-task benefit relative to single-task; negative values indicate a dual-task cost relative to single-task performance. None of the main effects or interactions in the ANCOVA were significant for DTErt or DTEacc.

	DTErt (%)			DTEacc (%)		
	Self-selected	Fast comfortable	Fast obstacle	Self-selected	Fast comfortable	Fast obstacle
Stroop						
Young	−7.6 (−14.8, −0.4)	−0.5 (−8.1, 7.2)	−1.0 (−8.7, 6.6)	−0.1 (−6.0, 5.7)	−0.7 (−5.9, 4.6)	−0.5 (−5.4, 4.4)
Older	−3.7 (−12.4, 5.0)	−5.2 (−14.5, 4.0)	−4.2 (−13.4, 5.1)	−0.4 (−7.4, 6.7)	−1.2 (−7.5, 5.2)	0.2 (−5.6, 6.1)
Clock						
Young	4.7 (−3.0, 12.5)	18.4 (11.2, 25.7)	11.3 (3.8, 18.7)	−1.6 (−9.7, 6.6)	0.4 (−10.7, 11.5)	−1.8 (−9.4, 5.8)
Older	14.5 (5.1, 23.9)	14.7 (5.9, 23.5)	12.9 (3.8, 21.9)	−4.6 (−14.4, 5.3)	−2.4 (−15.9, 11.0)	−11.3 (−20.6, −2.1)

among older adults the attentional demands of performing a difficult cognitive task interfere with the attention processing requirements of negotiating an obstacle. Indeed, obstacle negotiation requires attention to spatial characteristics of gait in order to adjust strides and avoid hitting the obstacle. It is likely that the older adults slowed down as an adaptive safety strategy to avoid making motor errors when stepping over the obstacle, and that this effect was exaggerated when the added cognitive task demanded greater attentional resources.

Consistent with previous research [17], older adults demonstrated a significant dual-task decline in gait speed during the Stroop task whereas young adults did not. Young adults, however, experienced a significant dual-task decline in gait speed during the Stroop task in the fast-obstacle condition. This finding suggests that in more attention-demanding gait tasks such as obstacle avoidance, a relatively simple cognitive task can impact gait speed, even in healthy young adults. Whereas the Stroop task affected walking speed in the fast-obstructed condition but not the fast-unobstructed condition, the clock task significantly reduced gait speed in both fast-obstructed and fast-unobstructed walking conditions. Thus, more difficult cognitive tasks may amplify dual-task interference in gait speed in easier gait tasks. The three-way interaction on DTEg corroborates the findings for gait speed and provides evidence for differential effects of gait and cognitive task difficulty on cognitive-motor interference during walking between young and older adults.

We hypothesized that increasing the attentional demands of gait would reduce the dual-task costs on gait speed due to increased allocation of attentional resources required for the gait task. In contrast to our hypothesis, there was a tendency for dual-task effects on gait speed to increase with increasing gait task difficulty, although this was only significant for the older adults in the clock task in the FC condition (see Figure 1). It is possible that because we did not instruct the participants where to prioritize their attention during the dual-task conditions, they chose to slow down to optimize safety and/or to maintain performance on the cognitive task. The large variability in the dual-task effects however, especially for cognitive task performance, implies that participants used a range of strategies to perform the dual-tasks. Future research should concentrate on identifying whether personal characteristics influence how individuals spontaneously allocate their attention during gait-related dual-task situations and whether particular subgroups of older adults are vulnerable to the effects of task difficulty.

An important finding from this study was the effect that controlling for education had on the dual-task interference effects on cognition. Analysis of the unadjusted means showed that the dual-task cost on accuracy in the clock task was significantly greater during obstacle avoidance than in any of the other gait conditions, but only for older adults. However, after controlling for between-group differences in education, the Cognitive Task by Gait Task interaction for older adults was no longer significant. The lack of significant interaction effects for cognitive variables after controlling for education suggests that education may play an important role in counteracting dual-task costs on cognitive task performance, especially accuracy. It may be that more education leads to fewer errors in cognitive processing during dual-task walking, regardless of the difficulty of the gait or cognitive task. That is, greater education may increase cognitive reserve and thereby reduce susceptibility to dual-task interference. The idea that education contributes to cognitive reserve, and that increased cognitive reserve can limit clinical expression of cognitive changes is supported by strong evidence from the field of dementia research [29, 30].

Although we tried to simulate the challenges of real-world walking demands by adding elements of speed and obstacle negotiation to our gait tasks, a limitation of this study is that the research was still conducted in a quiet research laboratory. Thus, it remains unknown how real-world environmental factors (e.g., noise, distraction) affect dual-task interference. Furthermore, we assumed a hierarchical increase in gait task difficulty between walking at self-selected speed, walking at fastest comfortable speed, and walking fast while stepping over an obstacle. However, we did not ask the participants of their perceptions of the tasks. Finally, the findings from this study may be limited in their generalizability due to the small sample size and the predominance of women in the sample. Thus, the findings should be viewed as preliminary; investigations involving larger, more representative samples are needed to examine the interactions between age group, gait task difficulty, and cognitive task difficulty on cognitive-motor interference. In the future, manipulating the timing of the onset of the stimulus in the obstacle negotiation path may provide more insight into the interactions between attentional processing associated with obstacle avoidance and the attention processing of an additional cognitive task.

5. Conclusions

In conclusion, the results of this study suggest that obstacle negotiation at fast walking speed, such as when stepping up a curb to avoid traffic, is highly attention-demanding for older adults and significantly compromises the ability to maintain walking speed. This study provides evidence that gait task difficulty influences dual-task effects on gait speed, especially in older adults. Moreover, the effects of gait task difficulty on dual-task interference appear to be influenced by the difficulty of the cognitive task. Education and/or cognitive reserve may be an important factor influencing cognitive-motor interference, especially in terms of performance of the cognitive task.

Acknowledgments

The authors acknowledge the assistance of Colleen Dowd, Kevin Kinnard, and Carole Sullivan. Study funding was provided by Undergraduate Research Grants (Birken, Bonke, Furey) from Northeastern University.

References

[1] A. E. Patla and A. Shumway-Cook, "Dimensions of mobility: defining the complexity and difficulty associated with community mobility," *Journal of Aging and Physical Activity*, vol. 7, no. 1, pp. 7–19, 1999.

[2] E. Al-Yahya, H. Dawes, L. Smith, A. Dennis, K. Howells, and J. Cockburn, "Cognitive motor interference while walking: a systematic review and meta-analysis," *Neuroscience and Biobehavioral Reviews*, vol. 35, no. 3, pp. 715–728, 2011.

[3] A. Shumway-Cook, M. Woollacott, K. A. Kerns, and M. Baldwin, "The effects of two types of cognitive tasks on postural stability in older adults with and without a history of falls," *Journals of Gerontology Series A*, vol. 52, no. 4, pp. M232–M240, 1997.

[4] O. Bock, K. Engelhard, P. Guardiera, H. Allmer, and J. Kleinert, "Gerontechnology and human cognition," *IEEE Engineering in Medicine and Biology Magazine*, vol. 27, no. 4, pp. 23–28, 2008.

[5] V. Weerdesteyn, A. M. Schillings, G. P. van Galen, and J. Duysens, "Distraction affects the performance of obstacle avoidance during walking," *Journal of Motor Behavior*, vol. 35, no. 1, pp. 53–63, 2003.

[6] L. A. Brown, N. C. McKenzie, and J. B. Doan, "Age-dependent differences in the attentional demands of obstacle negotiation," *Journals of Gerontology Series A*, vol. 60, no. 7, pp. 924–927, 2005.

[7] H. C. Chen, A. B. Schultz, J. A. Ashton-Miller, B. Giordani, N. B. Alexander, and K. E. Guire, "Stepping over obstacles: dividing attention impairs performance of old more than young adults," *Journals of Gerontology Series A*, vol. 51, no. 3, pp. M116–M122, 1996.

[8] H. D. Kim and D. Brunt, "The Effect of a dual-task on obstacle crossing in healthy elderly and young adults," *Archives of Physical Medicine and Rehabilitation*, vol. 88, no. 10, pp. 1309–1313, 2007.

[9] L. A. Schrodt, V. S. Mercer, C. A. Giuliani, and M. Hartman, "Characteristics of stepping over an obstacle in community dwelling older adults under dual-task conditions," *Gait and Posture*, vol. 19, no. 3, pp. 279–287, 2004.

[10] C. Harley, R. M. Wilkie, and J. P. Wann, "Stepping over obstacles: attention demands and aging," *Gait and Posture*, vol. 29, no. 3, pp. 428–432, 2009.

[11] J. C. Menant, R. J. St George, R. C. Fitzpatrick, and S. R. Lord, "Impaired depth perception and restricted pitch head movement increase obstacle contacts when dual-tasking in older people," *Journals of Gerontology Series A*, vol. 65, no. 7, pp. 751–757, 2010.

[12] K. C. Siu, L. S. Chou, U. Mayr, P. van Donkelaar, and M. H. Woollacott, "Attentional mechanisms contributing to balance constraints during gait: the effects of balance impairments," *Brain Research*, vol. 1248, pp. 59–67, 2009.

[13] K. C. Siu, L. S. Chou, U. Mayr, P. van Donkelaar, and M. H. Woollacott, "Does inability to allocate attention contribute to balance constraints during gait in older adults?" *Journals of Gerontology Series A*, vol. 63, no. 12, pp. 1364–1369, 2008.

[14] K. C. Siu, V. Lugade, L. S. Chou, P. van Donkelaar, and M. H. Woollacott, "Dual-task interference during obstacle clearance in healthy and balance-impaired older adults," *Aging Clinical and Experimental Research*, vol. 20, no. 4, pp. 349–354, 2008.

[15] P. Plummer-D'Amato, G. Shea, and C. Dowd, "Motor versus cognitive dual-task effects on obstacle negotiation in older adults," *International Journal of Therapy and Rehabilitation*, vol. 19, no. 4, pp. 200–207, 2012.

[16] V. E. Kelly, A. A. Janke, and A. Shumway-Cook, "Effects of instructed focus and task difficulty on concurrent walking and cognitive task performance in healthy young adults," *Experimental Brain Research*, vol. 207, no. 1-2, pp. 65–73, 2010.

[17] P. Plummer-D'Amato, L. J. P. Altmann, and K. Reilly, "Dual-task effects of spontaneous speech and executive function on gait in aging: exaggerated effects in slow walkers," *Gait and Posture*, vol. 33, no. 2, pp. 233–237, 2011.

[18] M. F. Folstein, L. N. Robins, and J. E. Helzer, "The mini-mental state examination," *Archives of General Psychiatry*, vol. 40, no. 7, p. 812, 1983.

[19] A. Smith, *Symbol Digit Modalities Test (SDMT)*, Western Psychological Services, Los Angeles, Calif, USA, 1982.

[20] J. R. Stroop, "Studies of interference in serial verbal reactions," *Journal of Experimental Psychology*, vol. 18, no. 6, pp. 643–662, 1935.

[21] C. R. Reynolds, *Comprehensive Trail Making Test*, Pro-Ed, Austin, Tex, USA, 2002.

[22] L. E. Powell and A. M. Myers, "The activities-specific balance confidence (ABC) scale," *Journals of Gerontology Series A*, vol. 50, no. 1, pp. M28–M34, 1995.

[23] D. Podsiadlo and S. Richardson, "The timed "up and go": a test of basic functional mobility for frail elderly persons," *Journal of the American Geriatrics Society*, vol. 39, no. 2, pp. 142–148, 1991.

[24] K. C. Siu, R. D. Catena, L. S. Chou, P. van Donkelaar, and M. H. Woollacott, "Effects of a secondary task on obstacle avoidance in healthy young adults," *Experimental Brain Research*, vol. 184, no. 1, pp. 115–120, 2008.

[25] P. Plummer-D'Amato, L. J. P. Altmann, D. Saracino, E. Fox, A. L. Behrman, and M. Marsiske, "Interactions between cognitive tasks and gait after stroke: a dual task study," *Gait and Posture*, vol. 27, no. 4, pp. 683–688, 2008.

[26] L. Portney and M. Watkins, *Foundations of Clinical Research: Applications to Practice*, Pearson Education, Upper Saddle River, NJ, USA, 3rd edition, 2009.

[27] S. Joy, D. Fein, E. Kaplan, and M. Freedman, "Speed and memory in WAIS-R-NI digit symbol performance among healthy older adults," *Journal of the International Neuropsychological Society*, vol. 6, no. 7, pp. 770–780, 2000.

[28] T. M. Steffen, T. A. Hacker, and L. Mollinger, "Age- and gender-related test performance in community-dwelling elderly people: six-minute walk test, berg balance scale, timed up and go test, and gait speeds," *Physical Therapy*, vol. 82, no. 2, pp. 128–137, 2002.

[29] L. Fratiglioni and H. X. Wang, "Brain reserve hypothesis in dementia," *Journal of Alzheimer's Disease*, vol. 12, no. 1, pp. 11–22, 2007.

[30] X. Meng and C. D'Arcy, "Education and dementia in the context of the cognitive reserve hypothesis: a systematic review with meta-analyses and qualitative analyses," *PLoS ONE*, vol. 7, no. 6, Article ID e38268, 2012.

16

Food Access Patterns and Barriers among Midlife and Older Adults with Mobility Disabilities

Deborah L. Huang,[1] Dori E. Rosenberg,[2] Shannon D. Simonovich,[3] and Basia Belza[4]

[1] *Veterans Affairs Puget Sound Health Care System, Geriatric Research, Education and Clinical Center (S-182), 1660 South Columbian Way, Seattle, WA 98108, USA*
[2] *Group Health Research Institute, 1730 Minor Avenue, Suite 1600, Seattle, WA 98101, USA*
[3] *Department of Biobehavioral Nursing and Health Systems, School of Nursing, University of Washington, P.O. Box 357266, Seattle, WA 98195, USA*
[4] *Health Promotion Research Center, University of Washington, P.O. Box 357266, Seattle, WA 98195, USA*

Correspondence should be addressed to Deborah L. Huang, huangdx@uw.edu

Academic Editor: Joseph R. Sharkey

We examined where midlife and older adults with a mobility disability accessed food outside the home in King County, Washington, USA, how they travelled to these food destinations, and facilitators and barriers to food access using qualitative interviews. Thirty-five adults aged ≥50 years with a mobility disability (defined as use of an assistive device for mobility) were interviewed. Supplemental objective information was obtained from a Global Positioning System device worn by participants for 3 days. Participants primarily accessed food at grocery stores, restaurants, and coffee shops/cafés. The most common transportation modes were walking, obtaining a ride from friends, motorized chair/scooter, and public transit. Location and proximity of food destinations were factors affecting participants' ability to access these destinations. Adequate space, ease of entry, available amenities such as restrooms, and helpful people were facilitators for participants to access food outside the home.

1. Introduction

The ability to access food is essential to life and health. Food access is defined as "having sufficient resources to obtain appropriate foods for a nutritious diet" and is one dimension of food security (defined as "including both physical and economic access to food that meets people's dietary needs as well as their food preferences") [1]. The prevalence of food insecurity was 7.9% among U.S. households with elderly individuals in 2010 [2]. Difficulty accessing food may negatively affect the nutritional status and health outcomes [3], especially in older adults [4, 5]. Food insecurity was previously reported to be associated with functional impairments in U.S. older adults [6]. Accessing food is a complex process requiring a location to access food, adequate financial and transportation resources, and the cognitive ability to plan and carry out accessing food.

Older adults and adults with a disability may have more difficulty accessing food due to physical limitations [7], inability to drive, financial limitations, and environmental limitations, among other factors. Physical limitations are more common in older age: in 2009, 38.4% of adults ≥65 years reported physical limitations (difficulty in stooping, lifting, reaching, grasping, or walking, but no limitations in carrying out activities of daily living or instrumental activities of daily living) [8], and 60.8% of community-dwelling adults ≥65 years in 2010 reported difficulty with at least one basic action (defined as movement, emotional, sensory [seeing or hearing], or cognitive) [9]. Lower income is also more common in older age and in adults with disability [10]. As these physical and financial limitations increase, environmental limitations may be more difficult to overcome.

Available transportation is another important factor for food access, especially considering that reliance on cars is high in the U.S. [7, 11, 12]; adults may be less likely to drive with increasing age due to disability and cost. An Australian study reported that lack of car access was a barrier to accessing food, and that older adults were more likely to lack car access [11]. Another study of 16 Australian adults reported that they most commonly walked to food shops, but also used several other transportation modes [12]. The built environment (human-made structures, e.g., buildings, roads, etc.) of potential food access destinations may also impair the ability of older adults and adults with mobility disabilities to access food. One study of grocery and convenience stores in Chicago found that while 63% of stores had an accessible entrance, none of the stores met all accessibility criteria [13]. While transportation and accessibility are key concepts in food access research, the perceptions of these characteristics are not well described. To date, there are few studies that explore how the built environment impacts the ability of adults with a mobility disability to access food.

We hypothesize that midlife and older adults with a mobility disability may face difficulty in accessing food. Food access was defined as going outside the home to obtain or consume food. The purposes of this study were to (1) increase understanding of where midlife and older adults with a mobility disability access food; (2) how they travel to food access destinations; (3) facilitators and barriers (including built environment) to accessing food. We undertook a qualitative study using interviews of adults aged ≥50 years with a mobility disability (defined as requiring an assistive device for mobility). Qualitative methods were used due to the lack of available studies about how this population perceives the built environment and to obtain robust descriptions of facilitators and barriers to accessing food. This approach is not frequently used in studying food access.

2. Methods

The Built Environment, Accessibility, and Mobility Study (BEAMS) was a pilot study conducted from October 2010 through September 2011 in King County, Washington, USA. Study procedures were approved by the Institutional Review Board at the University of Washington. The primary goal of BEAMS was to better understand built environment facilitators and barriers to physical activity in midlife and older adults with mobility disability by obtaining their perspectives [14]. Two sets of questions were also asked about utilitarian activities for goods and services, including food destinations. We conducted a qualitative study utilizing in-depth individual interviews in addition to obtaining participant travel information from Global Positioning System (GPS) devices. We chose interviews as the best method to obtain detailed information from study participants about their perceptions of the built environment, since there are few published studies about this topic.

Study eligibility criteria were as follows: age ≥50 years, use an assistive device for mobility, leave home ≥3 days/week, reside in King County, Washington, speak and read English, and allow study researchers to visit their residence. Our target study enrollment was 25–40 participants with the goal of reaching theme saturation (i.e., no additional new themes or concepts are generated from additional participant interviews) [15]. Participants were purposefully recruited through study announcements in relevant organizational e-newsletters (e.g., senior center newsletters, Arthritis Foundation), as well as flyers distributed at senior centers, community events and other locations where older adults meet. Additionally, we recruited participants with a range of disability types, who used different assistive devices, and resided in diverse types of neighborhoods (e.g., walkability, income) in order to obtain a variety of perspectives.

Individuals who were interested in the study, met eligibility criteria, and gave verbal consent to participate were mailed a written consent form, GPS device (Qstarz BT-Q1000XT, Qstarz International Co., Ltd., Taipei, Taiwan), GPS instructions for use, and a prepaid return envelope. Participants wore a GPS device for 3 days (2 weekdays and 1 weekend day) prior to their interview to acquire objective information about where participants travelled to destinations. The home interview was conducted after the signed consent form and GPS device were returned by mail. Prior to the interview, study researchers printed color maps from the GPS device to serve as interview prompts.

Semistructured interviews were conducted at participant homes by two study researchers. One researcher interviewed the participant, while the other researcher took detailed notes using a laptop computer. The interviewer was in the participant's direct sight line, while the researcher taking notes sat to the side. Interviewers had a Bachelor's degree or higher in a health-related field (e.g., nursing, clinical psychology) and underwent a minimum of 5 hours of training, which included practicing with the interview protocol, conducting a formal practice interview with observation and feedback from the principal investigators (D. E. Rosenberg, B. Belza), and observing one of the primary investigators conduct an interview. The note takers were trained to use an Excel template in which they could quickly and easily fill in responses to each item of the interview guide. This training included being observed and provided with feedback during at least one-structured-practice interview session.

The interview protocol consisted of open-ended questions about facilitators and barriers to (1) accessing and using destinations while using the GPS device (up to 3 locations were discussed); (2) accessing utilitarian locations (e.g., grocery stores, shops) in the neighborhood (up to 10 locations discussed); (3) use of indoor and outdoor physical activity locations in the neighborhood (interview protocol available upon request from D.R.). In addition to assessing barriers and facilitators, we asked participants what transportation mode they used to travel to each location visited while wearing the GPS device. Immediately upon completion of the interview, the two study researchers who conducted the home visit debriefed about the interview and each confirmed the interview notes' content and accuracy.

Additional participant demographic and background data collected with a self-reported, written survey were age, race/ethnicity, checklist of health conditions, and checklist of assistive devices used. Census 2000 data were used to determine median household income at the census tract level. (Census tracts are small statistical subdivisions of counties with 2,500–8,000 persons, which are "designed to be homogeneous with respect to population characteristics, economic status, and living conditions." [16]). Census 2000 data were the most current census data available during the study period. Neighborhood walkability scores were generated using walkscore.com. Walkability is a measure of how easy it is to walk and live in an area [17]. Walkscore may be used to estimate proximity to walkable destinations [18]; scores range from 0 to 100 with higher scores signifying greater walkability. The U.S. Department of Agriculture's Food Desert Locator [19] was used to determine whether any study participants lived in food deserts. Food deserts are defined as "a low-income census tract [poverty rate ≥20% or median family income ≤80% of area's median family income] where a substantial number or share of residents has low access to a supermarket or large grocery store [≥500 people and/or ≥33% of census tract's population resides >1 mile from a supermarket or large grocery store]" [19].

For the purpose of this study, typed interview notes were specifically analyzed pertaining to accessing food outside the home. Content analysis (i.e., analyzing themes and concepts) was used to develop a start list of codes [20] using an inductive reasoning approach after review of the interview notes. Codes pertained to participants' reports of where they accessed food outside their home, how they travelled to food access destinations, their reasons for visiting food access destinations, and their perceptions of the indoor built environment at food access destinations. These codes were subcategorized into facilitators and barriers to accessing food destinations. Two study researchers (D. L. Huang, D. E. Rosenberg) reviewed the start list of codes and achieved consensus. As new themes were introduced by participants, codes were further refined during coding using both inductive and deductive reasoning approaches. An audit trail tracking the decision-making process was kept throughout the coding process. Coding was performed by two study team members (D. L. Huang, D. E. Rosenberg) and results were discussed to determine consensus for final coding. We achieved theme saturation as well as interrater agreement in coding. Descriptive analyses of demographic data and assistive device use were performed using SPSS version 19 (IBM, Armonk, NY, USA).

3. Results

Thirty-five participants were interviewed. Characteristics of study participants are shown in Table 1. Participants had a mean age of 66.8 years, were predominantly female and Caucasian, and used a variety of mobility assistive devices (some participants used more than one assistive device). The majority of participants reported not driving. Two participants lived in food deserts [19], and four participants lived in retirement facilities that provided food on-site in a dining room. These facilities were not counted as an out-of-home location or place to obtain food for home consumption.

TABLE 1: Characteristics of study participants (n = 35).

Characteristic	Value
Age in years, mean ± SD (range)	66.8 ± 9.4 (50–86)
Sex, n (%)	
Male	9 (25.7)
Female	26 (74.3)
Race/ethnicity, n (%)	
Caucasian	30 (85.7)
African-American	2 (5.7)
Asian	1 (2.9)
≥1 race	1 (2.9)
Walkscore, mean (range)	67 (18–98)
Household income, median (range)	\$46,199 (\$25,821–\$94,179)
Reside in low-income (< \$35,000) census tract, n (%)	9 (25.7)
Reside in food desert, n (%)	2 (5.7)
Participants living in facilities that provide meals, n (%)	4 (11.4)
Type of assistive device, n (%)	
Cane	20 (57.1)
Walker (2- or 4-wheeled)	20 (57.1)
Electric wheelchair or scooter	9 (25.7)
Manual wheelchair	7 (20)
Other	4 (11.4)
Participants who drive, n (%)	7 (20)

3.1. Types of Food Access Locations. Participants accessed a variety of locations to obtain food (Figure 1). Grocery stores were the most commonly accessed out-of-home food location by study participants. Several participants reported accessing 2 or more different grocery stores. Participants also visited food banks, warehouse stores, farmers markets, convenience stores, corner stores, and drugstores to obtain food (see Figure 1 for the number of participants who reported going to various types of food locations). Destinations accessed for food consumed outside the home included restaurants (both full-service and fast food), cafés/coffee shops, senior centers, and shopping malls. Most participants went to more than one type of destination to access food. Participants who lived in facilities that provided on-site meals also accessed food outside the home at locations such as grocery stores and restaurants. Three participants reported that family members regularly brought food to their homes (e.g., family purchased groceries for participant).

3.2. Types of Transportation to Food Access Destinations. Transportation used by participants included active (e.g., walking) and passive (e.g., using a motorized chair or scooter, paratransit) modes to access food locations (Figure 1). The majority of participants reported using one transportation mode, but others reported using 2 or more modes of transportation to access food. These participants used combinations of walking, public transit, paratransit, rides from friends or family, and vans or shuttle services provided either by their residence or an organization (e.g., senior center).

3.3. Factors Impacting Choice of Food Destinations. Reasons for visiting (or not visiting) food access destinations were categorized into three major themes: destination factors,

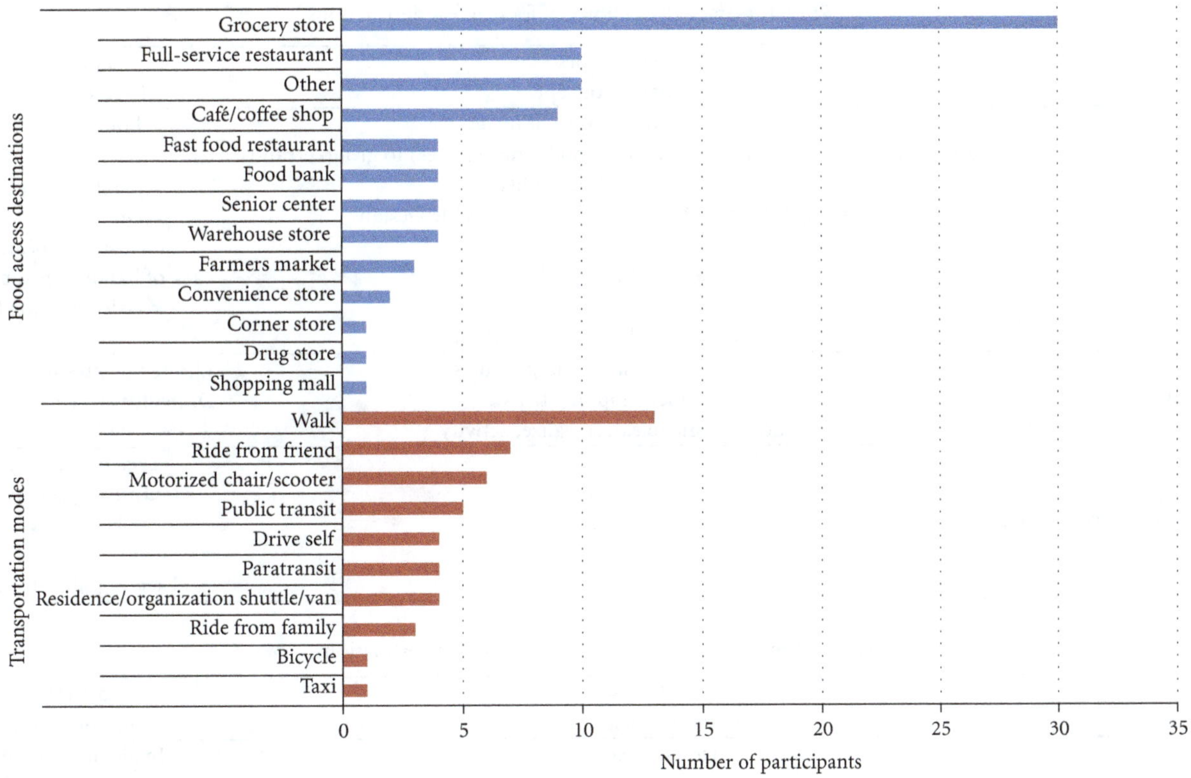

FIGURE 1: Counts of food access destinations and transportation modes used by study participants.

participant factors, and outdoor built environment (Table 2). Barriers to accessing food destinations included all three themes; facilitators to access included destination and participant factors.

3.3.1. Destination Factors. Location and proximity were frequent destination factor subthemes. Some participants reported visiting food destinations because of their proximity to other locations with goods and services, such as drugstores and banks. Cost was another common subtheme of destination factors: participants chose where they shopped for groceries and ate meals outside the home (e.g., restaurants, senior centers) based on cost.

3.3.2. Participant Factors. Subthemes included participants' preference for certain stores, usually based on product availability and selection. Some participants also reported going to food access destinations in order to socialize and stay active.

3.3.3. Outdoor Built Environment. Outdoor built environment characteristics were primarily perceived as (1) barriers to accessing certain food destinations and (2) transportation barriers to food destinations. These included lack of sidewalks, obstructed roads (e.g., parked vehicles, construction), hills and lack of public transit to food destinations.

3.4. Facilitators and Barriers of Food Access Destinations. Four themes emerged as key facilitators and barriers for visiting food access locations (Table 3). These included (1) space, (2) entry/accessibility, (3) amenities, (4) people.

3.4.1. Theme 1: Space. This theme included participants' general perceptions of (a) adequacy of space to carry out their intended activity (e.g., grocery shopping, drinking coffee at a coffee shop) while using a mobility assistive device, (b) ease or difficulty navigating the destination, and (c) general destination features. Participants reported that wide, unobstructed aisles facilitated shopping in grocery stores, while a common barrier was narrow aisles. Obstructed aisles, including displays in aisles and other shoppers' carts, were also commonly reported barriers to navigating grocery stores. Other examples of barriers included crowds and closely spaced tables and chairs at restaurants. Additional facilitators to navigating food destinations included elevators to access different floors, no stairs (destination on a single level), and stable product layouts. Built environment barriers to navigating destinations included escalators or stairs to access different floors, small elevators, changes in product layouts (e.g., items periodically moved to different locations in store), a large number of store aisles, and poor signage. General features that participants reported to be facilitators included clean flooring (slippery or uneven flooring were barriers), adequate light, and whether the destination followed the American with Disabilities Act Standards for Accessible Design.

3.4.2. Theme 2: Entry/Accessibility. Ease of entry to the food destination was a common theme among participants.

TABLE 2: Factors impacting choice of food access destinations.

Factors	Facilitators Theme/concept	Barriers Theme/concept
Location	Close proximity/ease of travel Proximity to other locations (e.g., other goods and services) to group errands Lower cost/affordability Facility follows ADA Standards for Accessible Design Larger size of location Product availability and selection	Long distance Higher cost Difficult entry Small size of location Lack of handicapped parking Crowded parking lot
Participant	Preference for store and products Smaller shopping trips Leave home to eat, socialize, activity	Limited by product selection Difficulty carrying purchases
Outdoor built environment		Lack of sidewalks Obstructed roads Highways Hills Lack of public transit

TABLE 3: Facilitators and barriers of food access destinations.

Theme	Facilitators Concept/theme	Barriers Concept/theme
Space	Adequate space Ease of navigation Helpful general features	Inadequate space Navigation difficulty Unhelpful general features
Entry/accessibility	Ease of entering destination	Difficulty entering destination
Amenities	Seating available Restrooms Drinking fountains Shopping cart as assistive device for mobility Availability of electric shopping carts	Seating unavailable Restroom features inadequate Lack of electric shopping carts
People	Good service Helpful family, friends, and caregivers	Poor/suboptimal service Inattentive fellow customers

Doors and entries were the two subthemes. Facilitators were automatic doors, lightweight doors, entries that were conveniently located, flat, at street level, and without an entry ramp or stairs. Barriers were heavy doors, doors that opened outward, two sets of entry doors, raised thresholds and door mats, poorly located entries, and the presence of stairs. One participant reported that an entry ramp was a barrier, because it was difficult to simultaneously open the entry door and control her assistive device on the ramp.

3.4.3. Theme 3: Amenities. A number of participants reported using shopping carts as an assistive device for support and mobility in stores. Participants also stated that the availability of electric shopping carts was a facilitator to food shopping and the lack of these carts was a barrier. Participants reported availability of seating and accessible restrooms as facilitators for accessing and utilizing food destinations. Lack of available seating to rest was a barrier. Seat height (which affects the ability to sit down and rise from seating) and space to sit with an assistive device were subthemes. Accessible restrooms with adequate space and doors that were easy to open were facilitators for use. Restrooms without accessibility features were reported as barriers to use. One participant specifically mentioned poor placement of grab bars affected his ability to transfer to and from the toilet, as well as urinals not designed for those using wheelchairs. An additional amenity facilitator was the availability of accessible drinking fountains.

3.4.4. Theme 4: People. The major theme was quality of service given by food access destination staff/employees. Poor or suboptimal service was reported by a few participants, though typically not at grocery stores: one participant reported rude volunteers at a food bank. Examples of suboptimal service included long waiting times for service and unavailability of table service. One participant mentioned avoiding certain food destinations because table service was not available; she preferred going to destinations with table service due to difficulty carrying food to a table while using an assistive device. Good service was a facilitator reported by several participants, which included destination staff/employees, and paratransit and shuttle service drivers. Examples of good service included assistance with bringing groceries to the participant's vehicle, reaching items on high shelves, and opening doors. Some participants reported visiting certain grocery stores because employees knew them. Another theme noted was having helpful family, friends, or caregivers to access food destinations (facilitator); inattentive fellow customers were a barrier. One participant mentioned nearly being knocked over by another customer's shopping cart.

4. Discussion

Midlife and older adults with mobility disability in our study accessed a variety of food destinations and utilized several different modes of transportation to these destinations. Many participants accessed more than one type of food destination and used more than one transportation mode. This included participants who lived in facilities that provided on-site meals; these participants also obtained groceries from facility "field trips" to grocery stores or from family members who brought groceries to their home. Additionally, many of those who accessed grocery stores reported going to more than one store. This demonstrates how our study participants adapted to carrying out these instrumental activities of daily living (shopping and transportation), despite their mobility and transportation limitations. While most participants used passive forms of transport (e.g., by automobile) to food destinations, thirteen participants reported walking to food destinations. This indicates that having food locations in proximity to where older adults live can promote physical activity as well as food access among people with mobility disabilities. An interesting concept that was not fully captured in these interviews was the amount of time some participants spent accessing food. For example, some participants reported devoting a certain day of the week to obtain food; one participant reported regularly visiting more than one food bank.

Location and proximity of food access destinations were important factors for our study participants. Interestingly, some participants reported accessing food in combination with carrying out other utilitarian activities such as going to the bank or to the doctor. One participant reported that she preferred to visit the grocery stores near a senior center (not in her neighborhood), because it was close to several other locations with goods and services. The two participants who lived in food deserts also spoke about the importance of location and proximity of food access destinations. Cost was another important factor for study participants in determining where they chose to access food. This is not surprising given that older adults are more likely to have a fixed income. Some participants also reported travelling farther from their residence to access food at a lower-cost destination. Preference for certain food access destinations was also important, but location, proximity, and cost seemed to carry greater weight in where our study participants chose to access food.

The perceived indoor built environment barriers and facilitators pertained to adequate space, ease of accessing multiple levels at destinations, ease of entry, and available amenities at food access destinations. Door features were frequently noted by our study participants, particularly doors that were difficult to open due to heavy weight and location (e.g., located at top of entry ramp). Amenities such as available seating and accessible restrooms were also important to participants. An interesting nonbuilt environment finding was the impact of helpful people on accessing food destinations. Participants appreciated friendly employees at these destinations and availability of extra assistance. Additionally, participants liked the extra help they received from paratransit and shuttle/van drivers. For example, one participant reported that the van driver for a senior center carried her groceries from the store to the van and from the van to her home.

Our findings must be couched within the context of the study limitations. A limitation of our study was that we did not audio record and transcribe the interviews due to participant concerns. Early in the recruitment process, our target population voiced concerns about being audio recorded. Many participants received government assistance for housing and transportation, and were concerned about the potential implications of being audio recorded for receiving these benefits. However, the credibility of our findings was enhanced by our training procedures for both interviewing and taking interview notes. In addition, the coders achieved consensus during the coding process even with their differing levels of interview involvement (D.H. was not involved in participant interviews, D. E. Rosenberg either conducted or took notes for approximately one-third of the interviews) and their different disciplinary backgrounds (geriatric medicine, clinical psychology, and public health).

An additional limitation of this study was that BEAMS' primary focus was to understand the impact of built environment on physical activity, though participants were interviewed about utilitarian activities (including food access). This likely influenced the depth of participant responses about food access, though accessing food was a topic initiated by many of our study participants. However, accessing food was one of the most important utilitarian activities that our participants needed to accomplish, and food locations were the most common destination visited while participants wore the GPS device. This finding must be cautiously interpreted given that 3 days is a relatively short time period to monitor mobility, but it illustrates the importance of addressing food access among this population of midlife and older adults with mobility disabilities. Other limitations of the study include that we specifically recruited participants who leave their homes at least 3 days per week, so we did not obtain the perspectives of those who are home-bound and likely face additional challenges to accessing food. Additionally, our participants were fairly culturally homogeneous (predominantly Caucasian and female).

The key strengths of our study are that it provides insightful information about where midlife and older adults with mobility disability accessed food, how they travelled to these destinations, reasons for accessing particular food destinations, and their perceptions of the indoor built environment and other factors at these destinations. Our use of qualitative methods allowed us to obtain information that would be otherwise difficult to capture using other research methods. Our findings are difficult to compare to previous studies, because these studies have not examined the types of destinations older adults with disabilities access for food, or many of the facilitators or barriers to food access. Since there is a lack of previous studies available about this topic, we feel our findings provide useful information.

Accessing food is essential to life and can become more difficult with older age and mobility disability. Consideration needs to be given to how our aging population will access food, principally where grocery stores are located and proximity to different modes of transportation (especially public transit where available). Urban planning should particularly consider proximity of food access destinations to other destinations with goods and services, as this may help older adults continue to live independently in the community. Attention to easy pedestrian access (e.g., short, well-marked, and protected routes) would facilitate visiting multiple destinations. Food access destinations should also take into account the needs of this population, especially the need for adequate space and ease of entry while using an assistive device. Future studies should include determining how food access can be better understood and improved in order to prepare for the growing population of adults aging with a mobility disability. Improved understanding of how the types of food destinations relate to caloric intake and diet quality among older adults with mobility disabilities would also be helpful for future research efforts. Overall, further research of maintaining food access for adults aging with mobility disability would ideally impact public policy, urban planning, and businesses to help older adults function and thrive in their communities.

Funding

This work was supported by the CDC Prevention Research Centers Program, through a Grant to the University of Washington Health Promotion Research Center (cooperative agreement no. U48-DP001911), The Built Environment, Accessibility and Mobility Study, Basia Belza and Dori Rosenberg, coprincipal investigators. This material is the result of work supported by resources from the VA Puget Sound Health Care System in Seattle, WA. Dr. D. L. Huang receives salary support from the Department of Veterans Affairs Advanced Fellowship in Geriatrics. The contents of this paper are the responsibility of the authors and do not necessarily represent the official view of the funders.

Acknowledgments

The authors thank Abinnet Ainalem, Steven Simpkins, and Amy Tseng for their assistance with recruitment and data collection. Results of this paper were presented at the American Geriatrics Society Annual Scientific Meeting, Seattle, WA, in May 2012.

References

[1] World Health Organization, "Food security," 2012, http://www.who.int/trade/glossary/story028/en/.

[2] Economic Research Service, "Food Security in the United States: Key Statistics and Graphs," Washington, DC: U.S. Department of Agriculture, 2012, http://www.ers.usda.gov/Briefing/FoodSecurity/stats_graphs.htm.

[3] M. Ahern, C. Brown, and S. Dukas, "A national study of the association between food environments and county-level health outcomes," *Journal of Rural Health*, vol. 27, no. 4, pp. 367–379, 2011.

[4] J. S. Lee and E. A. Frongillo, "Nutritional and health consequences are associated with food insecurity among U.S. Elderly persons," *Journal of Nutrition*, vol. 131, no. 5, pp. 1503–1509, 2001.

[5] J. S. Lee and E. A. Frongillo Jr., "Understanding needs is important for assessing the impact of food assistance program participation on nutritional and health status in U.S. elderly persons," *Journal of Nutrition*, vol. 131, no. 3, pp. 765–773, 2001.

[6] J. S. Lee and E. A. Frongillo Jr., "Factors associated with food insecurity among U.S. elderly persons: importance of functional impairments," *Journals of Gerontology. Series B, Psychological Sciences and Social Sciences*, vol. 56, no. 2, pp. S94–S99, 2001.

[7] W. S. Wolfe, E. A. Frongillo, and P. Valois, "Understanding the experience of food insecurity by elders suggests ways to improve its measurement," *Journal of Nutrition*, vol. 133, no. 9, pp. 2762–2769, 2003.

[8] Centers for Disease Control and Prevention (CDC), "National Center for Health Statistics. Health Data Interactive," 2012, http://www.cdc.gov/nchs/hdi.htm.

[9] National Center for Health Statistics, "Health, United States, 2010: With Special Feature on Death and Dying. Hyattsville, MD," http://www.cdc.gov/nchs/data/hus/hus10.pdf#054, 2011.

[10] C. Denavas-Walt, B. D. Proctor, and J. C. Smith, "Income, poverty, and health insurance coverage in the United States: 2010," Current Population Reports P60-239, U.S. Census Bureau, Washington, DC, USA, 2011, http://www.census.gov/prod/2011pubs/p60-239.pdf.

[11] C. Burns, R. Bentley, L. Thornton, and A. Kavanagh, "Reduced food access due to a lack of money, inability to lift and lack of access to a car for food shopping: a multilevel study in Melbourne, Victoria," *Public Health Nutrition*, vol. 14, no. 6, pp. 1017–1023, 2010.

[12] J. Coveney and L. A. O'Dwyer, "Effects of mobility and location on food access," *Health and Place*, vol. 15, no. 1, pp. 45–55, 2009.

[13] M. C. Mojtahedi, P. Boblick, J. H. Rimmer, J. L. Rowland, R. A. Jones, and C. L. Braunschweig, "Environmental barriers to and availability of healthy foods for people with mobility disabilities living in urban and suburban neighborhoods," *Archives of Physical Medicine and Rehabilitation*, vol. 89, no. 11, pp. 2174–2179, 2008.

[14] D. E. Rosenberg, D. L. Huang, S. D. Simonovich, and B. Belza, "Outdoor built environment barriers and facilitators to activity among midlife and older adults with mobility disabilities," *The Gerontologist*. In press.

[15] M. Sandelowski, "Sample size in qualitative research.," *Research in Nursing & Health*, vol. 18, no. 2, pp. 179–183, 1995.

[16] U. S. Census Bureau, "Census tracts and block numbering areas," Tech. Rep., U.S. Department of Commerce, Washington, DC, USA, 2000, http://www.census.gov/geo/www/cen_tract.html.

[17] Federal Highway Administration, "A resident's guide for creating safe and walkable communities," Tech. Rep., U.S.

Department of Transportation, Washington, DC, USA, 2012, http://safety.fhwa.dot.gov/ped_bike/ped_cmnity/ped_walk-uide/about.cfm.

[18] L. J. Carr, S. I. Dunsiger, and B. H. Marcus, "Validation of Walk Score for estimating access to walkable amenities," *British Journal of Sports Medicine*, vol. 45, no. 14, pp. 1144–1148, 2011.

[19] Economic Research Service, "About the food desert locator," Tech. Rep., U.S. Department of Agriculture, Washington, DC, USA, 2011, http://www.ers.usda.gov/Data/FoodDesert/about.html#Defined.

[20] M. B. Miles and A. M. Huberman, *Qualitative Data Analysis: an Expanded Sourcebook*, Sage Publications, Thousand Oaks, Calif, USA, 2nd edition, 1994.

17

The Impact of Body Mass Index and Weight Changes on Disability Transitions and Mortality in Brazilian Older Adults

Flávia Cristina Drumond Andrade,[1] Ahmad Iqmer Nashriq Mohd Nazan,[2] Maria Lúcia Lebrão,[3] and Yeda Aparecida de Oliveira Duarte[4]

[1] *Department of Kinesiology and Community Health, University of Illinois at Urbana-Champaign, 1206 South 4th Street, Champaign, IL 61820, USA*

[2] *Zilber School of Public Health, University of Wisconsin-Milwaukee, 1240 N. 10th Street, Milwaukee, WI 53205, USA*

[3] *School of Public Health, Departament of Epidemiology, University of São Paulo, Avenida Dr. Arnaldo, 715 Pinheiros, 01246-904 São Paulo, SP, Brazil*

[4] *School of Nursing, Department of Medical-Surgical Nursing, University of São Paulo, Avenida Dr. Enéas de Carvalho Aguiar, 419 3o. andar, Sala 318, Cerqueira Cesar, 05403-000 São Paulo, SP, Brazil*

Correspondence should be addressed to Flávia Cristina Drumond Andrade; fandrade@illinois.edu

Academic Editor: Heather Keller

The aim of this study was to examine the association between body mass index and weight changes on disability transitions and mortality among Brazilian older adults. Longitudinal data from the Health, Well-Being, and Aging in Latin America and the Caribbean Study conducted in São Paulo, Brazil (2000 and 2006), were used to examine the impact of obesity on disability and mortality and of weight changes on health transitions related to disability. Logistic and multinomial regression models were used in the analyses. Individuals who were obese were more likely than those of normal weight to have limitations on activities of daily living (ADL), instrumental activity of daily living (IADL), and Nagi's limitations. Obesity was associated with higher incidence of ADL and IADL limitations and with lower recovery from Nagi's limitations. Compared to those who maintained their weight, those who gained weight experienced higher incidence of ADL and Nagi's limitations, even after controlling for initial body mass index. Higher mortality among overweight individuals was only found when the reference category was "remaining free of Nagi limitations." The findings of the study underline the importance of maintaining normal weight for preventing disability at older ages.

1. Introduction

Brazil is among the 25 countries in the world with the fastest aging rates [1, 2]. In 1950, 2.6 million (4.9%) Brazilians were older than 60 years of age, and this number has increased to 20.6 million people (10.8%) according to the 2010 census [3]. Improvements in medical care and living standards have been shown to translate into higher life expectancy. In 1950, for example, life expectancy at birth in Brazil was 50.9 years, but the figure increased to 72.2 years in 2010 [3]. However, the number of disabled people is expected to increase in the coming years, given the rapid growth rate of the elderly population and the rise in the prevalence of obesity and chronic diseases [4].

Fast changes in the population's nutritional intake that have occurred in Brazil in recent decades [5] have resulted in an increase in the prevalence of obesity [6, 7]. In the past three decades, obesity rates in Brazil tripled among men and almost doubled among women [6]. With the exception of higher-income urban women [8], the prevalence of obesity is higher among women than among men.

Few studies focus on the impact of BMI on mortality and disability in the Latin American and the Caribbean (LAC) region. Based on the baseline for the Health, Well-Being, and Aging in Latin America and the Caribbean Study (SABE), Al Snih and colleagues [4] showed that obese individuals were 1.6 times more likely to face difficulties performing activities of daily living (ADL) than those with normal BMI [4]. Corona and colleagues [9] found that older adults who were underweight (BMI ≤ 23 kg/m^2) and obese (BMI ≥ 30 kg/m^2) were more likely to develop limitations on instrumental activity of daily living (IADL), but their analysis did not explore BMI associations with mortality or recovery from disability. Monteverde and colleagues [10] found that, based on relative cutoffs (quintiles), heavier older adults in Mexico face higher mortality risks than those in the United States. However, when BMI was categorized following the traditional World Health Organization cutoffs, no excess mortality was found among overweight and obese subjects [10]. In fact, coefficients for overweight and obesity were not in the expected direction [10]. However, none of these studies jointly examined the association between BMI, disability transitions, and mortality. This paper addresses this gap in the literature. We examine the association between body mass index and weight changes on disability transitions and mortality.

1.1. Association between BMI and Disability. Obesity has been associated with higher prevalence of disability in cross-sectional and longitudinal studies [4, 11–13]. This positive association has been found among middle- and older-aged adults [13–15], and it appears that this association has not changed over time [16, 17]. Additionally, the association between body mass index (BMI) and disability is strongest among those who are underweight (BMI < 18.5 kg/m^2) and among obese subjects (BMI > 30 kg/m^2) [4, 11]. Obese women face higher prevalence of mobility impairment than men [13]. In the United States, severe functional limitations are higher among older adults who gain or lose weight after age 50 compared to those with stable weight [18]. Emerging evidence supports the proposition that BMI is an important predictor of the onset of mobility limitations [13]. Older adults in the United States who gain weight over time have higher incidence of mobility limitations than those who maintain their weight [19].

1.2. Association between BMI and Mortality. Large systematic reviews have shown that the relationship between BMI and mortality seems to follow a J-shaped (sometimes U-shaped) curve [17, 20–22]. All-cause mortality appears to be lowest at BMI levels between 20 and 24.9 kg/m^2 [20, 22], with obese individuals facing higher mortality risks than their normal-weight counterparts [20, 22, 23]. Recent studies, however, show that overweight individuals have higher life expectancy than individuals of normal weight or those who are obese [12], whereas other studies have an L-shape (see [24], for a short review). Higher mortality at low levels of BMI has been associated primarily with lung cancer and respiratory diseases [22]. At older ages, results from a systematic review and meta-analysis indicated that BMI in the overweight range of 25–29.9 kg/m^2 is not associated with increased mortality [25], whereas other studies have shown that the burden of obesity on mortality seems to be reduced or eliminated among older adults [11, 12, 26–30].

The use of BMI categories has been criticized for not reproducing well the complexities of the BMI and mortality relationship [31–33]. These authors have suggested that the use of alternative models to assess this association. Gronniger [33] used semiparametric models and found that men in the mild-obese category (BMIs of 30–35 kg/m^2) had similar mortality than those of normal weight, but among women BMI levels above 27 kg/m^2 were associated with higher mortality in the U.S. Wong and colleagues [31] used multivariable fractional polynomials to explore the association between BMI and mortality in a sample of adults in the UA They found that the best fitting model contained the powers −1 and −2 for BMI [31]. Their results indicated that the nadir of the BMI mortality curve was in the normal range for women but overweight range for men [31]. Zajacova and Burgard [32] used generalized additive models and found that the nadir was at BMIs 23 to 26, which is also in the normal overweight range. However, they point out that there are important differences depending on the cause of death. For example, the association between BMI and diabetes mortality increases monotonically, but, for all-cause mortality, it followed more a V-shape [32]. However, even though these alternative models often provide better fit to the data, the results of these studies are often interpreted making references for traditional cutoffs as they are more easily understood by the general audience and health practitioners. The use of BMI and BMI categories have also been criticized because it can be related to underlying health status [17]. For example, individuals may be underweight based on their BMI because they have health conditions such as cancer, thyroid problems, infectious, or digestive diseases that lead to low body weight. One approach to address this limitation has been to take into account body weight changes [17].

Our study uses data a large cohort study conducted in São Paulo, Brazil, to examine the association between BMI and body weight changes on disability transitions and mortality, while controlling for a series of demographic, socioeconomic, and health determinants. We investigate these associations on three types of disability (activities of daily living, instrumental activities of daily living, and Nagi's limitations) transitions.

2. Materials and Methods

Data from the two waves (2000 and 2006) of the SABE cohort study conducted in São Paulo, Brazil, were used in this study. SABE is a multicenter survey with respondents in seven major cities throughout LAC countries that have been investigating the health and well-being of older adults (age 60 and over). The study was approved by the Institutional Review Boards at the collaborating institutions [34, 35], and the participants provided consent to have their data used for research purposes.

The baseline sample was obtained using a two-stage stratified sampling based on the 1995 National Household Survey master sampling frame. The data in the first wave were collected in two stages. The first stage was a household interview conducted by a single interviewer using a standardized questionnaire that included several questions about the living conditions and health status of the subjects. The second stage of data collection consisted of a household visit by a pair of interviewers who completed anthropometric and physical-performance measurements. At baseline, the response rates reached 84.6% in São Paulo. In the first stage, information on 2,143 individuals was collected. Additional characteristics of the baseline data collection process have been described elsewhere [36–38].

In 2006, to reestablish contact, trained interviewers visited the addresses and neighborhoods of surviving participants from the 2000 survey. For those not found during these visits, interviewers used the additional contact information collected at baseline (e.g., telephone numbers of children or other relatives) to obtain further information about the subjects' current location. In 2006, researchers collected data via face-to-face interviews using a standardized questionnaire. The 2006 questionnaire was very similar to the one used in 2000 but included additional questions that complemented the previous study. Vital statistics records were used to identify subjects who had died between 2000 and 2006. The search was based on the names, sex, dates of birth, and addresses listed in the 2000 database.

Of the 2,143 participants in the first wave of SABE São Paulo, 355 (16.6%) had missing data on selected variables. Most of them ($n = 347$) had missing data on BMI measure. Those with missing data were older (75.1 years) than those with complete data (72.9 years) ($P = 0.0001$), but there were no sex differences. The prevalence of all measures of disability was higher among those with missing data ($P < 0.001$). The final sample is composed of 1,788 individuals, with a subset of 961 with weight change included in the analyses. There were 473 participants who died between the baseline and the followup in 2006.

2.1. Measures. Self-reported disability in six ADL measures (dressing, bathing, eating, getting in and out of a bed, toileting, and getting across a room) were used to measure disability. Individuals were given the following introduction: "Here are a few everyday activities. Please tell me if you have any difficulty with these because of a health problem. Exclude any difficulties you expect to last less than three months." After this introduction, they were asked "Do you have difficulty...?" And the possible answers were: "yes," "no," "does not know," and "no response" for each one of the six ADL measures. Participants who answered "does not know" and "no response" were classified as missing. IADL questions followed the ADL ones. No additional introduction was made. Individuals were asked "Do you have difficulty...?" The IADL items included were preparing a hot meal, managing money, shopping, using of transportation within the community, ability to use the telephone, and responsibility for one's own medications. The possible answers were "yes," "no," "cannot do it," "does not know," and "no response." Those who answered "cannot do it" were classified as having difficulty performing the activity, whereas those answering "does not know" and "no response" were classified as missing. The Nagi physical performance measure included lifting or carrying objects that weighed five kilograms or more; lifting a coin; pulling or pushing a large object, such as a living-room chair; stooping, kneeling, or crouching; and reaching or extending the arms above shoulder level. Each of the three disability measures was converted into binary form, in which respondents scored "0" if they did not indicate any limitations and "1" if they reported having difficulty performing one or more activity in the scale.

Body weight and height were measured without shoes and with light clothing by trained examiners. BMI was calculated as kg/m^2. Four BMI categories were defined according to the criteria adopted by the Pan American Health Organization for the SABE study [38]: underweight ($BMI \leq 23.0$), normal ($BMI > 23$ and < 28), overweight ($BMI \geq 28.0$ and < 30), and obese ($BMI \geq 30$). Change in BMI was calculated as BMI in 2006 minus the BMI at baseline. This difference was divided by the baseline BMI and then recoded into three categories: (a) an increase of 5% or more; (b) a decrease of 5% or more; and (c) changes within 5% of the baseline weight (reference category) [19, 39].

The following sociodemographic characteristics were included in the analysis: age (in years), gender, smoking status (never, former, or current smoker), schooling (in years of formal education), and household arrangement (living alone or accompanied). All regression analysis also included a measure of number of chronic conditions at the baseline. Health status based on the number of self-reported chronic conditions included diabetes, hypertension, cardiovascular disease, stroke, cancer, arthritis, and osteoporosis.

STATA S.E. 12.1 for Windows (StataCorp, College Station, TX) was used for all the statistical analyses. Descriptive statistics were conducted first. Weighted logistic regressions were then used to assess the influence of BMI on disability prevalence. Multinomial logistic regressions were used to assess the influence of BMI on disability transitions and mortality. For those free of disability, four outcomes were considered in the multinomial logistic regressions: remained free of disability (reference category), became disabled (incidence), died, or were lost to followup. For those who were disabled at the baseline, four outcomes were included in the multinomial logistic regressions: remained disabled (reference category), recovered from disability, died, or were lost to followup. Multinomial logistic regressions were used to analyze the role of weight change on health transitions as discussed above, excluding mortality, as we do not have information on weight change prior to death in between waves.

In the baseline, there were 1,420 individuals free of ADL and 368 individuals with ADL. In 2006, among those free of ADL, 606 individuals had remained free of ADL, 226 had developed ADL, 329 had died, and 259 were lost in the followup or had missing data on ADL status. Among those who had ADL in the baseline, 99 remained with ADL, 75 recovered from ADL, 144 died and 50 were lost in the followup or had missing data on ADL in 2006. For IADL limitations, 1,207 were free of IADL, and 581 had IADL in the baseline. Among those who were free of IADL in the baseline, 491 remained free of limitations, 257 developed IADL, 230 had died, and 229 were lost in the followup or had missing data on IADL in the second wave. Among those with IADL in the baseline, 220 remained with IADL, 36 recovered from IADL, 243 had died, and 82 were lost in the followup or had missing data on IADL status in 2006. Regarding the Nagi, 654 participants were free of it in 2000, and 1,134 had at least one Nagi limitation. Among those free of Nagi, 192 remained free of it, 210 developed Nagi, 129 died, and 123 were lost in the followup or had missing data on the Nagi variable in 2006. Among those who had at least one Nagi limitation in 2000, 539 remained with Nagi's limitations, 70 recovered from Nagi's limitations, 344 died, and 181 were lost in the followup or had missing data on Nagi's limitations in the second wave.

3. Results

In the final sample, 23.4% were underweight, 43.3% had normal weight, 12.4% were overweight, and 21.1% of the participants were classified as obese. Table 1 presents the prevalence estimates of disability according to measures of ADL, IADL, and Nagi's limitations by sex and BMI category at baseline. Prevalence of ADL and Nagi's limitations was highest among obese individuals, whereas prevalence of IADL was highest among underweight older adults. Weighted estimates indicated that 16.7% of the sample in São Paulo had difficulty performing at least one ADL. Prevalence of IADL reached 24.4%, and most (57.8%) of the older Brazilian adults reported Nagi's limitations. In logistic regressions, after adjusting for age and sex (not shown), individuals who were underweight did not differ from those of normal weight on their likelihood of reporting having ADL, IADL, or Nagi in the baseline. Obese individuals were more likely than normal weight participants to report having at least one ADL (OR = 1.8, 95% CI = 1.2, 2.6) and Nagi's limitations (OR = 2.5, 95% CI = 1.8, 3.6). There were no statistical differences between normal weight and obese participants regarding IADL prevalence at baseline. There were no statistical differences between normal and overweight subjects regarding ADL and IADL prevalence at baseline, but overweight individuals were more likely than those of normal weight to have Nagi's limitations (OR = 1.6, 95% CI = 1.1, 2.2). Women were more likely than men to report having ADL, IADL, and Nagi's limitations at baseline ($P < 0.05$).

Table 2 shows the multinomial logistic regression results of the disability transitions and mortality between 2000 and 2006 among those who were free of disability in the baseline. Compared to normal weight individuals, obese individuals were more likely to develop ADL (RRR = 2.1) and IADL (RRR = 2.4), whereas individuals who were underweight were more likely to develop IADL (RRR = 1.9). Mortality risks were higher among those who were overweight (RRR = 2.5) compared to those of normal weight in the Nagi model in which the reference category was remaining free of Nagi's limitations. For all measures of disability, the risk of becoming disabled increased with age. As expected, older age was associated with higher mortality. Women were more likely to develop ADL and Nagi's limitations, but not IADL, between waves. Women had lower mortality in the ADL and IADL models. Higher number of chronic conditions was associated with higher mortality and higher incidence of ADL and IADL.

Table 3 shows the multinomial logistic regression results of the disability transitions and mortality between 2000 and 2006 among those who had disability in the baseline. Being obese was also associated with lower recovery from Nagi (RRR = 0.46) versus remaining with at least one Nagi limitation. Older age and higher number of chronic conditions were negatively associated with recovery.

In the last set of analyses, we focus on the role of weight gain between waves on disability transitions (Table 4). The analyses are restricted to those who have survived between waves. The results presented in Table 4 indicate that those who gained weight between waves were more likely to develop ADL (RRR = 2.3) and Nagi's limitations (RRR = 2.2) than those who maintained their weight, even after controlling for initial BMI categories and other covariates. Higher age was also associated with higher incidence of disability. Women faced higher incidence of ADL (RRR = 1.8) and Nagi (RRR = 2.4) than men. Obesity was associated with higher incidence of ADL and IADL. Underweight individuals were more likely to develop IADL. Individuals with more chronic conditions also faced higher incidence of ADL and IADL limitations. When the analyses focused on those who had disability in the baseline, we found that weight gain was associated with lower recovery from ADL (RRR = 0.18). Older age was negatively associated with recovery from disability. A higher number of chronic conditions were associated with lower recovery of ADL and Nagi. Obesity was negatively associated with recovery from Nagi's limitations.

4. Discussion

Most previous studies have focused on the association between BMI and disability [4, 9, 13, 15, 16] or BMI and mortality [10, 20–29, 31–33], but few have analyzed the effect of BMI on both disability and mortality [11, 12, 14, 30]. Using three disability measures and data from a large cohort study, this study contributes to the literature by exploring the impact of BMI and weight changes on disability status transitions and on mortality. This study confirmed the negative effects of obesity on disability in São Paulo, Brazil. Higher levels of Nagi's limitations were also found among those who were overweight at baseline. Most longitudinal studies have found that obese older adults are more likely to have experienced incidence of disability in the followup than those of normal weight [13, 14, 40], and our study confirmed these findings. Older adult Brazilians who were obese at baseline faced higher risks of becoming disabled with ADL or IADL limitations compared to those of normal weight. However, being overweight was not associated with higher incidence of disability after controls were included in the analysis, which is consistent with previous findings [41]. In terms of recovery, we also found that obese individuals were less likely to recover (versus remaining disabled in the followup), as other studies have also found [40].

There is growing interest in the role of weight changes on health transitions [13, 18, 19, 42]. Studies have shown that weight gain in older adults is associated with decreased physical function and role limitations [18, 19]. We found similar findings in which older adults who gained weight between waves were more likely to develop ADL and Nagi's limitations than those who maintained their weight, even after controlling for initial BMI categories. Al Snih and colleagues [19]

Table 1: Prevalence of ADL, IADL, and Nagi's limitations, by sex and BMI categories, São Paulo, 2000 (weighted estimates).

	Total	Underweight	Normal	Overweight	Obese	P
Total	$n = 1{,}788$	$n = 419$	$n = 775$	$n = 217$	$n = 377$	
ADL	16.7	14.7	13.9	18.2	23.4	**
IADL	24.4	28.9	21.0	25.0	26.7	**
Nagi	57.8	52.7	50.7	61.5	74.9	***
Females	$n = 1{,}062$	$n = 212$	$n = 415$	$n = 130$	$n = 305$	
ADL	19.8	14.8	17.2	22.2	25.4	**
IADL	30.5	36.5	26.7	33.8	30.4	
Nagi	67.2	59.7	60.5	73.9	78.3	***
Males	$n = 726$	$n = 207$	$n = 360$	$n = 87$	$n = 72$	
ADL	12.3	14.5	10.3	13.4	15.7	
IADL	15.6	19.9	14.6	13.9	12.7	
Nagi	44.1	44.4	39.6	45.9	61.8	**

ADL: activities of daily living; IADL: instrumental activities of daily living.
$^{***}P < 0.001$; $^{**}P < 0.05$; $^{*}P < 0.10$.

also reported higher ADL incidence among individuals who had weight gain of more than 5% between waves. Studies have reported contradictory findings related to weight loss. Some studies have indicated that weight loss is associated with improvements in mobility and functioning [13], whereas others have reported increased ADL disability [19]. Weight-loss therapy among obese older adults seems to be beneficial for improving quality of life and physical functioning [43]. Ritchie and colleagues [42] found that intentional weight loss was not associated with functional decline; however, those who unintentionally lost weight faced higher rates of functional decline, regardless of the initial BMI. In our study, we found no differences between those who lost weight and those who maintained weight on disability transitions after controlling for initial BMI. Given the lack of data on intent related to weight changes, further studies are necessary to explore the impact of weight change on mortality and disability in Latin American countries.

In additional analyses (not shown and available upon request), we have explored additional models to test whether BMI and weight changes influence changes in the number of disabilities over time. We found that obesity was associated with the increases in the number of Nagi's limitations. Weight loss and weight gain were associated with an increase in the number of ADL and Nagi's limitations over time. Changes in the number of IADL limitations were not statistically associated with BMI categories or weight changes. As expected, older age was associated with the increases in the number of ADL, IADL, and Nagi's limitations over time. A higher number of chronic conditions were also associated with an increase in the number of ADL, IADL and Nagi's limitations over time. Being female was also positively associated with increases in the number of Nagi limitations. We also tested fractional polynomial models following the approach suggested by Wong and colleagues [31] to examine the relationship between BMI, disability and mortality (results available upon request), and our main conclusions remain the same, which indicates that findings are robust to different model specifications.

The only mortality differential by BMI categories was found among overweight participants who were more likely to die than to remain free of Nagi's limitations. In further analyses (not shown), results from a logistic regression that controlled for the same covariates included in this study, revealed no differences in mortality among underweight, normal weight, overweight, and obese participants. This is consistent with previous studies suggesting that the association between BMI and mortality becomes less U-shaped at older ages [44], and others that suggest that higher BMI may not be detrimental for mortality at older ages [12]. Monteverde and colleagues [10] also did not find statistical differences in mortality among older adults between higher BMI categories (overweight and obese) and normal subjects when using traditional BMI cutoffs, though they reported statistical differences when BMI was categorized in relative terms. However, some studies allude to the fact that the association between BMI and mortality is differential between individuals who are healthy versus those with chronic conditions [45]. The obesity paradox literature indicates that excess weight is actually protective among patients with chronic disease [45]. In our sample, there were no mortality differentials by BMI categories among those with chronic conditions, but overweight individuals free of chronic conditions had lower mortality than those of normal weight (results available upon request).

Our findings also contribute to a growing debate in the field about whether greater life expectancy implies better health for the expanding surviving elderly female population in Latin America [37, 46–51]. We found that Brazilian women experience higher levels of disability than men, which is consistent with previous studies [52, 53]. Previous studies have indicated that Brazilian women face lower mortality than their male counterparts [37, 54], and this study confirms these findings.

Aging is related to the increase of fat mass, and there is growing evidence of the detrimental impact of obesity on disability at older ages. There is evidence as well that changes in lifestyle, such as walking, have positive effects on preventing

TABLE 2: Relative risk ratios of the impact of body mass index categories on disability transitions and mortality among those who were free of disability in the baseline, São Paulo, Brazil—2000–2006.

Variables	ADL		P	IADL		P	NAGI		P
	RRR[a]	95% CI		RRR	95% CI		RRR	95% CI	
Incidence of disability									
Age	1.10	[1.07, 1.13]	***	1.11	[1.08, 1.14]	***	1.05	[1.01, 1.09]	**
Female	1.70	[1.06, 2.73]	*	1.48	[0.86, 2.54]		2.37	[1.40, 4.02]	**
Smoking status									
Former smoker	0.94	[0.60, 1.46]		1.15	[0.68, 1.94]		1.36	[0.80, 2.32]	
Current smoker	1.58	[0.88, 2.85]		1.52	[0.73, 3.16]		0.93	[0.52, 1.65]	
Number of chronic conditions	1.56	[1.33, 1.83]	***	1.33	[1.12, 1.58]	**	1.23	[0.94, 1.62]	
Schooling	0.95	[0.86, 1.04]		0.91	[0.82, 1.00]		0.88	[0.79, 0.98]	*
Live alone	0.81	[0.50, 1.31]		0.61	[0.35, 1.06]		0.93	[0.39, 2.24]	
BMI categories									
Underweight	1.16	[0.66, 2.01]		1.92	[1.21, 3.03]	**	1.03	[0.56, 1.89]	
Overweight	0.93	[0.49, 1.75]		1.57	[0.84, 2.96]		1.86	[0.89, 3.87]	
Obese	2.07	[1.21, 3.57]	**	2.42	[1.65, 3.53]	***	1.19	[0.63, 2.26]	
Mortality									
Age	1.11	[1.08, 1.14]	***	1.13	[1.10, 1.16]	***	1.11	[1.07, 1.16]	***
Female	0.60	[0.38, 0.95]	*	0.41	[0.25, 0.65]	***	0.68	[0.34, 1.36]	
Smoking status									
Former smoker	1.25	[0.82, 1.90]		1.17	[0.67, 2.03]		0.90	[0.46, 1.77]	
Current smoker	2.89	[1.66, 5.03]	***	2.69	[1.36, 5.33]	**	2.68	[1.13, 6.37]	*
Number of chronic conditions	1.40	[1.16, 1.68]	***	1.41	[1.17, 1.69]	***	1.82	[1.25, 2.64]	**
Schooling	0.95	[0.89, 1.02]		0.94	[0.87, 1.02]		0.93	[0.82, 1.07]	
Live alone	1.01	[0.62, 1.63]		1.16	[0.64, 2.12]		1.36	[0.66, 2.79]	
BMI categories									
Underweight	1.21	[0.79, 1.85]		1.22	[0.71, 2.09]		1.87	[0.95, 3.66]	
Overweight	1.30	[0.78, 2.14]		1.41	[0.80, 2.48]		2.50	[1.01, 6.15]	*
Obese	1.07	[0.65, 1.75]		1.29	[0.77, 2.18]		0.68	[0.22, 2.07]	
Lost to followup or missing disability status in 2006									
Age	1.03	[1.00, 1.05]	*	1.05	[1.02, 1.08]	***	1.03	[0.99, 1.08]	
Female	1.38	[0.99, 1.94]		1.24	[0.84, 1.83]		2.19	[1.37, 3.52]	**
Smoking status									
Former smoker	1.36	[0.90, 2.06]		1.54	[1.00, 2.38]		2.01	[1.10, 3.70]	*
Current smoker	1.05	[0.60, 1.84]		1.02	[0.53, 1.98]		1.32	[0.61, 2.89]	
Number of chronic conditions	1.12	[0.96, 1.31]		1.12	[0.94, 1.34]		1.22	[0.94, 1.58]	
Schooling	1.02	[0.92, 1.13]		1.01	[0.91, 1.12]		0.99	[0.85, 1.16]	
Live alone	1.37	[0.84, 2.22]		1.42	[0.84, 2.40]		0.93	[0.38, 2.30]	
BMI categories									
Underweight	1.58	[0.97, 2.59]		2.07	[1.24, 3.45]	**	1.44	[0.70, 2.98]	
Overweight	1.25	[0.69, 2.26]		1.33	[0.78, 2.26]		1.41	[0.59, 3.35]	
Obese	1.36	[0.87, 2.12]		1.55	[1.02, 2.37]	*	1.32	[0.56, 3.14]	
N	1,420			1,207			654		
BIC$'$	−104.55			−82.451			47.73		

ADL: activities of daily living; IADL: instrumental activities of daily living; RRR: relative risk ratio; CI: confidence interval; BMI: body mass index.
[a]Remaining free of disability is the reference category. Normal weight is the reference category for BMI, living accompanied is the baseline category for household arrangement, and never smoked is the reference category for smoking status.
$^{***}P < 0.001$; $^{**}P < 0.05$; $^{*}P < 0.10$.

Table 3: Relative risk ratios of the impact of body mass index categories on disability transitions and mortality among those who had disability in the baseline, São Paulo, Brazil—2000–2006.

Variables	ADL		P	IADL		P	NAGI		P
	RRR[a]	95% CI		RRR	95% CI		RRR	95% CI	
Recovery from disability									
Age	0.93	[0.88, 0.97]	**	0.92	[0.87, 0.98]	**	0.96	[0.92, 1.00]	*
Female	0.65	[0.25, 1.73]		0.39	[0.13, 1.17]		0.56	[0.30, 1.07]	
Smoking status									
Former smoker	0.39	[0.11, 1.33]		1.04	[0.42, 2.57]		1.54	[0.72, 3.27]	
Current smoker	1.43	[0.49, 4.18]		0.55	[0.11, 2.79]		1.01	[0.41, 2.49]	
Number of chronic conditions	0.72	[0.52, 0.99]	*	0.93	[0.68, 1.27]		0.59	[0.44, 0.79]	***
Schooling	1.03	[0.83, 1.27]		0.99	[0.76, 1.28]		1.05	[0.89, 1.25]	
Live alone	0.55	[0.17, 1.74]		1.11	[0.31, 3.92]		3.24	[1.59, 6.57]	**
BMI categories									
Underweight	0.37	[0.10, 1.34]		0.14	[0.01, 1.45]		0.62	[0.25, 1.58]	
Overweight	1.01	[0.35, 2.97]		0.80	[0.22, 2.88]		0.82	[0.29, 2.28]	
Obese	0.48	[0.21, 1.08]		0.77	[0.28, 2.17]		0.46	[0.22, 0.97]	*
Mortality									
Age	1.12	[1.07, 1.18]	***	1.07	[1.04, 1.10]	***	1.10	[1.08, 1.12]	***
Female	0.40	[0.18, 0.90]	*	0.65	[0.30, 1.38]		0.48	[0.30, 0.77]	**
Smoking status									
Former smoker	1.33	[0.57, 3.09]		1.75	[0.92, 3.34]		1.75	[1.13, 2.69]	*
Current smoker	3.35	[1.06, 10.64]	*	3.09	[1.35, 7.07]	**	2.30	[1.29, 4.09]	**
Number of chronic conditions	0.87	[0.67, 1.14]		0.97	[0.79, 1.19]		0.98	[0.86, 1.13]	
Schooling	0.98	[0.82, 1.17]		1.04	[0.93, 1.16]		0.95	[0.89, 1.02]	
Live alone	1.03	[0.42, 2.50]		0.88	[0.53, 1.45]		1.23	[0.77, 1.97]	
BMI categories									
Underweight	0.97	[0.44, 2.12]		1.28	[0.74, 2.21]		0.9	[0.57, 1.44]	
Overweight	0.35	[0.11, 1.14]		0.75	[0.41, 1.39]		0.79	[0.45, 1.38]	
Obese	0.54	[0.22, 1.35]		0.66	[0.36, 1.19]		0.78	[0.51, 1.22]	
Lost to followup or missing disability status in 2006									
Age	1.00	[0.94, 1.06]		1.00	[0.96, 1.04]		1.01	[0.97, 1.04]	
Female	0.50	[0.18, 1.39]		1.40	[0.48, 4.08]		0.93	[0.54, 1.60]	
Smoking status									
Former smoker	0.40	[0.13, 1.21]		0.69	[0.23, 2.04]		1.09	[0.60, 1.99]	
Current smoker	0.62	[0.08, 4.53]		0.86	[0.30, 2.48]		0.66	[0.36, 1.19]	
Number of chronic conditions	0.73	[0.53, 1.01]		0.88	[0.66, 1.16]		0.88	[0.76, 1.03]	
Schooling	1.16	[0.97, 1.40]		1.07	[0.92, 1.24]		1.03	[0.93, 1.15]	
Live alone	1.73	[0.53, 5.57]		1.43	[0.68, 3.01]		2.38	[1.34, 4.24]	**
BMI categories									
Underweight	1.67	[0.47, 5.89]		1.42	[0.72, 2.82]		1.85	[1.09, 3.14]	*
Overweight	0.43	[0.12, 1.54]		0.90	[0.36, 2.27]		1.27	[0.63, 2.53]	
Obese	0.92	[0.32, 2.63]		1.14	[0.49, 2.65]		1.24	[0.75, 2.04]	
N		368			581			1,134	
BIC′		30.33			62.47			−42.91	

ADL: activities of daily living; IADL: instrumental activities of daily living; RRR: relative risk ratio; CI: confidence interval; BMI: body mass index.

[a]Remaining with disability is the reference category. Normal weight is the reference category for BMI, living accompanied is the baseline category for household arrangement, and never smoked is the reference category for smoking status.

$^{***}P < 0.001$; $^{**}P < 0.05$; $^{*}P < 0.10$.

TABLE 4: Relative risk ratios of the impact of body mass index categories and body mass index changes on disability transitions, São Paulo, Brazil—2000–2006.

Variables	ADL		P	IADL		P	NAGI		P
	RRR[a]	95% CI		RRR	95% CI		RRR	95% CI	
Incidence of disability (reference = remain free of disability)									
Age	1.10	[1.07, 1.13]	* * *	1.11	[1.08, 1.15]	* * *	1.05	[1.01, 1.09]	*
Female	1.75	[1.04, 2.94]	*	1.53	[0.88, 2.65]		2.44	[1.44, 4.12]	* *
Smoking status									
Former smoker	0.85	[0.53, 1.38]		1.14	[0.67, 1.95]		1.47	[0.87, 2.50]	
Current smoker	1.38	[0.71, 2.70]		1.45	[0.67, 3.16]		0.97	[0.56, 1.69]	
Number of chronic conditions	1.56	[1.32, 1.86]	* * *	1.33	[1.12, 1.59]	* *	1.25	[0.92, 1.68]	
Schooling	0.97	[0.88, 1.07]		0.92	[0.82, 1.03]		0.90	[0.80, 1.01]	
Live alone	0.85	[0.50, 1.44]		0.60	[0.34, 1.08]		1.01	[0.42, 2.41]	
BMI categories									
Underweight	0.92	[0.48, 1.77]		1.73	[1.05, 2.84]	*	0.93	[0.49, 1.79]	
Overweight	0.72	[0.36, 1.44]		1.39	[0.67, 2.88]		1.87	[0.87, 3.99]	
Obese	1.99	[1.10, 3.57]	*	2.38	[1.61, 3.52]	* * *	1.22	[0.66, 2.27]	
BMI change									
Loss	1.23	[0.76, 2.00]		0.99	[0.62, 1.60]		0.85	[0.49, 1.48]	
Gain	2.30	[1.03, 5.12]	*	1.97	[0.97, 4.01]		2.15	[1.20, 3.85]	*
N		800			737			389	
BIC′		27.46			9.40			28.56	
Recovery from disability (reference = remain with disability)									
Age	0.92	[0.87, 0.98]	*	0.93	[0.88, 0.99]	*	0.95	[0.91, 0.99]	*
Female	0.43	[0.13, 1.47]		0.41	[0.11, 1.58]		0.53	[0.28, 1.01]	
Smoking status									
Former smoker	0.34	[0.09, 1.30]		1.40	[0.60, 3.29]		1.46	[0.74, 2.87]	
Current smoker	1.11	[0.29, 4.17]		0.69	[0.10, 4.70]		0.97	[0.38, 2.44]	
Number of chronic conditions	0.64	[0.45, 0.90]	*	0.94	[0.68, 1.29]		0.60	[0.46, 0.80]	* * *
Schooling	1.05	[0.87, 1.28]		1.05	[0.82, 1.34]		1.03	[0.87, 1.22]	
Live alone	0.50	[0.12, 2.02]		1.03	[0.22, 4.85]		3.27	[1.63, 6.57]	* *
BMI categories									
Underweight	0.49	[0.12, 2.04]		0.16	[0.02, 1.40]		0.71	[0.26, 1.88]	
Overweight	0.89	[0.27, 2.88]		0.76	[0.18, 3.20]		0.86	[0.31, 2.36]	
Obese	0.42	[0.17, 1.05]		0.68	[0.22, 2.07]		0.43	[0.21, 0.86]	*
BMI change									
Loss	0.52	[0.23, 1.19]		0.53	[0.21, 1.35]		1.07	[0.61, 1.89]	
Gain	0.18	[0.05, 0.68]	*	0.64	[0.15, 2.73]		0.53	[0.21, 1.37]	
N		161			224			572	
BIC′		31.87			91.45			85.22	

ADL: activities of daily living; IADL: instrumental activities of daily living; RRR: relative risk ratio; CI: confidence interval; BMI: body mass index.
[a]Relative risk ratios were adjusted by smoking status. Remaining free of disability is the reference category for those who started without disability, and remaining with disability is the reference category for those who had disability in the baseline. Normal weight is the reference category for BMI. Stable weight is the baseline category for weight change. Results for lost in the followup were omitted (available upon request).
***$P < 0.001$; **$P < 0.05$; *$P < 0.10$.

mobility limitations [55]. A large proportion of older adults, however, do not engage in physical activity. In a study based on an urban sample in Brazil, for example, 71% of older adults reported living sedentary lives [56]. When asked about neighborhood characteristics related to concerns of leaving home to go out, most (78%) reported fear of being robbed, while almost half (48.2%) said that they were afraid of falling because of sidewalk defects [56]. Fear of falling due to poor sidewalk conditions was associated with a 62% increase in the expected number of ADL conditions [56]. Therefore, investments aimed at improving urban infrastructure and safety may be effective in addressing the health conditions of older adults in Brazil.

This study advances the literature on the impact of body weight and body weight changes on disability and mortality. This study, however, has some limitations. First, the data used in the study on disability measures were self-reported. Although this could be a possible source of bias, methodological studies have shown that self-reported data on functional disability are consistent with medical diagnoses [57]. Second, the use of BMI as a measure for body weight composition among older adults is very controversial as it does not take into account body fat distribution [17]. In addition, BMI at baseline can be associated with health status [16, 17]. Therefore, it is important to control for weight changes, which we accomplished in this study. Some authors have argued that waist circumference or waist-to-hip ratio could be better predictors of disability and mortality [10]; however, most studies to date have focused on the use of BMI and the categories used here. Other scholars have indicated that, at least for developed countries, information on BMI, waist circumference, or waist-to-hip ratio do not necessarily improve prediction of mortality due to cardiovascular disease; instead, they suggest using information on systolic blood pressure, diabetes status, and lipids when those are available [58]. And still others argue that—in addition to BMI—waist circumference and waist-to-hip ratio can be useful in better understanding mortality risks [59, 60]. In Brazil, as in other developing countries, data on blood pressure and lipids are often lacking, so the use of anthropometric measures, such as waist circumference, may improve our understanding of the impact of body composition changes on mortality and disability. Third, the first wave of SABE focuses on the civilian population not residing in institutions. As a result, estimates may be biased if one expects institutionalized individuals, particularly those residing in nursing homes, to be more likely to have a higher prevalence of disability than the non-institutionalized population. However, because the institutionalized population in Brazil is relatively small [61], this possible bias is likely not to be very significant.

5. Conclusion

This study confirms previous studies that have found obesity to be associated with increased disability in Brazilian older adults. Historically, Brazil has mainly been concerned with curbing malnutrition; however, in recent years, new policies have targeted the marketing of highly processed and unhealthy foods [5]. Owing to the fact that obesity rates in Brazil have been increasing drastically for the past three decades [6], our findings have important implications for policy makers in Brazil with regard to curbing disability risk by promoting the use of effective preventive measures to reduce body weight, thereby making healthy aging a reality.

Author's Contribution

F. C. D. Andrade planned the study, supervised the data analysis, and wrote the paper. A. I. N. M. Nazan contributed to the paper writing. M. L. Lebrão and Y. A. de O. Duarte collected the data, helped plan the study, including instrumentation, and revised the paper.

Acknowledgments

This study was supported by grants from FAPESP/Brazil, the Brazilian Ministry of Health, and the Lemann Institute for Brazilian Studies at the University of Illinois at Urbana-Champaign. The authors gratefully acknowledge the feedback received at the 2012 Population Association of America Annual Meeting. They also thank Fernão Dias de Lima for the careful management of the database.

References

[1] D. Cotlear, *Population Aging? Is Latin America Ready?* World Bank, Washington, DC, USA, 2011.

[2] K. Kinsella and W. He, *An Aging World: 2008*, Government Printing Office, Washington, DC, USA, 2009.

[3] Population Division of the Department of Economic and Social Affairs of the United Nations Secretariat, *World Population Prospects: The 2010 Revision*, United Nations, New York, NY, USA, 2011.

[4] S. Al Snih, J. E. Graham, Y. F. Kuo, J. S. Goodwin, K. S. Markides, and K. J. Ottenbacher, "Obesity and disability: relation among older adults living in latin america and the caribbean," *American Journal of Epidemiology*, vol. 171, no. 12, pp. 1282–1288, 2010.

[5] B. M. Popkin, L. S. Adair, and S. W. Ng, "Global nutrition transition and the pandemic of obesity in developing countries," *Nutrition Reviews*, vol. 70, no. 1, pp. 3–21, 2012.

[6] C. A. Monteiro, W. L. Conde, and B. M. Popkin, "Income-specific trends in obesity in Brazil: 1975–2003," *American Journal of Public Health*, vol. 97, no. 10, pp. 1808–1812, 2007.

[7] C. A. Monteiro, W. L. Conde, and B. M. Popkin, "The burden of disease from undernutrition and overnutrition in countries undergoing rapid nutrition transition: a view from Brazil," *American Journal of Public Health*, vol. 94, no. 3, pp. 433–434, 2004.

[8] C. A. Monteiro, W. L. Conde, and B. M. Popkin, "Independent effects of income and education on the risk of obesity in the Brazilian adult population," *Journal of Nutrition*, vol. 131, no. 3, pp. 881S–886S, 2001.

[9] L. P. Corona, T. R. Pereira de Brito, D. P. Nunes et al., "Nutritional status and risk for disability in instrumental activities of daily living in older Brazilians," *Public Health Nutrition*, vol. 13, pp. 1–6, 2012.

[10] M. Monteverde, K. Noronha, A. Palloni, and B. Novak, "Obesity and excess mortality among the elderly in the United States and Mexico," *Demography*, vol. 47, no. 1, pp. 79–96, 2010.

[11] S. Al Snih, K. J. Ottenbacher, K. S. Markides, Y. F. Kuo, K. Eschbach, and J. S. Goodwin, "The effect of obesity on disability versus mortality in older Americans," *Archives of Internal Medicine*, vol. 167, no. 8, pp. 774–780, 2007.

[12] I. M. Majer, W. J. Nusselder, J. P. MacKenbach, and A. E. Kunst, "Life expectancy and life expectancy with disability of normal weight, overweight, and obese smokers and nonsmokers in Europe," *Obesity*, vol. 19, no. 7, pp. 1451–1459, 2011.

[13] H. K. Vincent, K. R. Vincent, and K. M. Lamb, "Obesity and mobility disability in the older adult," *Obesity Reviews*, vol. 11, no. 8, pp. 568–579, 2010.

[14] I. A. Lang, D. J. Llewellyn, K. Alexander, and D. Melzer, "Obesity, physical function, and mortality in older adults," *Journal of the American Geriatrics Society*, vol. 56, no. 8, pp. 1474–1478, 2008.

[15] S. Larrieu, K. Pérès, L. Letenneur et al., "Relationship between body mass index and different domains of disability in older persons: the 3C study," *International Journal of Obesity*, vol. 28, no. 12, pp. 1555–1560, 2004.

[16] D. E. Alley and V. W. Chang, "The changing relationship of obesity and disability, 1988–2004," *Journal of the American Medical Association*, vol. 298, no. 17, pp. 2020–2027, 2007.

[17] D. E. Alley, L. Ferrucci, M. Barbagallo, S. A. Studenski, and T. B. Harris, "A research agenda: the changing relationship between body weight and health in aging," *Journals of Gerontology Series A*, vol. 63, no. 11, pp. 1257–1259, 2008.

[18] A. P. Carson, D. N. Holmes, and D. L. Howard, "Weight change and functional limitations among older adults in North Carolina," *Journal of Community Health*, vol. 35, no. 6, pp. 586–591, 2010.

[19] S. Al Snih, M. A. Raji, K. S. Markides, K. J. Ottenbacher, and J. S. Goodwin, "Weight change and lower body disability in older Mexican Americans," *Journal of the American Geriatrics Society*, vol. 53, no. 10, pp. 1730–1737, 2005.

[20] A. B. De Gonzalez, P. Hartge, J. R. Cerhan et al., "Body-mass index and mortality among 1.46 million white adults," *New England Journal of Medicine*, vol. 363, no. 23, pp. 2211–2219, 2010.

[21] L. C. Hwang, S. C. Chen, J. J. Tjung, H. Y. Chiou, C. J. Chen, and C. H. Tsai, "Body mass index as a predictor of mortality in older people in Taiwan," *International Journal of Gerontology*, vol. 3, no. 1, pp. 39–46, 2009.

[22] Prospective Studies Collaboration, "Body-mass index and cause-specific mortality in 900 000 adults: collaborative analyses of 57 prospective studies," *The Lancet*, vol. 373, no. 9669, pp. 1083–1096, 2009.

[23] A. Peeters, J. J. Barendregt, F. Willekens et al., "Obesity in adulthood and its consequences for life expectancy: a life-table analysis," *Annals of Internal Medicine*, vol. 138, no. 1, pp. 24–32, 2003.

[24] A. C. Tsai and M. Hsiao, "The association of body mass index (BMI) with all-cause mortality in older Taiwanese: results of a national cohort study," *Archives of Gerontology and Geriatrics*, vol. 55, no. 2, pp. 217–220, 2012.

[25] I. Janssen and A. E. Mark, "Elevated body mass index and mortality risk in the elderly," *Obesity Reviews*, vol. 8, no. 1, pp. 41–59, 2007.

[26] R. Bender, K. H. Jöckel, C. Trautner, M. Spraul, and M. Berger, "Effect of age on excess mortality in obesity," *Journal of the American Medical Association*, vol. 281, no. 16, pp. 1498–1504, 1999.

[27] K. M. Flegal, B. I. Graubard, D. F. Williamson, and M. H. Gail, "Excess deaths associated with underweight, overweight, and obesity," *Journal of the American Medical Association*, vol. 293, no. 15, pp. 1861–1867, 2005.

[28] R. Huxley, F. Barzi, and M. Woodward, "Excess risk of fatal coronary heart disease associated with diabetes in men and women: meta-analysis of 37 prospective cohort studies," *British Medical Journal*, vol. 332, no. 7533, pp. 73–76, 2006.

[29] M. Reuser, L. Bonneux, and F. Willekens, "The burden of mortality of obesity at middle and old age is small. A life table analysis of the US Health and Retirement Survey," *European Journal of Epidemiology*, vol. 23, no. 9, pp. 601–607, 2008.

[30] S. L. Reynolds, Y. Saito, and E. M. Crimmins, "The impact of obesity on active life expectancy in older American men and women," *Gerontologist*, vol. 45, no. 4, pp. 438–444, 2005.

[31] E. Wong, B. Wang, L. Garrison et al., "Examining the BMI-mortality relationship using fractional polynomials," *BMC Medical Research Methodology*, vol. 11, no. 1, article 175, 2011.

[32] A. Zajacova and S. A. Burgard, "Shape of the BMI-mortality association by cause of death, using generalized additive models: NHIS 1986–2006," *Journal of Aging and Health*, vol. 24, no. 2, pp. 191–211, 2012.

[33] J. T. Gronniger, "A semiparametric analysis of the relationship of body mass index to mortality," *American Journal of Public Health*, vol. 96, no. 1, pp. 173–178, 2006.

[34] A. Palloni, G. Pinto-Aguirre, and M. Pelaez, "Demographic and health conditions of ageing in Latin America and the Caribbean," *International Journal of Epidemiology*, vol. 31, no. 4, pp. 762–771, 2002.

[35] R. Wong, M. Peláez, A. Palloni, and K. Markides, "Survey data for the study of aging in Latin America and the Caribbean: selected studies," *Journal of Aging and Health*, vol. 18, no. 2, pp. 157–179, 2006.

[36] C. Albala, M. L. Lebrão, E. M. L. Diaz et al., "Salud, Bienestar y Envejecimiento (SABE): metodologia de la encuesta t perfil de la población estudiada," *Pan American Journal of Public Health*, vol. 17, no. 5-6, pp. 307–322, 2005.

[37] F. C. D. Andrade, P. E. Guevara, M. L. Lebrão, Y. A. de Oliveira Duarte, and J. L. F. Santos, "Gender differences in life expectancy and disability-free life expectancy among older adults in São Paulo, Brazil," *Women's Health Issues*, vol. 21, no. 1, pp. 64–70, 2011.

[38] M. L. Lebrão and R. Laurenti, "Saúde, bem-estar e envelhecimento: o estudo SABE no município de São Paulo," *Revista Brasileira De Epidemiologia*, vol. 8, no. 2, pp. 127–141, 2005.

[39] F. C. D. Andrade, I. Vazquez-Vidal, and T. Flood, "One-year follow-up changes in weight are associated with changes in blood pressure in young Mexican adults," *Public Health*, vol. 126, no. 6, pp. 535–540, 2012.

[40] S. Walter, A. Kunst, J. MacKenbach, A. Hofman, and H. Tiemeier, "Mortality and disability: the effect of overweight and obesity," *International Journal of Obesity*, vol. 33, no. 12, pp. 1410–1418, 2009.

[41] H. Dong, M. Unosson, E. Wressle, and J. Marcusson, "Health consequences associated with being overweight or obese: a Swedish population-based study of 85-year-olds," *Journal of the American Geriatrics Society*, vol. 60, no. 2, pp. 243–250, 2012.

[42] C. S. Ritchie, J. L. Locher, D. L. Roth, T. McVie, P. Sawyer, and R. Allman, "Unintentional weight loss predicts decline in activities of daily living function and life-space mobility over 4 years among community-dwelling older adults," *Journals of Gerontology Series A*, vol. 63, no. 1, pp. 67–75, 2008.

[43] D. T. Villareal, C. M. Apovian, R. F. Kushner, and S. Klein, "Obesity in older adults: technical review and position statement of the American Society for Nutrition and NAASO, The Obesity Society," *American Journal of Clinical Nutrition*, vol. 82, no. 5, pp. 923–934, 2005.

[44] M. Thinggaard, R. Jacobsen, B. Jeune, T. Martinussen, and K. Christensen, "Is the relationship between bmi and mortality increasingly u-shaped with advancing age? A 10-year follow-up of persons aged 70–95 years," *Journals of Gerontology Series A*, vol. 65, no. 5, pp. 526–531, 2010.

[45] J. P. Curtis, J. G. Selter, Y. Wang et al., "The obesity paradox: body mass index and outcomes in patients with heart failure," *Archives of Internal Medicine*, vol. 165, no. 1, pp. 55–61, 2008.

[46] B. E. Alvarado, M. V. Zunzunegui, F. Béland, M. Sicotte, and L. Tellechea, "Social and gender inequalities in depressive symptoms among urban older adults of Latin America and the Caribbean," *Journals of Gerontology Series B*, vol. 62, no. 4, pp. S226–S237, 2007.

[47] F. C. Andrade, "Measuring the impact of diabetes on life expectancy and disability-free life expectancy among older adults in Mexico," *The Journals of Gerontology Series B*, vol. 65, no. 3, pp. 381–389, 2010.

[48] M. C. S. Camargos, C. J. Machado, and R. Do Nascimento Rodrigues, "Disability life expectancy for the elderly, city of São Paulo, Brazil, 2000: gender and educational differences," *Journal of Biosocial Science*, vol. 39, no. 3, pp. 455–463, 2007.

[49] M. C. S. Camargos, C. J. Machado, and R. N. Rodrigues, "Life expectancy among elderly Brazilians in 2003 according to different levels of functional disability," *Cadernos de Saude Publica*, vol. 24, no. 4, pp. 845–852, 2008.

[50] S. Reyes-Beaman, C. Jagger, C. Garcia-Peña, O. Muñoz, P. E. Beaman, and B. Stafford, "Active life expectancy of older people in Mexico," *Disability and Rehabilitation*, vol. 27, no. 5, pp. 213–219, 2005.

[51] C. A. Reyes-Ortiz, G. V. Ostir, M. Pelaez, and K. J. Ottenbacher, "Cross-national comparison of disability in Latin American and Caribbean persons aged 75 and older," *Archives of Gerontology and Geriatrics*, vol. 42, no. 1, pp. 21–33, 2006.

[52] R. O. Guerra, B. E. Alvarado, and M. V. Zunzunegui, "Life course, gender and ethnic inequalities in functional disability in a Brazilian urban elderly population," *Aging*, vol. 20, no. 1, pp. 53–61, 2008.

[53] J. L. F. Santos, M. L. Lebrão, Y. A. O. Duarte, and F. D. De Lima, "Functional performance of the elderly in instrumental activities of daily living: an analysis in the municipality of São Paulo, Brazil," *Cadernos de Saude Publica*, vol. 24, no. 4, pp. 879–886, 2008.

[54] M. F. Lima-Costa, S. V. Peixoto, D. L. Matos, J. O. A. Firmo, and E. Uchôa, "Predictors of 10-year mortality in a population of community-dwelling Brazilian elderly: the Bambuí cohort study of aging," *Cadernos De Saúde Pública*, vol. 27, pp. s360–s369, 2011.

[55] N. M. de Vries, C. D. van Ravensberg, J. S. Hobbelen, M. G. Olde Rikkert, J. B. Staal, and M. W. Nijhuis-van der Sanden, "Effects of physical exercise therapy on mobility, physical functioning, physical activity and quality of life in community-dwelling older adults with impaired mobility, physical disability and/or multi-morbidity: a meta-analysis," *Ageing Research Reviews*, vol. 11, no. 1, pp. 136–149, 2012.

[56] F. R. Ferreira, C. C. César, V. P. Camargos, M. F. Lima-Costa, and F. A. Proietti, "Aging and urbanization: the neighborhood perception and functional performance of elderly persons in belo horizonte metropolitan area-Brazil," *Journal of Urban Health*, vol. 87, no. 1, pp. 54–66, 2010.

[57] M. V. Zunzunegui, B. E. Alvarado, F. Béland, and B. Vissandjee, "Explaining health differences between men and women in later life: a cross-city comparison in Latin America and the Caribbean," *Social Science and Medicine*, vol. 68, no. 2, pp. 235–242, 2009.

[58] D. Wormser, S. Kaptoge, E. Di Angelantonio et al., "Separate and combined associations of body-mass index and abdominal adiposity with cardiovascular disease: collaborative analysis of 58 prospective studies," *The Lancet*, vol. 377, no. 9771, pp. 1085–1095, 2011.

[59] T. Pischon, H. Boeing, K. Hoffmann et al., "General and abdominal adiposity and risk of death in Europe," *New England Journal of Medicine*, vol. 359, no. 20, pp. 2105–2120, 2008.

[60] T. Pischon, "Commentary: use of the body mass index to assess the risk of health outcomes: time to say goodbye?" *International Journal of Epidemiology*, vol. 39, no. 2, pp. 528–529, 2010.

[61] A. A. Camarano and S. Kanso, "As instituições de longa permanência para idosos no Brasil," *Revista Brasileira de Estudos de População*, vol. 27, no. 1, pp. 232–235, 2010.

18

Sleep Environment and Insomnia in Elderly Persons Living at Home

Jonathan Desaulniers,[1] **Sophie Desjardins**,[1] **Sylvie Lapierre**,[1] **and Alain Desgagné**[2]

[1]*Department of Psychology, Université du Québec à Trois-Rivières, C.P. 500, Trois-Rivières, Québec, Canada G9A 5H7*
[2]*Department of Mathematics, Université du Québec à Montréal, C.P. 8888, Succursale Centre-ville, Montréal, Québec, Canada H3C 3P8*

Correspondence should be addressed to Sophie Desjardins; sophie.desjardins@uqtr.ca

Academic Editor: Jean-Francois Grosset

The aim of this study was to draw a portrait of the sleep environment of elderly persons living in private households and to determine its relationship with the presence of insomnia. A sample of 599 individuals aged 70 years and older responded to questions about the comfort of their pillow and mattress and the noise level and brightness of their bedroom at night and in the morning. They were also asked whether or not they shared their bed or bedroom with a sleep partner. The Insomnia Severity Index was used to assess insomnia severity. Over 40% of the study participants were using a pillow that was not very comfortable, and almost 30% said that their bedroom was not completely quiet. Binomial logistic regression results revealed that two variables were significantly associated with insomnia symptoms: a pillow rated as moderately comfortable to very uncomfortable and a bedroom that was not completely quiet. No other sleep environment characteristics considered in this study were associated with the risk of insomnia. These results indicate that a nonnegligible proportion of the elderly population endures a suboptimal sleep environment. Although it is difficult to predict the real impact of changes to the sleep environment, this study supports the proposal that simple, minor changes to the bedroom can promote sleep in the elderly.

1. Introduction

The frequency of self-reported sleep problems increases with age. Whereas 40% of individuals who consult a general physician complain of significant sleep problems, the proportion rises to 63% for individuals aged 60 years and over, and to 67% if they are living in a long-term care residence [1–3]. As life expectancies rise in the vast majority of industrialized countries [4, 5], sleep problems will become a growing concern.

Although certain physiological changes that affect sleep quality are considered normal with increasing age, cognitive behavioral therapy (CBT) is used as a standard first-line treatment to reduce many sleep-related symptoms in the elderly [6, 7]. Such treatment generally involves recommendations for good sleep hygiene, including changes to the sleep environment. Elderly persons are at greater risk for nocturnal awakenings and sleep fragmentation compared with the general population [8]. Consequently, they are at greater risk for being affected by an inadequate sleep environment, namely, a bedroom that is insufficiently quiet, dark, or comfortable.

Because the brain processes auditory stimuli in both the awake and asleep state, sleep quality can be affected by auditory pollution [9]. When the noise level is within the range from 40 to 55 dB or approximately the volume of light road traffic, people generally try to adapt their environment to preserve adequate sleep quality. At noise levels above 55 dB or approximately the volume of two people having a conversation, sleep problems become more frequent, depending on whether hearing acuity is preserved [10].

Exposure to nocturnal light is another risk factor for sleep problems. Nocturnal light inhibits the secretion of melatonin, a hormone involved in sleep regulation [11, 12].

Moreover, in the elderly, nocturnal light can promote the development of depressive symptoms [13], raise blood pressure [14], and contribute to the development of carotid stenosis [15]. Conditions such as advanced or delayed sleep phase disorder can also impair sleep quality in this population [16].

Pillow comfort can also affect sleep quality [17] because a properly designed pillow allows greater surface contact with the neck, for a more even distribution of pressure on the cervical (neck) muscles [18]. Although the shape, thickness, and material of commercially available pillows vary, consumers continue to choose based largely on personal preferences [19]. However, for the general population, feather pillows may be less performant than those made of other materials [17, 20]. Considering that the prevalence of chronic pain ranged from 23.9 to 31.3% in Canadians aged 65 years and older from 1994 to 2008 [21], studies have examined the use of pillows designed to alleviate cervical pain. Although the specifications for these pillows vary across studies, a simple change of pillow can improve the sleep of elderly persons [22, 23]. Still, the findings of the most recent meta-analysis on this topic do not allow recommending the use of a cervical pillow to improve sleep quality in a population presenting chronic cervical pain [24].

Mattress comfort can also affect sleep quality by making it easier to change position during the night to prevent muscular stiffness [25]. Studies conducted in adults with chronic pain underscore the benefits of a moderately firm mattress to optimize sleep in this population, independently of age [26, 27]. In addition, variations in weight and height can affect perceptions of comfort [28]. However, the current state of knowledge does not allow specifying the mattress characteristics that are likely to promote sleep in the elderly [29–31].

Given the prevalence of sleep problems in the elderly and the difficulty of access to healthcare specialists, including lengthy wait times, researchers should delve more deeply into the specific contribution of the sleep environment. The results could help empower older individuals to manage sleep problems with no demonstrable organic cause. Currently, the individual influences of environmental factors that could improve sleep quality remain unknown [32], and the same goes for the typical sleep environment of elderly persons. In order to fill this research gap, the present study aims, on the one hand, to draw a portrait of the sleep environment of elderly persons, and on the other hand, to determine whether the presence (or not) of a partner in the same bed or bedroom, the noise and brightness of the bedroom, and pillow and mattress comfort allow distinguishing between elderly persons who present insomnia and those who do not.

2. Materials and Methods

The participants initially took part in the longitudinal Québec Survey on Seniors' Health (Enquête sur la santé des aînés), which addressed a representative sample (n = 2798) of elderly persons living in the community (i.e., in private households) [33]. These individuals were recontacted by mail and invited to participate in the present study. Once the study objective was explained and the participants had given their informed consent to participate, they filled out questionnaires on sociodemographic characteristics, sleep environment characteristics, and sleep quality. The participation rate for the present study was over 20%. This rate is satisfactory given that it can be explained not only by refusal, but also by mortality, disability, and loss of contact. This study was approved by the Research Ethics Committees of the Université du Québec à Trois-Rivières (UQTR) and the Institut universitaire de gériatrie de l'Université de Sherbrooke (IUGS).

Insomnia symptoms were assessed with the Insomnia Severity Index (ISI) [34, 35]. This questionnaire contains seven questions on participants' perceptions of the type, severity, and impact of insomnia within the past month, for a total score ranging from 0 to 28. A score from 0 to 7 indicates absence of insomnia, from 8 to 14 mild insomnia, from 15 to 21 moderate insomnia, and 22 and higher severe insomnia. Cronbach's alpha for the questionnaire items varies from 0.74 to 0.78 [34]. Content validity was demonstrated by principle component analysis, which identified three components: impact of insomnia, insomnia severity, and satisfaction with sleep. Despite some overlap between these components, they allow capturing an insomnia diagnosis as defined by the DSM-IV [34]. An ISI score of 14 demonstrates 94% sensitivity and 94% specificity to distinguish individuals presenting a diagnosis of primary insomnia from good sleepers in a control group. The psychometric properties of the questionnaire have been demonstrated for the English version and the French translated version [34, 35].

The sleep environment was explored with a set of seven questions referring to the past month, as follows: "How comfortable was your pillow?"; "How comfortable was your mattress?"; "What was the level of noise in your bedroom at night?"; "What was the level of noise in your bedroom in the morning?"; "How bright was your bedroom at night?"; and "How bright was your bedroom in the morning?" Responses were rated on a four-point Likert scale. For pillow and mattress comfort, the response choices were "Very uncomfortable," "Not very comfortable," "Moderately comfortable," and "Very comfortable," with 1 for lowest and 4 for greatest comfort. Similarly, for noise level, the choices were "Very loud," "Moderately loud," "Not very quiet," and "Completely quiet," and for brightness, the choices were "Very bright," "Moderately bright," "Moderately dark," and "Very dark." Participants were also asked if a partner shared the same bed or same bedroom: "Did you share your bed or your bedroom with a partner?" The four response choices were: "I did not share my bed or my bedroom with a partner," "My partner or roommate slept in a separate room," "My partner slept in my bedroom but in a separate bed," and "I slept in the same bed as my partner."

First, descriptive analyses were performed. T-tests and Pearson's correlations were calculated to examine associations with the variables. Participants who scored a total of 8 or more on the ISI (n = 245) were classified into the Insomnia group and those who scored less than 8 (n = 343)

Table 1: Descriptive statistics according to the presence or absence of insomnia.

Variable	Total	Insomnia	Absence of insomnia	p
Age	79.29 (4.87)	79.17 (4.68)	79.38 (5.01)	0.603
Sex				0.119
Male	179 (30.4)	66 (36.9)	113 (63.1)	
Female	409 (69.6)	179 (43.8)	230 (56.2)	
Body mass index (BMI)	26.21 (4.41)	26.08 (4.16)	26.31 (4.58)	0.553
Civil status				0.482
Living alone	330 (56.3)	141 (42.7)	189 (57.3)	
Living as a couple	256 (43.7)	102 (39.8)	154 (60.2)	
Highest education level				0.646
Zero to 12 years	338 (58.5)	140 (41.4)	198 (58.6)	
College to university degree	240 (41.5)	104 (43.4)	136 (56.7)	
Partner sleeps in the same bed or bedroom				0.306
Sleeps alone in the bedroom	394 (69.1)	168 (42.6)	226 (57.4)	
Partner sleeps in the same bedroom	176 (30.9)	67 (38.1)	109 (61.9)	
Pillow comfort				<0.001
Very uncomfortable to moderately comfortable	273 (47.2)	138 (50.5)	135 (49.5)	
Very comfortable	306 (52.8)	104 (34.0)	202 (66.0)	
Mattress comfort				0.023
Very uncomfortable to moderately comfortable	244 (42.2)	115 (47.1)	129 (52.9)	
Very comfortable	334 (57.8)	126 (37.7)	208 (62.3)	
Nocturnal bedroom noise				0.001
Very loud to not very loud	171 (29.5)	89 (52.0)	82 (48.0)	
Completely quiet	408 (70.5)	152 (37.3)	256 (62.7)	
Morning bedroom noise				0.030
Very loud to not very loud	216 (37.6)	102 (47.2)	114 (52.8)	
Completely quiet	358 (62.4)	136 (38.0)	222 (62.0)	
Bedroom brightness at night				0.667
Very bright to moderately bright	71 (12.3)	28 (39.4)	43 (60.6)	
Moderately dark to very dark	508 (87.7)	214 (42.1)	294 (57.9)	
Bedroom brightness in the morning				0.452
Very bright to moderately bright	259 (44.8)	104 (40.2)	155 (59.8)	
Moderately dark to very dark	319 (55.2)	138 (43.3)	181 (56.7)	

Data are presented as mean (standard deviation) or number of participants (percentage).

were classified into the No-insomnia group. A binomial logistic regression followed by model adjustment of all the study variables were then performed to estimate the probability of belonging to the Insomnia group according to the sleep environment and sociodemographic variables. The assumptions of multicollinearity were met. The analyses were performed using SPSS Statistics 24 at a significance level of 5%.

3. Results

3.1. Participant Characteristics. Participants (N = 599) were 79.3 years old on average (range = 70.0–94.6 years). All lived at home. Women accounted for 69.6% of the sample. Of the women, 3.1% were below normal weight, 41.2% normal weight, 34.8% overweight, and 20.9% obese. Of the men, 1.7% were underweight, 35.1% normal weight, 48.9% overweight, and 14.3% obese. Almost 40% of participants were married and lived as a couple. Only 24.1% had completed a university degree, and 42% of participants had an average annual income less than $25,000.

Table 1 presents the descriptive statistics according to the presence (or not) of insomnia. With respect to comfort, 52.8% of participants reported sleeping with a very comfortable pillow and 57.8% on a very comfortable mattress. The bedroom was quiet at night for 70.5% of participants and quiet for 62.4% in the morning. The bedroom was moderate to very dark for 8.7% of participants at night and in the morning for 55.2%. Almost 70% of participants slept alone in a separate bedroom.

3.2. Comparison of Participants with and without Insomnia. Elderly persons who slept with a very uncomfortable pillow or mattress experienced insomnia significantly more often than those who reported their pillow or mattress as from not very comfortable to very comfortable. Similarly, insomniac participants slept significantly more often in a bedroom that was not completely quiet, both at night and in the morning. Table 2 presents the binomial logistic regression results. The adjusted model indicates that the probability of suffering from insomnia is twice as great when the pillow was rated from moderately comfortable to very uncomfortable and the bedroom was rated as not completely quiet at night. No other sleep environment characteristic was associated with a higher risk of insomnia while accounting for the other variables. The percentage of variance explained by the model is between 5.5% and 7.4%, suggesting that other variables not considered in this study would be more influential.

Table 2: Odds ratio and confidence intervals for the predictive variables for the presence or absence of insomnia.

Variables	Insomnia vs. absence of insomnia[a] OR	CI 95 %
Age	1.03	0.99–1.07
Sex		
Male	1.44	0.94–2.21
Female	1.00	
Body mass index (BMI)	1.00	0.96–1.05
Civil status		
Living along	1.06	0.62–1.81
Living as a couple	1.00	
Highest education level		
Zero to 12 years	0.78	0.53–1.15
College to university degree	1.00	
Partner sleeps in the same bed or bedroom		
Sleeps alone in the bedroom	1.01	0.57–1.81
Partner sleeps in the same bedroom	1.00	
Pillow comfort		
Very uncomfortable to moderately comfortable	2.00**	1.27–3.17
Very comfortable	1.00	
Mattress comfort		
Very uncomfortable to moderately comfortable	0.97	0.61–1.53
Very comfortable	1.00	
Nocturnal bedroom noise		
Very loud to not very loud	2.20**	1.26–3.82
Completely quiet	1.00	
Morning bedroom noise		
Very loud to not very loud	0.70	0.41–1.18
Completely quiet	1.00	
Bedroom brightness at night		
Very bright to moderately bright	0.88	0.48–1.62
Moderately dark to very dark	1.00	
Bedroom brightness in the morning		
Very bright to moderately bright	0.95	0.64–1.42
Moderately dark to very dark	1.00	

[a]Reference group. OR, odds ratio; CI, confidence interval. ** $p < 0.01$. Model $\chi^2_{(12)} = 28.70$, $p < 0.004$. $R^2 = 0.055$ (Cox and Snell), 0.074 (Nagelkerke).

4. Discussion

Our results indicate that a nonnegligible proportion of the elderly population endures a suboptimal sleep environment. Two components are significantly associated with insomnia symptoms: a pillow rated as moderately comfortable to very uncomfortable and a bedroom that was rated as not completely quiet.

These findings highlight the fact that many elderly persons sleep with a pillow that is uncomfortable to some extent and that these individuals are more likely to be insomniacs. Almost half of the participants reported that their pillow was not very comfortable. Given the relatively affordable cost of a new pillow, we might wonder what would justify hanging on to an uncomfortable one. Perhaps the vast choice of materials, shapes, and sizes available on the market [19, 23] combined with a lack of guidelines for consumers [20] would discourage some elderly persons from making a change. In fact, the study participants appeared to have had trouble finding a pillow that met their needs. These results support studies that have found that many people continue using an uncomfortable pillow, even when they wake up in pain [36]. Further studies are needed to understand the factors that influence pillow choice, as well as the pillow features that can provide comfort, diminish pain upon awakening, and promote good sleep quality in the elderly. At the same time, many cohort studies have found evidence to support a reciprocal relationship between sleep problems and chronic pain [37]. Because chronic pain was not measured in the present study, it is possible that some results could be partly attributable to the absence of control for pain in this sample. Given that the cervical region grows more vulnerable with age, it becomes all the more important to choose a good pillow [25].

Second, our results add to the evidence on increased symptoms of insomnia in the elderly when exposed to nocturnal noise [9, 38–41]. Almost 30% of our participants reported that they slept in a room that was not completely quiet at night. It is probable that some elderly persons ignore or play down the consequences of nocturnal noise. Because the elderly are at greater risk for nocturnal awakenings and sleep fragmentation than the general population [8], they would be at greater risk for suffering the consequences of a loud sleep environment, insofar as their hearing acuity is preserved. However, [42] demonstrated that simply using earplugs reduced noise by 7 to 12 dB, thereby promoting deep sleep. Furthermore, insulating the bedroom walls and replacing windows reduced noise by an average of 7 dB [43].

Over 40% of our participants reported that their mattress was not very comfortable. Despite the available information on sleep ergonomics, notably the importance of a good mattress to support the natural curvature of the spine, these findings indicate that insomnia was not associated with mattress discomfort. In view of the significant association found for pillow discomfort, this result is intriguing. It is possible that insomniac individuals tend to attribute certain symptoms to pillow discomfort rather than mattress discomfort. Because changes in position during nocturnal awakenings result in postural changes that affect the neck more than other parts of the body, the mattress may be perceived as playing a lesser role. Furthermore, the cost of a new mattress combined with the physical effort required to manoeuver it onto the bed could also influence how elderly persons perceive its impact on the sleep environment. This cognitive bias could steer complaints toward a factor that is more easily controlled, which could explain why the pillow was blamed more readily than the mattress. Although perceptions of mattress comfort could also be influenced by individual morphology, our finding showed no significant association between body mass index (BMI) and insomnia.

Approximately 12% of participants reported sleeping in a bedroom that was moderately or very bright at night. Although this proportion is small, making a room darker is a simple and affordable fix, and the reluctance to do so is puzzling. The normal deterioration of vision and the higher risk of falling in the elderly might threaten feelings of safety, whence the desire to keep the room at least dimly lighted at night. However, our results contradict studies that demonstrated a significant association between insomnia and exposure to nocturnal light in elderly populations [44, 45]. Although exposure to nocturnal light disrupts melatonin secretion and can consequently delay sleep, there is insufficient evidence in the literature to support a direct association between exposure to nocturnal light and insomnia. Nevertheless, it would be advisable to limit nocturnal light exposure in order to maintain a balanced circadian rhythm and prevent the development of disorders associated with an asynchronous circadian rhythm.

Compared with loud noise in the bedroom at night, loud noise in the morning was not associated with higher risk of insomnia. This could be explained by the systematic finding that elderly persons wake up earlier than the general population [46]. It is therefore possible that morning noise would be interpreted as time to get up. Rather than considering the noise as a problem, some individuals would simply get up and begin their day.

Almost 70% of participants slept alone in a separate bedroom, even though 44% lived as a couple. This practice could be partly explained by the high prevalence of unsatisfactory unions in the elderly population found in some studies [47]. The fragmented sleep of one member of the couple would probably lead to separate sleeping arrangements to preserve the sleep quality of the unaffected partner. In the population of middle-aged men, 17.5% snore loudly, and this proportion rises with age [48] to 33% of men and 19% of women aged 65 years and over [49]. It is reasonable to believe that some partners would prefer to sleep in a separate room to escape loud snoring. Separate rooms could also be explained by certain physical conditions, such as restless legs syndrome, which increases in prevalence with age and affects from 7 to 23% of individuals aged 40 years and over [50].

Among the limitations of this study, it is important to mention the impossibility of establishing a causal relationship between insomnia and either pillow comfort or nocturnal noise. Due to the cross-sectional study design, the relationships between the environmental factors and insomnia could be two directional. Thus, it is possible that a suboptimal sleep environment causes insomnia, which does not exclude the possibility that insomnia could lead to perceptions that certain aspects of the sleep environment are disturbing. The subjective measures used in this study would have been improved by the addition of objective measures to allow comparison with other studies. Considering that depression is an important risk factor for the development of sleep problems [51], and given the known association between these two conditions [52], it would have been relevant to assess the presence of depressive symptoms in our sample. In addition, pain assessments would have been useful to distinguish between insomnia that was primarily associated (or not) with physical pain. Hearing acuity could also have been determined, and earplug use could have been controlled for. These additional measures would allow further isolating the influence of sleep environment variables.

Despite these limitations, our results are based on a large sample of 600 elderly persons aged 70 years and over. All participants lived at home, which provided greater choice in arranging the sleep environment. The statistical analyses enabled assessing the contribution of each variable while taking into account the overall sleep environment, resulting in the identification of two sleep environment variables that were significantly associated with insomnia in our sample.

In a field that has received little attention, our results testify to the fact that a nonnegligible proportion of the elderly population endures a suboptimal sleep environment. The significant associations found between insomnia and pillow comfort as well as nocturnal noise point to future research avenues. To date, no studies to our knowledge have measured the impact of noise reduction at night on the sleep of elderly persons with insomnia. More studies are also needed to explore the impact of pillow replacement on elderly insomniacs. We do not know which factors contribute to the choice of a new pillow or the decision to continue using an uncomfortable pillow or mattress. Future studies could also look at the average age of pillows and mattresses used by elderly persons to determine the influence of wear and tear on insomnia. Although our study supports the research that demonstrates the harmful effect of nocturnal noise, more studies are needed to better target the consequences for sleep in the aging population. Similarly, the consequences of and the underlying reasons for the widespread practice of sleeping in a separate room remain unclear. Considering that it is preferable to use a combination of objective and subjective measures to examine sleep in the elderly [53], we recommend that future studies take advantage of a variety of available measures to gain a deeper understanding of the sleep experience in this population. Finally, pharmaceutical trials and CBT clinical trials should routinely measure or control for environmental factors when studies are done in the home. This environmental information might be used as covariates to improve signal detection of the primary intervention.

5. Conclusion

Although it is difficult to predict the actual impact of changes in the sleep environment of elderly persons, this study lends credibility to the hypothesis that simple, minor, and easily managed changes can promote sleep. Weighed against the minimal to nonexistent risks associated with such environmental changes, the potential benefits for the physical and psychological health of the elderly are substantial.

Conflicts of Interest

The authors declare that there are no conflicts of interest regarding the publication of this paper.

Acknowledgments

This work was supported by the Fonds de recherche du Québec–Société et culture (FRQSC) (2011-NP-137991).

References

[1] O. P. Almeida and J. J. Pfaff, "Sleep complaints among older general practice patients: association with depression," *British Journal of General Practice*, vol. 55, pp. 864–866, 2005.

[2] E. J. Haesler, "Effectiveness of strategies to manage sleep in residents of aged care facilities," *International Journal of Evidence-Based Healthcare*, vol. 2, no. 4, pp. 115–183, 2004.

[3] G. E. Simon and M. VonKorff, "Prevalence, burden, and treatment of insomnia in primary care," *The American Journal of Psychiatry*, vol. 154, no. 10, pp. 1417–1423, 1997.

[4] F. Breyer, J. Costa-Font, and S. Felder, "Ageing, health, and health care," *Oxford Review of Economic Policy*, vol. 26, no. 4, pp. 674–690, 2010.

[5] M. V. Vitiello, "The effective assessment and management of sleep disturbances in community-dwelling and institutionalized older adults," in *Introduction to Modern Sleep Technology*, D. R. P.-Y. Chiang, S.-C. Kang, R. P.-Y. Chiang, and S.-C. Kang, Eds., pp. 245–259, Springer Science+Business Media, New York, NY, USA, 2012.

[6] L. Bélanger, M. Leblanc, and C. M. Morin, "Cognitive behavioral therapy for insomnia in older adults," *Cognitive and Behavioral Practice*, vol. 19, no. 1, pp. 101–115, 2012.

[7] J. E. Maglione and S. Ancoli-Israel, "Sleep disorders in the elderly," in *The Oxford Handbook of Sleep and Sleep Disorders*, D. C. M. Morin, C. A. Espie, C. M. Morin, and C. A. Espie, Eds., pp. 769–786, Oxford University Press, New York, NY, USA, 2012.

[8] S. Koch, E. Haesler, A. Tiziani, and J. Wilson, "Effectiveness of sleep management strategies for residents of aged care facilities: findings of a systematic review," *Journal of Clinical Nursing*, vol. 15, no. 10, pp. 1267–1275, 2006.

[9] A. Muzet, "Environmental noise, sleep and health," *Sleep Medicine Reviews*, vol. 11, no. 2, pp. 135–142, 2007.

[10] R. Kim and M. van den Berg, "Summary of night noise guidelines for Europe," *Noise and Health*, vol. 12, no. 47, pp. 61–63, 2010.

[11] D. M. Berson, F. A. Dunn, and M. Takao, "Phototransduction by retinal ganglion cells that set the circadian clock," *Science*, vol. 295, no. 5557, pp. 1070–1073, 2002.

[12] C. Cajochen, "Alerting effects of light," *Sleep Medicine Reviews*, vol. 11, no. 6, pp. 453–464, 2007.

[13] K. Obayashi, K. Saeki, J. Iwamoto, Y. Ikada, and N. Kurumatani, "Exposure to light at night and risk of depression in the elderly," *Journal of Affective Disorders*, vol. 151, no. 1, pp. 331–336, 2013.

[14] K. Obayashi, K. Saeki, J. Iwamoto, Y. Ikada, and N. Kurumatani, "Association between light exposure at night and nighttime blood pressure in the elderly independent of nocturnal urinary melatonin excretion," *Chronobiology International*, vol. 31, no. 6, pp. 779–786, 2014.

[15] K. Obayashi, K. Saeki, and N. Kurumatani, "Light exposure at night is associated with subclinical carotid atherosclerosis in the general elderly population: the HEIJO-KYO cohort," *Chronobiology International*, vol. 32, no. 3, pp. 310–317, 2015.

[16] L. Zhu and P. C. Zee, "Circadian rhythm sleep disorders," *Neurologic Clinics*, vol. 30, no. 4, pp. 1167–1191, 2012.

[17] S. J. Gordon and K. Grimmer-Sommers, "How well does your own pillow perform?," *Journal of Musculoskeletal Pain*, vol. 19, no. 2, pp. 87–94, 2011.

[18] H.-L. Chen and D. Cai, "Body dimension measurements for pillow design for Taiwanese," *Work (Reading, Mass)*, vol. 41, no. S1, pp. 1288–1295, 2012.

[19] S.-F. Liu, Y.-L. Lee, and J.-C. Liang, "Shape design of an optimal comfortable pillow based on the analytic hierarchy process method," *Journal of Chiropractic Medicine*, vol. 10, no. 4, pp. 229–239, 2011.

[20] S. J. Gordon, K. Grimmer-Somers, and P. Trott, "Pillow use: the behaviour of cervical pain, sleep quality and pillow comfort in side sleepers," *Manual Therapy*, vol. 14, no. 6, pp. 671–678, 2009.

[21] M. L. Reitsma, J. E. Tranmer, D. M. Buchanan, and E. G. Vandenkerkhof, "The prevalence of chronic pain and pain-related interference in the Canadian population from 1994 to 2008," *Chronic Diseases and Injuries in Canada*, vol. 31, no. 4, pp. 157–164, 2011.

[22] M. Bernateck, M. Karst, S. Merkesdal, M. J. Fischer, and C. Gutenbrunner, "Sustained effects of comprehensive inpatient rehabilitative treatment and sleeping neck support in patients with chronic cervicobrachialgia: a prospective and randomized clinical trial," *International Journal of Rehabilitation Research*, vol. 31, no. 4, pp. 342–346, 2008.

[23] L. Persson, "Neck pain and pillows—A blinded study of the effect of pillows on non-specific neck pain, headache and sleep," *Advances in Physiotherapy*, vol. 8, no. 3, pp. 122–127, 2006.

[24] N. Shields, J. Capper, T. Polak, and N. Taylor, "Are cervical pillows effective in reducing neck pain?," *New Zealand Journal of Physiotherapy*, vol. 34, no. 1, pp. 3–9, 2006.

[25] L. Torii, J. Taylor, M. Rooney et al., "Effect of mattresses and pillow designs on promoting sleep quality, spinal alignment and pain reduction in adults: systematic reviews of controlled trials," Available from ProQuest Dissertations & Theses Full Text, 2016-26520-068, 2016.

[26] B. H. Jacobson, A. Boolani, G. Dunklee, A. Shepardson, and H. Acharya, "Effect of prescribed sleep surfaces on back pain and sleep quality in patients diagnosed with low back and shoulder pain," *Applied Ergonomics*, vol. 42, no. 1, pp. 91–97, 2010.

[27] M. Monsein, T. P. Corbin, P. D. Culliton, D. Merz, and E. A. Schuck, "Short-term outcomes of chronic back pain patients on an airbed vs innerspring mattresses," *Medscape General Medicine*, vol. 2, no. 3, p. E36, 2000.

[28] B. H. Jacobson, H. A. Gemmell, B. M. Hayes, and T. S. Altena, "Effectiveness of a selected bedding system on quality of sleep, low back pain, shoulder pain, and spine stiffness," *Journal of Manipulative and Physiological Therapeutics*, vol. 25, no. 2, pp. 88–92, 2002.

[29] G. G. Bader and S. Engdal, "The influence of bed firmness on sleep quality," *Applied Ergonomics*, vol. 31, no. 5, pp. 487–497, 2000.

[30] W. V. McCall, N. Boggs, and A. Letton, "Changes in sleep and wake in response to different sleeping surfaces: a pilot study," *Applied Ergonomics*, vol. 43, no. 2, pp. 386–391, 2012.

[31] L. Tonetti, M. Martoni, and V. Natale, "Effects of different mattresses on sleep quality in healthy subjects: an actigraphic study," *Biological Rhythm Research*, vol. 42, no. 2, pp. 89–97, 2011.

[32] L. A. Irish, C. E. Kline, H. E. Gunn, D. J. Buysse, and M. H. Hall, "The role of sleep hygiene in promoting public health: a review of empirical evidence," *Sleep Medicine Reviews*, vol. 22, pp. 23–36, 2015.

[33] M. Préville, R. Boyer, S. Grenier et al., "The epidemiology of psychiatric disorders in Quebec's older adult population," *Canadian Journal of Psychiatry*, vol. 53, no. 12, pp. 822–832, 2008.

[34] C. H. Bastien, A. Vallières, and C. M. Morin, "Validation of the Insomnia Severity Index as an outcome measure for insomnia research," *Sleep Medicine*, vol. 2, no. 4, pp. 297–307, 2001.

[35] F. C. Blais, L. Gendron, V. Mimeault, and C. M. Morin, "Évaluation de l'insomnie: validation de trois questionnaires," *L'Encéphale: Revue de psychiatrie clinique biologique et thérapeutique*, vol. 23, no. 6, pp. 447–453, 1997.

[36] S. J. Gordon and K. Grimmer-Somers, "Your pillow may not guarantee a good night's sleep or symptom-free waking," *Physiotherapy Canada*, vol. 63, no. 2, pp. 183–190, 2011.

[37] P. H. Finan, B. R. Goodin, and M. T. Smith, "The association of sleep and pain: an update and a path forward," *Journal of Pain*, vol. 14, no. 12, pp. 1539–1552, 2013.

[38] J. I. Halonen, J. Vahtera, S. Stansfeld et al., "Associations between nighttime traffic noise and sleep: the Finnish public sector study," *Environmental Health Perspectives*, vol. 120, no. 10, pp. 1391–1396, 2012.

[39] H. M. E. Miedema and H. Vos, "Associations between self-reported sleep disturbance and environmental noise based on reanalyses of pooled data from 24 studies," *Behavioral Sleep Medicine*, vol. 5, no. 1, pp. 1–20, 2007.

[40] E. Öhrström, E. Hadzibajramovic, M. Holmes, and H. Svensson, "Effects of road traffic noise on sleep: studies on children and adults," *Journal of Environmental Psychology*, vol. 26, no. 2, pp. 116–126, 2006.

[41] L. Stosić, G. Belojević, and S. Milutinović, "Effects of traffic noise on sleep in an urban population," *Journal of Institute for Medical Research and Occupational Health*, vol. 60, no. 3, pp. 335–342, 2009.

[42] H. Xie, J. Kang, and G. H. Mills, "Clinical review: the impact of noise on patients' sleep and the effectiveness of noise reduction strategies in intensive care units," *Critical Care*, vol. 13, no. 208, pp. 1–8, 2009.

[43] A. H. Amundsen, R. Klæboe, and G. M. Aasvang, "Long-term effects of noise reduction measures on noise annoyance and sleep disturbance: the Norwegian facade insulation study," *Journal of the Acoustical Society of America*, vol. 133, no. 6, pp. 3921–3928, 2013.

[44] K. Obayashi, K. Saeki, J. Iwamoto et al., "Effect of exposure to evening light on sleep initiation in the elderly: a longitudinal analysis for repeated measurements in home settings," *Chronobiology International*, vol. 31, no. 4, pp. 461–467, 2014.

[45] K. Obayashi, K. Saeki, and N. Kurumatani, "Association between light exposure at night and insomnia in the general elderly population: the HEIJO-KYO cohort," *Chronobiology International*, vol. 31, no. 9, pp. 976–982, 2014.

[46] M. M. Ohayon, M. A. Carskadon, C. Guilleminault, and M. V. Vitiello, "Meta-analysis of quantitative sleep parameters from childhood to old age in healthy individuals: developing normative sleep values across the human lifespan," *Sleep*, vol. 27, no. 7, pp. 1255–1273, 2004.

[47] K. Margelisch, K. A. Schneewind, J. Violette, and P. Perrig-Chiello, "Marital stability, satisfaction and well-being in old age: variability and continuity in long-term continuously married older persons," *Aging and Mental Health*, vol. 21, no. 4, pp. 389–398, 2015.

[48] D. Teculescu, L. Benamghar, B. Hannhart, and J.-P. Michaely, "Habitual loud snoring. A study of prevalence and associations in 850 middle-aged French males," *Respiration International Review of Thoracic Diseases*, vol. 73, no. 1, pp. 68–72, 2006.

[49] P. L. Enright, A. B. Newman, P. W. Wahl, T. A. Manolio, E. F. Haponik, and P. J. Boyle, "Prevalence and correlates of snoring and observed apneas in 5,201 older adults," *Sleep*, vol. 19, no. 7, pp. 531–538, 1996.

[50] M. M. Ohayon, R. O'Hara, and M. V. Vitiello, "Epidemiology of restless legs syndrome: a synthesis of the literature," *Sleep Medicine Reviews*, vol. 16, no. 4, pp. 283–295, 2012.

[51] M. Fok, R. Stewart, A. Besset, K. Ritchie, and M. Prince, "Incidence and persistence of sleep complaints in a community older population," *International Journal of Geriatric Psychiatry*, vol. 25, no. 1, pp. 37–45, 2010.

[52] I. Jaussent, J. Bouyer, M.-L. Ancelin et al., "Insomnia and daytime sleepiness are risk factors for depressive symptoms in the elderly," *Sleep*, vol. 34, no. 8, pp. 1103–1110, 2011.

[53] G. J. Landry, J. R. Best, and T. Liu-Ambrose, "Measuring sleep quality in older adults: a comparison using subjective and objective methods," *Frontiers in Aging Neuroscience*, vol. 7, no. 166, pp. 1–10, 2015.

19

Self-Rated Health Trajectories among Married Americans: Do Disparities Persist over 20 Years?

Terceira A. Berdahl[1] **and Julia McQuillan**[2]

[1]Division of Research and Modeling, Center for Financing, Access and Cost Trends, Agency for Healthcare Research and Quality, 5600 Fishers Lane, Rockville, MD 20852, USA
[2]University of Nebraska-Lincoln, 709 Oldfather Hall, Lincoln, NE 68588-0324, USA

Correspondence should be addressed to Terceira A. Berdahl; terceira.berdahl@ahrq.hhs.gov

Academic Editor: F. R. Ferraro

The purpose of this study is to understand self-rated health (SRH) trajectories by social location (race/ethnicity by gender by social class) among married individuals in the United States. We estimate multilevel models of SRH using six observations from 1980 to 2000 from a nationally representative panel of married individuals initially aged 25–55 (Marital Instability Over the Life Course Study). Results indicate that gender, race/ethnicity, and social class are associated with initial SRH disparities. Women are less healthy than men; people of color are less healthy than whites; lower educated individuals are less healthy than higher educated individuals. Women's health declined slower than men's but did not differ by race/ethnicity or education. Results from complex intersectional models show that white men with any college had the highest initial SRH. Only women with any college had significantly slower declines in SRH compared to white men with any college. For married individuals of all ages, most initial SRH disparities persist over twenty years. Intersecting statuses show that education provides uneven health benefits across racial/ethnic and gender subgroups.

1. Introduction

There are well-documented disparities in health by race/ethnicity, gender, and social class in the United States. Less is known about the combined advantages and disadvantages at the intersection of race/ethnicity, gender, and social class. Questions also remain regarding whether or not initial self-rated health disparities exacerbate or diminish over time. It is important to estimate, and not assume, whether social class effects on health are similar for men and women and white and nonwhite Americans. To advance knowledge of patterns of health disparities in the United States, we estimate self-rated health (SRH) trajectories over 20 years using six waves (observations) from a panel study of married individuals who were aged 25–55 in 1980 at the time of the first interview.

2. Background

2.1. Intersectionality and Health Disparities. A growing number of researchers are calling for more nuanced analyses of health inequality to acknowledge diverse outcomes of individuals who occupy different positions in social structural hierarchies [1–3]. One useful approach is the intersectionality paradigm [4–6], which emphasizes how social structures intersect to create the axis of advantage and disadvantage in multiplicative rather than only in separate or additive ways. For example, there is evidence that the experiences of women of color cannot be adequately understood by studying race/ethnicity or gender in isolation [1, 7–9]. To assess particular policies or laws, it can be appropriate to study only one axis of inequality; but to gain a more comprehensive understanding of overall changes in health with aging, comparing subgroups created by assessing multiple axes of stratification simultaneously (e.g., social class, race/ethnicity, and gender) is fruitful [10–12].

Prior work on health disparities finds that indicators of social location (e.g., race, gender, and education) contribute to health inequality [10, 13]. Men have worse mortality than women but spend fewer years with comorbidity and disability [10, 14]. Compared to whites, racial-ethnic minorities continue to face lower life expectancy and worse health outcomes from birth until death [14]. Studies of educational disparities find that people with lower education have worse health and faster health declines with aging compared to people with higher education [15, 16]. Recent studies have examined the intersections of gender and social class or race/ethnicity and social class and find that these intersections matter for health changes associated with aging [10].

Most longitudinal studies of aging include people as young as 25 and follow people for decades in small geographic areas with little racial diversity. We know of no studies that simultaneously analyze the intersections of class, race/ethnicity, and gender for twenty years. Instead, most studies focus on older and elderly adults. The current study focuses on people who were married at the start of the study. It is possible that the health protective effects of marriage could minimize gender, education, and race/ethnicity health disparities [17, 18]. Yet, recent research highlighting the long reach of inequality from grandparents and from early life suggests that even among the married, disparities are likely to persist with aging [19–21].

2.2. Health Protective Effects of Marriage. Marital status is a social resource that can protect against steep health declines associated with aging. Among people who are married, the influence of depressive symptoms and chronic conditions on subsequent functional limitations is weaker compared to nonmarried [22]. The end of a marriage is also associated with higher allostatic load (an indicator of biological risk for worse health) [23]. The physiological impact of marital disruption is larger for widowhood than divorce, as indicated by comparisons of inflammatory, metabolic, and cardiovascular functioning compared to those who remain married [23].

Rates of marriage, like health disparities, vary by race and social class. Marriage rates and duration are lower among people with lower education and racial/ethnic minorities compared to people who have higher education and who are white [24]. Therefore, health differences by race/ethnicity and education could be smaller among the married than the nonmarried because of selection into a status with privileges [25]. In 1980, the difference in ever-married rates among white women (95%) and black women (87%) was smaller than that in 2012 (87% for white women and 63% for black women) [24]. Because marriage was ubiquitous in 1980, it is unclear if there will be health disparities in this more narrow group than the general population, yet we argue that it is important to find out, because marriage is sometimes promoted as a way to reduce social problems, even though there is evidence that marriage does not have the same privileges for all [26].

3. Current Study

In the present study, we advance understanding of health disparities by answering two important questions: In the United States, are there health disparities among people who are married that are created by disadvantaged social locations due to the intersections of gender, race, and education? If yes, do disparities persist over decades? To answer these questions, we examined self-rated health trajectories of a random sample of individuals who were married in 1980 and followed over twenty years. We restricted the sample to adults who were initially aged 25–55 years. We categorized individuals by gender (men or women), race/ethnicity (white or nonwhite), and level of education (up to less than a high school degree, a high school degree, or any level of college education), thus creating twelve subgroups with varying advantages and disadvantages.

4. Data and Methods

For the current study, we used data from the *Marital Instability Over the Life Course (MIOLC)* study, a six-wave panel study of a national sample of initially married persons in the United States [27]. Respondents were interviewed by telephone in 1980, 1983, 1988, 1992, 1997, and 2000 (*waves 1–6*). Only the wife or the husband was included in the study; the participant was selected by random assignment. During the first wave of the study, the survey involved random digit dialing and screening of individuals for inclusion in the study. The inclusion criteria required that individuals had to be married and between the ages of 18 and 55. Among eligible households, the rate of completed interviews for the initial wave of the study was 65%, yielding a sample size of 2,034. The response rates varied among subsequent waves of data collection (in the order: 78%, 84%, 88%, 90%, and 82%). The analytical sample for this study includes those between the ages of 25 and 55 at the initial interview in order to ensure that they were likely to have finished their education. Multilevel models incorporate data from as many waves as participants completed; as with all longitudinal studies, there was attrition over time. Comprehensive information about the data set and how well it represents the U.S. married population of 1980 and comparisons with formerly married adults in 2000 is provided in the methodology report [28].

4.1. Variables/Measures

4.1.1. Self-Rated Health (SRH). We measure self-rated health, the dependent variable, with the following question: "Now I have some questions about your health. In general, would you say your own health is excellent (3), good (2), fair (1), or poor (0)?" This single-item measure has a strong association with mortality, suggesting that it is a valid indicator of health [29]. Self-rated health is measured in every wave of data collection in the same way.

4.1.2. Wave/Trajectory. To measure the changes in self-rated health, we include a variable that indicates the wave of observation. This variable is coded as 0 for the first interview in 1980 and 5 for the last interview in 2000, with consecutive numbers in between. There were about three years between interviews. With this variable in the model, the intercept indicates the average initial self-rated health, and the coefficient for "wave" indicates the average change in self-rated health between observations, or the trajectory of change in health. The variance component for this variable indicates the amount of spread around the average trajectory.

4.1.3. Age. We included age (measured in years) as an individual level characteristic to adjust for differences in initial health status. We mean center age so that the intercept represents participants with the average age for the sample.

4.1.4. Social Location. We measure social class using education, a common practice in health research [30]. We use only the initial value of education because very few people add years of education beyond age 25 in the 1980s. Education was measured in years of completed formal education. We converted years into three categories. Because a high school degree is a requirement for many jobs and a college degree is required for another set of jobs, we divided years into less than a high school degree (<12 years) (LTHS), high school (12 years) (HS), and any college (13+ years). The three-category measure of education helped to make meaningful subgroups for the intersectionality analysis by combining education with *gender* (what is your sex? male/female) and *race/ethnicity* (what race do you consider yourself to be? recoded into white and nonwhite) to create 12 total subgroups.

4.2. Analysis Strategy. We use multilevel models to estimate the trajectories of self-rated health. The multilevel model trajectory approach appropriately estimates the nesting of observations within individuals and attrition [31]. All models are estimated with random effects for the intercept (initial status) and slope parameters using HLM 7.03. Additionally, we control for initial age because the rate of health decline is likely to be steeper for those closer to 55 than to 25. The time variable is centered at the initial observation to facilitate meaningful interpretation of the constant (e.g., average initial self-rated health) [32].

Our analysis begins with a brief discussion of the sample in 1980 (see Tables 1 and 2). After presenting these descriptive statistics, we move to the HLM analysis. In Table 3, we present Model 1, which includes the time variable and serves as a baseline trajectory model for self-rated health. This model contains an intercept and a slope for time (year) with random effects for these parameters as well as an overall Level 1 error term. Next, we present estimates from Model 2 (Table 3) which includes a variable capturing respondent age at the first year of the survey (initial age). In Models 3–5 (Table 4), we present separate models with gender (Model 3), race (Model 4), and education (Model 5) to evaluate the effects of these characteristics on the aging trajectories without other variables in the model. These models illustrate how gender, race, and education modify self-rated health over time. Finally, in Model 4, we explore the joint effects of gender, race, and education by constructing comparative categories to capture the three-way interaction of these variables (Table 5).

A conventional interaction approach would also generate eleven coefficients with a comparison to the intercept

TABLE 1: Sample descriptive statistics for MIOLC wave 1, aged 25–55.

	Mean (%)	SD
Self-rated health	2.26	0.75
Age (in years)	37.24	8.33
Race		
Nonwhite	11.9	—
White	88.1	—
Gender		
Men	41.5	—
Women	58.5	—
Education		
<HS	10.4	—
High school graduate	63.1	—
Any college	26.5	—

$N = 1{,}785$.

TABLE 2: Self-rated health by gender, race, and education for adults aged 25–55 in 1980.

			Mean	SD	N
Women	White	Less than high school	2.09	0.85	88
		High school graduate	2.30	0.72	371
		Any college	2.49	0.67	455
	Nonwhite	Less than high school	1.85	0.81	20
		High school graduate	2.15	0.70	52
		Any college	2.05	0.71	58
Men	White	Less than high school	1.88	1.00	57
		High school graduate	2.36	0.77	181
		Any college	2.55	0.62	420
	Nonwhite	Less than high school	2.10	0.89	21
		High school graduate	2.22	0.67	23
		Any college	2.31	0.73	39

MIOLC data, wave 1, $N = 1{,}785$.

and the need to rotate out the reference category using a "simple slope" approach to hypothesis testing to determine which groups are different from each other [33]. Yet, the conventional approach also requires solving equations to determine the total difference of each group from the others based upon the main effects, two-way interactions, and three-way interactions. We constructed indicator variables for the subgroups to provide a mathematically equivalent way to determine subgroup differences in SRH and simultaneously increase the ease of interpreting coefficients summarizing those differences [8]. We also estimated supplemental analyses by rotating the reference group to compare each subgroup (available from the author upon request). Our approach involves multiple significance tests, which in classical regression can increase the risk of Type 1 errors (finding a significant association when none exists). By using HLM with empirical Bayes estimation methods, we reduce the risk of Type 1 error [34]. There are practices for post hoc adjustments to reduce the risk of Type 1 error (e.g., Bonferroni adjustments), but there are arguments against this practice [35]. Because we also have some groups with small sample sizes (e.g., nonwhite

TABLE 3: Models 1-2: self-rated health by age and self-rated health aging trajectory.

	Model 1			Model 2		
	b	SE	p value	b	SE	p value
Initial SRH (intercept)	2.358	0.016	<0.001	2.358	0.016	<0.001
× initial age	—	—	—	−0.011	0.002	<0.001
SRH trajectory (time slope)	−0.061	0.005	0.005	−0.061	0.005	<0.001
× initial age	—	—	—	−0.001	0.001	0.034
Random effects	SD	VC	p value	SD	VC	p value
Initial SRH intercept, u_0	0.561	0.311	<0.001	0.551	0.301	<0.001
SRH trajectory slope, u_1	0.111	0.011	<0.001	0.111	0.011	<0.001
Level 1, r	0.511	0.261	—	0.511	0.261	—

Note. SD = standard deviation; VC = variance component; Level 2 MIOLC N = 1,785.

TABLE 4: Models 3–5: self-rated health trajectories by gender, race, and education.

	Model 3			Model 4			Model 5		
	b	SE	p value	b	SE	p value	b	SE	p value
Initial SRH (intercept)	2.410	0.025	<0.001	2.389	0.017	<0.001	2.462	0.020	<0.001
× initial age	−0.012	0.002	<0.001	−0.012	0.002	<0.001	−0.010	0.002	<0.001
Women (men = reference group)	−0.085	0.033	0.009	—	—	—	—	—	—
Nonwhite (white = reference group)	—	—	—	−0.266	0.050	<0.001	—	—	—
Less than HS (any college = reference group)	—	—	—	—	—	—	−0.440	0.065	<0.001
High school	—	—	—	—	—	—	−0.168	0.034	<0.001
SRH trajectory (time slope)	−0.083	0.008	<0.001	−0.064	0.005	<0.001	−0.062	0.006	<0.001
× initial age	−0.001	0.001	0.064	−0.001	0.001	0.041	−0.001	0.001	0.020
Women (men = reference group)	0.037	0.010	<0.001	—	—	—	—	—	—
Nonwhite (white = reference group)	—	—	—	0.022	0.020	0.289	—	—	—
Less than HS (any college = reference group)	—	—	—	—	—	—	0.021	0.024	0.392
High school	—	—	—	—	—	—	−0.007	0.010	0.496
Random effects	SD	VC	p value	SD	VC	p value	SD	VC	p value
Initial SRH intercept, u_0	0.546	0.298	<0.001	0.541	0.293	<0.001	0.532	0.282	<0.001
SRH trajectory slope, u_1	0.106	0.011	<0.001	0.108	0.012	<0.001	0.108	0.012	<0.001
Level 1, r	0.508	0.258	—	0.508	0.258	—	0.508	0.258	—

Note. SRH = self-rated health; VC = variance component; SD = standard deviation; Level 2 MIOLC N = 1,785.

women with less than a high school degree), we also risk making Type 2 errors (failing to find significance when there really is an association in the population). We therefore use the conventional 0.05 level of significance, focus on the size and meaning of differences, and use the significance tests as a heuristic for interpreting patterns of associations.

5. Results

5.1. Sample Descriptive Characteristics. We report sample descriptive statistics for the sample in Table 1. The mean age for the analytical sample was 37.24 (SD = 8.33) at the initial interview. Just over 10 percent of the sample is nonwhite (12%). Over half (58%) of the sample was women. Fewer participants have less than a high school degree (10%) than any college education (55%). On a scale from 0 to 3, with zero representing poor health and 3 representing excellent health, average initial self-rated health was above the midpoint (M = 2.26 and SD = 0.75).

In the initial survey, 1,785 participants responded to the variables in the analytical sample. Average self-rated health ranges from a low of 1.85 among nonwhite women with less than a high school degree (those with the most social disadvantages) to a high of 2.55 among white men with any college education (those with the most social advantages) (Table 2). For every race by the gender group, those with any college education are the largest group. Almost half of the sample consists of people who are white with any college education. The smallest groups are people who are nonwhite with less than a high school degree. Only nonwhite women do not have an education health gradient because those with any college education have lower self-rated health than those with a high school degree. For all other gender by race groups, higher education is associated with higher self-rated health.

5.2. Aging Trajectory Findings. We first describe the baseline model (no covariates; not shown in the table). The baseline

Table 5: Model 6: self-rated health trajectories by gender, race, and education.

	Model 6		
	b	SE	p value
Initial SRH (intercept)	2.52	0.03	<0.001
× initial age	−0.01	0.00	<0.001
Race by gender by education			
× nonwhite women LTHS	−0.67	0.14	<0.001
× nonwhite women HS	−0.42	0.08	<0.001
× nonwhite women any college	−0.47	0.09	<0.001
× nonwhite men LTHS	−0.32	0.18	0.07
× nonwhite men HS	−0.30	0.14	0.03
× nonwhite men any college	−0.22	0.12	0.06
× white women LTHS	−0.47	0.09	<0.001
× white women HS	−0.22	0.05	<0.001
× white women any college	−0.05	0.04	0.19
× white men LTHS	−0.54	0.13	<0.001
× white men HS	−0.19	0.06	0.00
SRH trajectory (time slope)	−0.082	0.010	<0.001
× initial age	−0.001	0.001	0.047
Race by gender by education			
× nonwhite women LTHS	0.057	0.128	0.653
× nonwhite women HS	0.042	0.035	0.226
× nonwhite women any college	0.096	0.035	0.006
× nonwhite men LTHS	0.064	0.070	0.361
× nonwhite men HS	−0.041	0.043	0.345
× nonwhite men any college	−0.045	0.051	0.383
× white women LTHS	0.050	0.030	0.099
× white women HS	0.022	0.014	0.105
× white women any college	0.029	0.013	0.022
× white men LTHS	0.015	0.045	0.745
× white men HS	−0.012	0.021	0.550
Random effects	SD	VC	p value
Initial SRH intercept, u_0	0.525	0.275	<0.001
SRH trajectory slope, u_1	0.106	0.011	<0.001
Level 1, r	0.508	0.258	—

Note. The reference group is white men with any college; LTHS = less than high school; HS = high school; AC = any college; Level 2 MIOLC N = 1,785.

model provides an estimate of the intercept and variance components. The intercept indicates that the average self-rated health across all participants and all waves is 2.252***, a value that is above the midpoint of the 0 to 3 range for the variable (3 indicates excellent health). Average self-rated health varies significantly between people (the variance component for the intercept in the baseline model is 0.267***, and for within people, the Level 1 error is 0.308). The variance components indicate that just under half of the variance in self-rated health is between individuals (47%, or (0.267/(0.267 + 0.307))) and just over half is within individuals over time (53%).

Model 1 in Table 3 provides an estimate of the aging trajectory in self-rated health, which is measured by the time variable (one unit is approximately three years). The trajectory measure has the value 0 for the first year, 1980, and 5 for the twentieth year, 2000. Therefore, the intercept for this model provides the average self-rated health in the first year of the study (1980). Initial self-rated health is 2.361***, slightly higher (better) than the average for all years in the baseline model. The SRH trajectory coefficient indicates that, on average, self-rated health declines between interviews ($b = -0.061$***). The standard deviation for self-rated health is 0.75. Therefore, over the six waves and twenty years, on average, self-rated health declines by −0.36 (−0.06 × 6), or almost half a standard deviation. The rate of decline in self-rated health varies across individuals, indicated by the significant variance component (variance components p value = 0.012***).

To adjust for the thirty-year range of initial ages, we included an indicator of initial age in Model 2 (Table 3). Consistent with the strong association between age and health, health declines with age ($b = -0.012$***), and the self-rated health aging trajectory is steeper for participants who were older at the start of the study (the coefficient is −0.001* larger for each additional year). The average age in the analytical sample is 37.24, with a standard deviation of 8.33 years. Therefore, the difference between a standard deviation below and above the mean age is 16.66 years translating into 24% of a standard deviation in initial self-rated health (−0.011 × 16.66 = −0.18/.75 = 24%). Initial self-rated health is arranged as we would expect, with those who are 25 reporting the best health and those age 55 the worst health. Twenty years later, all groups decline, but the decline is steeper for those who were initially older, resulting in larger differences between the age groups at the end of the study.

Building on the model with initial age and the self-rated health trajectory, we next separately explore if there are disparities by gender, race/ethnicity, or level of education for the initial or the aging trajectory of self-rated health (Table 4, Models 3–5). Women have lower average initial self-rated health ($b = -0.085$**, or 12% of a standard deviation lower), yet the decline in health for women is less steep than it is for men ($b = 0.037$***; therefore, the slope for women is −0.083*** + 0.037*** = −0.05). Women initially have worse health, but because their health declines more slowly, over time, they end up with better health than men twenty years later.

There is also an initial difference between nonwhite and white individuals (Table 4, Model 4). The race/ethnicity difference is larger than the gender effect ($b = -0.266$***). The declines in self-rated health are not as steep for nonwhite compared to white individuals (white = −0.064; nonwhite = −0.064*** + 0.022 = −0.040), yet this difference is not significant.

Consistent with prior research, there is a steep health gradient by education (Table 4, Model 5). Individuals with any college have the highest self-rated health (intercept = 2.462***). Those with a high school level of education have about a fifth of a standard deviation lower self-rated health ($b = -0.168$***), and the difference is even greater for those with less than a high school degree ($b = -0.440$***). Although education has strong associations with initial SRH, level of education does not modify the rate of decline, adjusted for age. Those who start the study in their older age do have slightly but significantly steeper declines in health (age $b = -0.001^{*}$ + trajectory coefficient $= -0.062^{***}$; therefore, for each additional year, the rate of decline is -0.001 larger).

The separate models of gender, race/ethnicity, and education also show that none of these indicators of social status alone explain the variance in initial self-rated health or in the change in self-rated health over time, indicated by the significant variance components in all of the models.

We next examine the combined effect of all three indicators of social location simultaneously (Table 5, Model 6). Most of the subgroups differ in initial self-rated health relative to white men with any college, the reference group. All groups have negative coefficients, indicating lower initial self-rated health. Three groups do not have significantly lower self-rated health than white men with any college (nonwhite men with less than a high school level of education and nonwhite men and white women with any college). The differences in initial self-rated health for most groups persist with age because the rate of decline is not significantly different from the most privileged group (white men with any college: $b = -0.08^{***}$). Two groups, however, did have significantly slower declines (positive coefficients) in self-rated health with age: nonwhite women ($b = 0.100^{**}$) and white women ($b = 0.029^{*}$) with any college.

In addition to the comparisons with the most privileged group (white men who have any college education), it is useful to determine if there are significant differences among the groups with varying levels of privilege and disadvantage as indicated by gender, race/ethnicity, and education. We therefore reran the final model and rotated the comparison group until we estimated all possible comparisons (detailed results available upon request). Unlike the story from the separate gender, race/ethnicity, and education models, all women are not different from all men. White women at any level of education do not differ from less-educated nonwhite men (less than HS and HS). Education does not have the same strong association with self-rated health among nonwhite men and women; there are no education differences among those who are nonwhite, but there is an education health gradient among those who are white. White men have higher levels of self-rated health than nonwhite women but only if they have at least a high school level of education. There are no gender differences in self-rated health between white men and women who have the same level of education. Therefore, the main effects of gender, race, and education do not hold among all of the subgroups.

6. Discussion

Most prior research on health disparities focuses on either racial-ethnic, gender, or social class as separate forms of social stratification and focuses on older adults. Our findings provide support for the value of recognizing multiple intersecting systems of advantage and disadvantage simultaneously [1, 5, 6, 11]. For example, similar to prior studies, we find strong associations of education and health [36]. We did not observe similar effects of education, however, across self-rated health trajectories for all racial/ethnic and gender groups. For lower educated women, declines in health are similar to higher educated white men. For higher educated women, there are slower declines in self-rated health compared to higher educated white men. Thus, the rate of decline in self-rated health is conditioned by gender and education. Similar to Liang et al. we find racial differences in the intercept, or average health at the beginning of the study, with nonwhites scoring significantly worse on health measures [19]. Additionally, that study found few significant racial differences in aging trajectories over time, which is also similar to our study (although not directly comparable because they did not evaluate racial effects across gender and education) [19]. Consistent with our study findings, another study of aging among African Americans found that in older adults, self-rated health did not decline significantly over time [37].

The current study provides evidence that among married individuals, there are several initial differences in self-rated health, and for all but higher educated women, those differences persist over twenty years. Consistent with other studies, older age was associated with worse health initially and a steeper decline in health over time. Not surprisingly, for all age groups, self-rated health declined with aging. We were surprised to find that even among married individuals, there are important disparities in health and persistence in disparities with declines in aging. Therefore, neither selection into nor the protective effects of marriage eliminate the effects of structural inequality on health.

Data limitations require some caution in overgeneralizing these results. One limitation is that the study was designed to focus on married individuals. We do not have a comparison group of unmarried individuals during the same time period. We cannot generalize beyond the ever-married population in 1980. This limitation is somewhat mitigated by historical context because marriage was more common for whites and blacks in 1980 [24]. We expect that health status, however, would be worse among unmarried individuals; therefore, these results should not be generalized beyond the married [17].

The MIOLC data set has smaller sample sizes for the sample of nonwhite men and women. Because of the smaller relative sample of nonwhites, it is possible our study lacks power to find statistically significant differences for subgroups with small samples in our data (more likely to have a type 2 error). As described above, there is a risk that we will falsely claim significance when nonexists with the many comparisons involved in subgroup analysis to model intersectionality.

In a recent study, Ferarro et al. reviewed several possible mechanisms for long-standing racial and ethnic health disparities (e.g., differential exposure to environmental hazards, poverty, higher rates of smoking, more dangerous jobs, less access to health care, accumulation of disadvantages, and weathering) [3]. A central idea in health disparities research is that differences between groups constructed from different locations in social hierarchies reflect modifiable characteristics potentially amenable to interventions. Even with our limitations, the current study provides valuable evidence that for most groups, health disparities persist with age, yet for women, higher education can be protective (but not for nonwhite men). In addition, we have an unusually wide range of ages and participants are followed for two decades, providing considerable data to estimate health trajectories. Many studies of aging tend to start when people are in the 50s, because most studies rely upon data sources such as the Health and Retirement Survey, which is limited to individuals aged 50 or older [19].

7. Conclusion

Our findings join the growing effort to provide more context for health inequality and to address groups that have been historically marginalized (e.g., women of color). This approach also allows us to compare groups that are simultaneously advantaged and disadvantaged, such as lower educated white men and women, groups recently receiving increased research and policy attention [38, 39]. As urged by Bauer, our study illustrates how using an intersectionality framework can further disparities research, especially among married individuals [2]. Future studies should evaluate whether or not health advantages for married individuals intersect with race, gender, and education to explain the effect of marital status on health. Our findings suggest that policy efforts to promote marriage are not likely to reduce health disparities, but discovering if disparities exist even among the married will add to efforts to reduce disparities by focusing efforts on factors that matter the most [26]. In addition to healthier people "selecting into" marriage, there is also evidence that marriage has health benefits [18], particularly for men [40]. However, this benefit may not extend to nonwhite men given lower marriage and higher cohabitation rates among African Americans compared to white Americans [24].

Examining multiple subgroups with varying levels of privilege and disadvantage reveals that the most structurally advantaged group did indeed have the best initial self-rated health. Most, but not all, subgroups declined in health at similar rates. Therefore, we cannot expect that health disparities will diminish with time, as would occur if age was a leveler [15, 16]. Instead, gaps persist, and therefore efforts to improve health disparities by gender, race, and class are still needed.

Conflicts of Interest

The authors declare that there are no conflicts of interest regarding the publication of this paper.

References

[1] L. Bowleg, "The problem with the phrase women and minorities: intersectionality—an important theoretical framework for public health," *American Journal of Public Health*, vol. 102, no. 7, pp. 1267–1273, 2012.

[2] G. R. Bauer, "Incorporating intersectionality theory into population health research methodology: challenges and the potential to advance health equity," *Social Science & Medicine*, vol. 110, pp. 10–17, 2014.

[3] K. F. Ferraro, B. R. Kemp, and M. M. Williams, "Diverse aging and health inequality by race and ethnicity," *Innovation in Aging*, vol. 1, no. 1, pp. 1–11, 2017.

[4] P. H. Collins, "Toward a new vision: race, class, and gender as categories of analysis and connection," *Race, Sex & Class*, vol. 1, no. 1, pp. 25–45, 1993.

[5] K. Crenshaw, "Demarginalizing the intersection of race and sex: a black feminist critique of antidiscrimination doctrine, feminist theory and antiracist politics," *University of Chicago Legal Forum*, vol. 1989, p. 139, 1989.

[6] P. H. Collins, *Black Feminist Thought: Knowledge, Consciousness, and the Politics of Empowerment*, Routledge, New York, NY, USA, 2002.

[7] L. McCall, *Complex Inequality: Gender, Class, and Race in the New Economy*, Psychology Press, New York, NY, USA, 2001.

[8] L. McCall, "The complexity of intersectionality," *Signs*, vol. 30, no. 3, pp. 1771–1800, 2005.

[9] I. Browne and J. Misra, "The intersection of gender and race in the labor market," *Annual Review of Sociology*, vol. 29, no. 1, pp. 487–513, 2003.

[10] T. M. Calasanti and K. F. Slevin, *Gender, Social Inequalities, and Aging*, AltaMira Press, Walnut Creek, CA, USA, 2001.

[11] T. M. Calasanti and K. F. Slevin, *Age Matters: Realigning Feminist Thinking*, Taylor & Francis, New York, NY, USA, 2006.

[12] S. W. Hinze, J. Lin, and T. E. Andersson, "Can we capture the intersections? Older Black women, education, and health," *Women's Health Issues*, vol. 22, no. 1, pp. e91–e98, 2012.

[13] D. R. Williams and C. Collins, "US socioeconomic and racial differences in health: patterns and explanations," *Annual Review of Sociology*, vol. 21, no. 1, pp. 349–386, 1995.

[14] United States Center for Disease Control NCHS, *Health, United States, 2015: With Special Feature on Racial and Ethnic Health Disparities*, CreateSpace Independent Publishing Platform, Hyattsville, MD, USA, 2016.

[15] M. E. Dupre, "Educational differences in age-related patterns of disease: reconsidering the cumulative disadvantage and age-as-leveler hypotheses," *Journal of Health and Social Behavior*, vol. 48, no. 1, pp. 1–15, 2007.

[16] D. Dannefer, "Cumulative advantage/disadvantage and the life course: cross-fertilizing age and social science theory," *Journals of Gerontology Series B: Psychological Sciences and Social Sciences*, vol. 58, no. 6, pp. S327–S337, 2003.

[17] L. J. Waite, "Does marriage matter?," *Demography*, vol. 32, no. 4, pp. 483–507, 1995.

[18] J. S. Wong and L. J. Waite, "Marriage, social networks, and health at older ages," *Journal of Population Ageing*, vol. 8, no. 1-2, pp. 7–25, 2015.

[19] J. Liang, A. R. Quiñones, J. M. Bennet et al., "Evolving self-rated health in middle and old age: how does it differ across Black, Hispanic, and White Americans?," *Journal of Aging and Health*, vol. 22, no. 1, pp. 3–26, 2010.

[20] B. J. Goosby, J. E. Cheadle, and T. McDade, "Birth weight, early life course BMI, and body size change: chains of risk to adult inflammation?," *Social Science & Medicine*, vol. 148, pp. 102–109, 2016.

[21] K. M. Walsemann, B. J. Goosby, and D. Farr, "Life course SES and cardiovascular risk: heterogeneity across race/ethnicity and gender," *Social Science & Medicine*, vol. 152, pp. 147–155, 2016.

[22] B. L. Kail, "Marital status as a moderating factor in the process of disablement," *Journal of Aging and Health*, vol. 28, no. 1, pp. 139–164, 2016.

[23] R. Sunshine and S. Rote, "Marital disruption and allostatic load in late life," *Journal of Aging and Health*, vol. 29, no. 4, pp. 688–707, 2016.
[24] R. K. Raley, M. M. Sweeney, and D. Wondra, "The growing racial and ethnic divide in US marriage patterns," *The Future of Children*, vol. 25, no. 2, pp. 89–109, 2015.
[25] K. Edin and J. M. Reed, "Why don't they just get married? Barriers to marriage among the disadvantaged," *The Future of Children*, vol. 15, no. 2, pp. 117–137, 2005.
[26] K. Edin and M. J. Kefalas, *Promises I Can Keep: Why Poor Women Put Motherhood before Marriage*, University of California Press, Berkeley, CA, USA, 2011.
[27] P. R. Amato, D. R. Johnson, A. Booth, and S. J. Rogers, "Continuity and change in marital quality between 1980 and 2000," *Journal of Marriage and Family*, vol. 65, no. 1, pp. 1–22, 2003.
[28] A. Booth and D. R. Johnson, "Tracking respondents in a telephone interview panel selected by random digit dialing," *Sociological Methods & Research*, vol. 14, no. 1, pp. 53–64, 1985.
[29] E. L. Idler and Y. Benyamini, "Self-rated health and mortality: a review of twenty-seven community studies," *Journal of Health and Social Behavior*, vol. 38, no. 1, pp. 21–37, 1997.
[30] I. Kawachi, B. P. Kennedy, K. Lochner, and D. Prothrow-Stith, "Social capital, income inequality, and mortality," *American Journal of Public Health*, vol. 87, no. 9, pp. 1491–1498, 1997.
[31] S. W. Raudenbush and A. S. Bryk, *Hierarchical Linear Models: Applications and Data Analysis Methods*, Vol. 1, Sage Publications, Thousand Oaks, CA, USA, 2002.
[32] J. D. Singer and J. B. Willett, *Applied Longitudinal Data Analysis: Modeling Change and Event Occurrence*, Oxford University Press, Oxford, UK, 2003.
[33] G. N. Holmbeck, "Post-hoc probing of significant moderational and mediational effects in studies of pediatric populations," *Journal of Pediatric Psychology*, vol. 27, no. 1, pp. 87–96, 2002.
[34] A. Gelman, J. Hil, and M. Yajima, "Why we (usually) don't have to worry about multiple comparisons," *Journal of Research on Educational Effectiveness*, vol. 5, no. 2, pp. 189–211, 2012.
[35] T. Perneger, "What's wrong with Bonferroni adjustments," *British Medical Journal*, vol. 316, no. 7139, pp. 1236–1238, 1998.
[36] J. Mirowsky and C. E. Ross, "Education, health, and the default American lifestyle," *Journal of Health and Social Behavior*, vol. 56, no. 3, pp. 297–306, 2015.
[37] F. D. Wolinsky, T. R. Miller, T. K. Malmstrom et al., "Self-rated health: changes, trajectories, and their antecedents among African Americans," *Journal of Aging and Health*, vol. 20, no. 2, pp. 143–158, 2008.
[38] J. K. Montez and A. Zajacova, "Why is life expectancy declining among low-educated women in the United States?," *American Journal of Public Health*, vol. 104, no. 10, pp. e5–e7, 2014.
[39] A. Case and A. Deaton, "Rising morbidity and mortality in midlife among white non-Hispanic Americans in the 21st century," *Proceedings of the National Academy of Sciences*, vol. 112, no. 49, pp. 15078–15083, 2015.
[40] R. M. Stolzenberg and K. Williams, "Gendered reciprocity: work discontent and the household production of health," *Social Science Research*, vol. 37, no. 1, pp. 180–201, 2008.

20

The Association between Sleep Problems, Sleep Medication use, and Falls in Community-Dwelling Older Adults: Results from the Health and Retirement Study 2010

Yaena Min, Pramit A. Nadpara, and Patricia W. Slattum

Department of Pharmacotherapy and Outcomes Science, School of Pharmacy, Virginia Commonwealth University, Richmond, VA 23298-0533, USA

Correspondence should be addressed to Patricia W. Slattum; pwslattu@vcu.edu

Academic Editor: Barbara Shukitt-Hale

Background. Very few studies have assessed the impact of poor sleep and sleep medication use on the risk of falls among community-dwelling older adults. The objective of this study was to evaluate the association between sleep problems, sleep medication use, and falls in community-dwelling older adults. *Methods.* The study population comprised a nationally representative sample of noninstitutionalized older adults participating in the 2010 Health and Retirement Study. Proportion of adults reporting sleep problems, sleep medication use, and fall was calculated. Multiple logistic regression models were constructed to examine the impact of sleep problems and sleep medication use on the risk of falls after controlling for covariates. *Results.* Among 9,843 community-dwelling older adults, 35.8% had reported a fall and 40.8% had reported sleep problems in the past two years. Sleep medication use was reported by 20.9% of the participants. Older adults who do have sleep problems and take sleep medications had a significant high risk of falls, compared to older adults who do not have sleep problems and do not take sleep medications. The other two groups also had significantly greater risk for falls. *Conclusion.* Sleep problems added to sleep medication use increase the risk of falls. Further prospective studies are needed to confirm these observed findings.

1. Introduction

One-third of community-dwelling adults aged 65 years and older experience a fall per year [1]. Falls can cause both fatal and nonfatal injuries. It is also associated with reduced functioning and earlier admission to nursing homes [2, 3]. In 2010, approximately 21,700 of older adults died from unintentional fall injuries [4].

One potential risk factor for falls that needs further investigation is self-reported sleep problems [5]. Sleep complaints are common in older adults, as 50% of community-dwelling older adults report poor sleep [6, 7], and studies have shown that sleep problems increase the risk of falls in older adults [5, 8–10]. Additionally, the consumption of medications to aid sleep, like sedative hypnotics, is common in older adults [11], and studies have shown such medication use to be associated with risk of falls [11, 12]. A meta-analysis found that sedatives and hypnotics (OR = 1.47; 95% CI = 1.35–1.62), antidepressants (OR = 1.68; 95% CI = 1.47–1.91), and benzodiazepines (OR = 1.57; 95% CI = 1.43–1.72) have a significant association with falls in older adults [12]. In another study with community-dwelling older adults, use of anxiolytics and sedatives hypnotics significantly increased the risk of falls in men (OR = 1.43; 95% CI = 1.22–1.67) and in women (OR = 1.33; 95% CI = 1.22–1.46), when they used the drug up to 85 days before the fall [13]. However, these studies did not consider reported sleep problems as a potential confounder when assessing the relationship.

One study has assessed the association between insomnia and hypnotics use on risk of falls among institutionalized population [14]. This study found that older adults with insomnia but who did not take hypnotics as well as those who have insomnia and who did use hypnotics had a greater risk of falls compared to those who did not have insomnia and did not use hypnotics [14]; thus it remains to be seen if such an association exists among community-dwelling older adults. There is clearly a lack of literature on whether the underlying sleep problems cause falls in older adults who take medications for sleep. Therefore, we conducted a study to evaluate if sleep problems and sleep medication use were associated with risk of falls, injurious falls, and recurrent falls in community-dwelling adults aged 65 years or older. Identifying whether sleep problems, sleep medication use, or both increase the risk of falls may further help healthcare decision-makers to better treat older adults with poor sleep and who are already at risk of falling.

2. Methods

2.1. Data Source and Study Sample. This study was a cross-sectional analysis of the 2010 Health and Retirement Study (HRS) dataset. Health and Retirement Study (HRS) is a longitudinal panel study that surveys more than 22,000 Americans every two years and it is conducted by the University of Michigan [15]. The most recent wave of 2010 data at the time was used in the study. In this study, we included all community-dwelling adults aged 65 years or older from the HRS dataset. We excluded those respondents who (1) resided in nursing homes during year 2010, (2) did not respond in the year 2010 survey, or (3) had missing values on any of the variables.

2.2. Outcome Variable. Falls were assessed in the HRS by asking the question, "Have you fallen down in the last two years?" The response to this question was categorized as "yes" or "no" and was used to define the outcome variable in this study. If the participants responded "yes," they were further asked the number of times they had fallen and whether they had been injured seriously enough to need medical treatment in any of the falls.

2.3. Predictor Variables. In the HRS, respondents were asked about their sleep problems through four questions: (1) "How often do you have trouble falling asleep?" (2) "How often do you have trouble with waking up during the night?" (3) "How often do you have trouble with waking up too early and not being able to fall asleep again?" (4) "How often do you feel really rested when you wake up in the morning?" The responses were categorized as "most of the time," "sometimes," and "rarely or never." Since the questions about sleep are asked as part of a questionnaire about their current health status, the responses reflect their current sleep issues. For this study, participants were defined as having a sleep problem, if the respondents answered "most of the time" in any of the first three questions or "rarely or never" on the fourth question [5, 16]. This approach was appropriate since the questions and responses were mostly the same with the past literature.

Sleep medication use by respondents was assessed in HRS with the question: "In the past two weeks, have you taken any medications or used other treatments to help you sleep?" The responses were categorized as "yes" or "no" and were used to identify respondents that used sleep medications in this study.

2.4. Covariates. Based on previous studies, the covariates that are recognized as a risk factor for falls were included in this study. Demographic variables of interest in this analysis were age, sex, race, education level, and marital status. Other variables of interest included smoking status, alcohol use, health status, number of comorbidities, limitation in activities of daily living (ADL), limitation in instrumental activities of daily living (IADL), limitation in mobility, self-rated eyesight, and presence of incontinence [17–19]. Age was categorized as "65–74 years," "75–84 years," and "85 years or older." Sex was categorized as "male" and "female," race as "Caucasian" and "others," and marital status as "married" and "others." Education level was estimated by the years of education and categorized as "no education," "less than high school," "high school," and "more than high school."

Smoking status was categorized as "current," "former," and "nonsmokers." Use of alcohol was classified as "drinker" and "nondrinker." Health status was self-reported and was categorized as "excellent/very good/good," "fair," and "poor." Based on previous studies using HRS data, the number of comorbidities was measured by the sum of the following self-reported conditions: high blood pressure, diabetes, lung disease, heart disease, stroke, emotional or psychiatric problems, arthritis, and Alzheimer's disease [20–22]. Comorbidities were then categorized as "none," "1-2," "3-4," or "5 or more."

Information about functional status was also taken into account because it is highly related to risk of falls [17, 23]. Activities of daily living (ADL) included bathing, dressing, toileting, eating, and transferring. The number of limitations in activities of daily living (ADL) was the sum of any difficulties on these five tasks. Instrumental activities of daily living (IADL) included ability to use the phone, shopping, preparing for food, responsibility for own medications, and ability to handle finances. The number of limitations in instrumental activities of daily living (IADL) was the sum of any difficulties on these five tasks [21, 24]. Limitations in mobility included difficulty in any of the following tasks such as walking one block, walking several blocks, waking across a room, climbing one flight of stairs, and climbing several flights of stairs. Each criterion of functional limitation was categorized as "0," "1-2," or "3–5." Self-rated eyesight was included because impaired vision has been reported to be a risk factor for falls [17, 23]. It was categorized as "excellent/very good/good/fair" and "poor/legally blind." The presence of incontinence, categorized as "yes" or "no," was also included [18].

2.5. Statistical Analysis. Using individual sampling weights, weighted descriptive statistics were generated and used to summarize the characteristics of the participants. Percentages were used to describe categorical variables, and mean and standard deviation (SD) were used to describe continuous variables. Chi-square analysis was conducted to determine the association among categorical variables of interest.

The effect of sleep problems and sleep medication use and their combined effect on falls were assessed by multiple logistic regression models. Multinominal logistic regression models were used to assess the association of recurrent falls or injurious falls with predictor variables with nonfallers as the reference group. The unadjusted relationship was calculated followed by adjusted relationship with all the covariates in the model. Collinearity among the covariates was assessed. In addition, the effect of each sleep problem ("trouble falling asleep," "trouble with waking up during the night," "trouble with waking up too early and not being able to fall asleep again," and "trouble feeling rested when waking up in the morning") on the risk of falls was assessed. Results were reported as odds ratios (OR) and 95% confidence intervals (CI). p value < 0.05 was considered significant. All statistical analyses were performed using SAS 9.4 statistical software (SAS Institute Inc., Cary, NC, USA).

3. Results

3.1. Population Characteristics. Based on our inclusion and exclusion criteria, we identified 10,354 older adults from the HRS 2010 dataset. Data from 511 respondents were excluded due to missing data, which is less than 5% of the respondents. Thus, the final dataset consisted of 9,843 participants.

Overall, 35.8% of the older adults reported a fall at least once in the last two years. Among those reporting a fall, 29.9% had serious injuries requiring medical treatment and 60.4% fell more than once. The proportion of older adults reporting sleep problems and sleep medication use was 40.8% and 20.9%, respectively.

Table 1 shows the characteristics of the participants by fallers and nonfallers. The proportion of participants with falls was higher among those aged 85 years or older and among females, compared to nonfallers. Similar results were seen in participants who self-reported their health as poor, had 5 or more comorbidities, had more activities of daily living (ADL), had instrumental activities of daily living (IADL) and mobility limitations, and self-reported their eyesight as poor/legally blind.

3.2. Associations between Sleep Problems, Sleep Medications, and Falls. Among individuals reporting falls, 43.3% (N = 1,515) reported no sleep problems and no use of sleep medications, 31.9% (N = 1,144) reported sleep problems but no use of sleep medications, 9.6% (N = 334) reported no sleep problems but still used sleep medications, and 15.2% (554) reported sleep problems and used sleep medications (Table 2).

Table 3 reports the unadjusted and adjusted associations between sleep problems, sleep medication use, and falls. Compared to participants reporting no sleep problems and no sleep medication use, those reporting sleep problems and sleep medication use had significantly increased risk of falls (OR = 1.79; 95% CI = 1.54–2.08). However, after adjusting for covariates, older adults with no sleep problems and sleep medication use had the highest increase in the risk of falls compared to the other groups. All of the associations were attenuated after adjusting for the covariates in the full model but remained significant.

3.3. Associations between Sleep Problems, Sleep Medications, and Injurious Falls. The falls were further categorized into injurious falls and noninjurious falls. Among the total sample, 10.7% experienced injurious falls while 25.1% experienced noninjurious falls. Greater proportion of injurious fallers (49.0%, N = 520) reported sleep problems than noninjurious fallers (46.4%, N = 1,178) and nonfallers (37.2%, N = 2,362). Similarly, greater proportion of injurious fallers (30.0%, N = 309) reported using sleep medications than noninjurious fallers (22.6%, N = 579) and nonfallers (18.8%, N = 1,140). Compared with nonusers, sleep medication users had a 40% higher risk of having injurious falls. All the groups were more likely to experience injurious falls compared with the group with no sleep problems and no use of sleep medications. However, the effect of sleep problems and sleep medication use did not increase the risk of noninjurious falls. Table 4 reports the relationship between sleep problems, sleep medication use, and injurious falls.

3.4. Associations between Sleep Problems, Sleep Medications, and Recurrent Falls. Recurrent falls were defined as falling more than once in the past two years. Among the total sample, 14.2% were single fallers, and 21.7% were recurrent fallers. Participants using medications or treatments for sleep were approximately 18.8% (N = 1,140) among nonfallers, 21.6% (N = 305) among single fallers, and 26.9% (N = 583) in recurrent fallers. Recurrent fallers had higher proportion of those with sleep problems (51.8%, N = 1,129) compared with single fallers (40.2%, N = 569) and nonfallers (37.2%, N = 2,362). After combining sleep problems and sleep medication use, recurrent fallers had a higher proportion of those with both sleep problems and sleep medication use (17.7%, N = 388) compared with single fallers (11.5%, N = 166) and nonfallers (10.8%, N = 649). Compared with participants with no sleep problems, those with sleep problems were 26% more likely to have recurrent falls. Similarly, compared with nonusers of sleep medications, users had 21% higher odds of having recurrent falls. However, sleep problems and sleep medication use did not affect the risk of nonrecurrent falls. In addition, the group with sleep problems and sleep medication use had a significantly higher risk of recurrent falls compared with the group with no sleep problems and no sleep medication use. Table 5 reports the relationship between sleep problems, sleep medication use, and recurrent falls.

3.5. Association between Type of Reported Sleep Problem and Falls. Among individuals reporting a fall, 16.9% (N = 624) reported having trouble falling asleep, 31.1% (N = 1,089) reported trouble waking up during the night, 15.6% (N = 565) reported trouble with waking up too early and not being able to fall asleep again, and 14.8% (N = 530) reported trouble feeling rested when waking up in the morning. Table 6 reports the relationship between type of sleep problem and the risk for falls. The risk of falls was higher among respondents reporting any of the four sleep problems in the unadjusted associations. However, after adjusting for covariates including sleep medication use, only respondents with "trouble falling asleep" had an increased risk of falls.

Table 1: Characteristics of community-dwelling older adults by reported sleep problems and sleep medication use and falls in the US, 2010.

Variable	Total N (%)	Fallers[a]				Nonfallers			
		Sleep problems[b], %		Sleep medication use[c], %		Sleep problems, %		Sleep medication use, %	
		Yes	No	Yes	No	Yes	No	Yes	No
Total	9843	1698	1849	888	2659	2362	3934	1140	5156
Age (years)[†]									
65–74	5112 (55.5)	47.8	51.1	47.5	50.2	55.8	60.7	56.4	59.4
75–84	3505 (32.3)	36.5	33.5	36.7	34.3	33.1	29.5	32.5	30.5
>85	1226 (12.2)	15.7	15.4	15.8	15.5	11.1	9.8	11.1	10.1
Sex[*]									
Male	4195 (43.7)	38.3	42.7	30.9	43.9	42.9	46.9	35.8	47.6
Female	5648 (56.3)	61.7	57.3	69.1	56.1	57.1	53.1	64.2	52.4
Race[†]									
Caucasian	8207 (89.9)	91.8	91.7	94.8	90.8	89.9	88.2	94.1	87.6
Others	1636 (10.1)	8.2	8.3	5.2	9.2	10.1	11.8	5.9	12.4
Marital status[†]									
Married	5594 (54.9)	48.2	51.9	51.1	49.8	54.3	59.5	56.0	57.9
Others	4249 (45.1)	51.8	48.1	48.9	50.2	45.7	40.5	44.0	42.1
Education									
No education	66 (0.4)	0.5	0.3	0.4	0.4	0.7	0.2	0.2	0.5
<High school	2329 (19.9)	24.5	18.4	21.4	21.2	21.6	17.7	16.5	19.8
High school	3448 (35.4)	32.6	38.2	34.8	35.8	35.3	35.3	34.0	35.5
>High school	4000 (44.3)	42.4	43.1	43.4	42.6	42.5	46.8	49.3	44.2
Smoking									
Current smoker	846 (9.4)	9.8	8.2	8.3	9.2	10.4	9.2	8.0	10.1
Former smoker	4769 (48.4)	49.9	48.6	50.7	48.7	49.7	46.8	46.8	48.1
Nonsmoker	4228 (42.2)	40.3	43.2	41.0	42.1	39.9	44.0	45.2	41.8
Alcohol[†]									
Current drinker	4698 (50.8)	45.6	48.5	43.4	48.4	50.3	54.4	53.3	52.8
Nondrinker	5145 (49.2)	54.4	51.5	56.6	51.6	49.7	45.6	46.7	47.2
Self-reported health[†]									
E/VG/G	7076 (74.5)	54.7	72.9	55.8	67.1	71.4	85.2	74.9	81.3
Fair	2022 (18.6)	28.6	20.7	26.8	23.7	21.3	11.9	18.1	14.8
Bad	745 (6.9)	16.7	6.4	17.4	9.2	7.3	2.8	7.0	3.9
Number of comorbidities[†]									
0	661 (7.6)	2.8	5.4	2.6	4.7	5.9	11.7	4.6	10.7
1-2	4730 (49.4)	36.3	47.8	35.2	44.7	48.7	56.1	51.7	53.7
3-4	3753 (36.2)	46.5	38.5	47.7	40.5	39.1	29.1	38.8	31.4
5 or more	699 (6.8)	14.4	8.3	14.5	10.1	6.3	3.1	4.9	4.2

Table 1: Continued.

Variable	Total N (%)	Fallers[a]				Nonfallers			
		Sleep problems[b], %		Sleep medication use[c], %		Sleep problems, %		Sleep medication use, %	
		Yes	No	Yes	No	Yes	No	Yes	No
ADL limitations†									
None	7964 (82.4)	64.2	77.5	63.8	73.6	84.0	91.5	87.0	89.1
1-2	1330 (12.6)	24.1	16.4	23.9	18.8	11.4	6.6	8.6	8.3
3–5	549 (5.0)	11.7	6.1	12.3	7.6	4.6	1.9	4.4	2.6
IADL limitations†									
None	8070 (83.4)	69.1	78.7	68.5	76.0	85.3	90.6	84.8	89.5
1-2	1254 (12.1)	21.4	15.3	21.8	17.0	11.7	7.0	11.7	8.0
3–5	519 (4.5)	9.5	6.0	9.7	7.0	3.0	2.4	3.5	2.5
Mobility limitations†									
None	4137 (44.3)	24.7	39.5	26.1	34.6	40.8	56.8	40.7	53.2
1-2	3485 (34.6)	35.2	35.8	34.0	36.0	38.2	31.7	39.9	32.8
3–5	2221 (21.1)	40.1	24.7	39.9	29.4	21.0	11.5	19.4	14.0
Self-reported eyesight†									
E/VG/G/fair	9161 (93.8)	87.6	92.8	88.1	91.1	94.2	96.6	94.6	95.9
Bad/legally blind	682 (6.2)	12.4	7.2	11.9	8.9	5.8	3.4	5.4	4.1
Incontinence†									
Yes	2806 (28.6)	45.3	30.0	43.1	35.3	31.2	19.4	33.4	21.6
No	7037 (71.4)	54.7	70.0	56.9	64.7	68.8	80.6	66.6	78.4

Note. Data source: 2010 HRS (RAND HRS data file and 2010 HRS core physical health file).
Results are reported in weighted percentages.

*Chi-test p value < 0.05; †< 0.0001.

[a]Fallers = participants who reported having a fall at least once in the previous two years.

[b]Sleep problems = participants who have trouble "most of the time" in any of sleep problems: "trouble falling asleep," "trouble with waking up during the night," and "trouble with waking up too early and not being able to fall asleep again," or "rarely or never" on sleep problem: "trouble feeling rested when waking up in the morning."

[c]Sleep medication use = participants who have reported taking any medications or using other treatments to help sleep.

ADL = activities of daily living; IADL = instrumental activities of daily living; E/VG/G = excellent/very good/good.

Table 2: Distribution of predictor variables against falls in community-dwelling older adults in the US, 2010.

Variables	Fallers N (%)	Nonfallers N (%)
Sleep problems		
Yes	1698 (47.2)	2362 (37.2)
No	1849 (52.8)	3934 (62.8)
Sleep medication use		
Yes	888 (24.8)	1140 (18.8)
No	2659 (75.2)	5156 (81.2)
Sleep problems + sleep medication use		
No sleep problem + no sleep med use[a]	1515 (43.3)	3443 (54.8)
No sleep problem + sleep med use[b]	334 (9.6)	491 (8.0)
Sleep problem + no sleep med use[c]	1144 (31.9)	1713 (26.4)
Sleep problem + sleep med use[d]	554 (15.2)	649 (10.8)

Note. Data source: 2010 HRS dataset (RAND HRS data file and 2010 HRS core physical health file). Results are reported in weighted percentages. Column percentages are significantly different by Rao-Scott chi-square test $p < 0.05$ and cannot be calculated based on raw numbers.
[a]No sleep problem + no sleep med use = participants who reported no sleep problems and no use of sleep medications.
[b]No sleep problem + sleep med use = participants who reported no sleep problems but use of sleep medications.
[c]Sleep problem + no sleep med use = participants who reported sleep problems and no use of sleep medications.
[d]Sleep problem + sleep med use = participants who reported sleep problems and use of sleep medications.

Table 3: Association between sleep problems, sleep medication use, and falls in community-dwelling older adults in the US, 2010.

Variables	Unadjusted odds ratios (95% CI)	Adjusted odds ratios[a] (95% CI)
Sleep problems		
Yes	1.51‡ (1.37–1.65)	1.13* (1.01–1.25)
No	Ref.	Ref.
Sleep medication use		
Yes	1.43‡ (1.26–1.62)	1.14 (1.00–1.31)
No	Ref.	Ref.
Sleep problems + sleep medication use		
No sleep problem + no sleep med use[b]	Ref.	Ref.
No sleep problem + sleep med use[c]	1.52‡ (1.31–1.78)	1.24† (1.05–1.47)
Sleep problem + no sleep med use[d]	1.53‡ (1.36–1.73)	1.16* (1.02–1.32)
Sleep problem + sleep med use[e]	1.79‡ (1.54–2.08)	1.19* (1.01–1.41)

Note. Data source: 2010 HRS dataset (RAND HRS data file and 2010 HRS core physical health file).
$^{*}p$ value < 0.05, $^{†}< 0.01$, and $^{‡}< 0.0001$.
Ref. = reference.
[a]Full model: adjusted for age, sex, education, marital status, race, self-reported health, alcohol, number of comorbidities, limitations in instrumental activities of daily living (IADL), limitations in activities of daily living (ADL), limitations in mobility, self-rated eyesight, and incontinence.
[b]No sleep problem + no sleep med use = participants who reported no sleep problems and no use of sleep medications.
[c]No sleep problem + sleep med use = participants who reported no sleep problems but use of sleep medications.
[d]Sleep problem + no sleep med use = participants who reported sleep problems and no use of sleep medications.
[e]Sleep problem + sleep med use = participants who reported sleep problems and use of sleep medications.

4. Discussion and Conclusion

The purpose of this study was to assess the effect of sleep problems and sleep medication use and their combined effect on the risk of falls, injurious falls, and recurrent falls in community-dwelling older adults. In a representative sample of community-dwelling older adults in 2010, this study showed that 35.8% of the participants had a fall at least once in the last two years. Similar percentage of older adults had fallen compared to the prior studies which reported that one in three community-dwelling older adults has a fall per year [25]. However, what constitutes a fall was not defined further in the survey. About 5–10% of falls in community-dwelling older adults result in severe head injury and joint dislocation and additional 5% in a fracture [26]. Approximately 30% of falls led to serious injuries in this study; thus it is possible that respondents were more likely to remember to report falls that required medical treatments. Additionally, this study found that 40.8% report sleep problems. The prevalence was similar compared to previous studies [6, 7]. Only 20.9% used medications or other treatments to help sleep in the past two weeks and among those who have sleep problems as we have defined in this study, only 30.4% used sleep medications. Many older adults may continue to take sleep

Table 4: Association between sleep problems, sleep medication use, and injurious falls in community-dwelling older adults in the US, 2010.

Variables	Noninjurious fallers Adjusted OR (95% CI)	Injurious fallers Adjusted OR[e] (95% CI)
Sleep problems		
Yes	1.12 (1.00–1.25)	1.16 (0.98–1.36)
No	Ref.	Ref.
Sleep medication use		
Yes	1.04 (0.89–1.22)	1.40† (1.15–1.71)
No	Ref.	Ref.
Sleep problems + sleep medication use		
No sleep problem + no sleep med use[a]	Ref.	Ref.
No sleep problem + sleep med use[b]	1.05 (0.86–1.30)	1.76‡ (1.40–2.20)
Sleep problem + no sleep med use[c]	1.13 (0.99–1.29)	1.25* (1.02–1.54)
Sleep problem + sleep med use[d]	1.12 (0.92–1.35)	1.40* (1.08–1.82)

Note. Data source: 2010 HRS dataset (RAND HRS data file and 2010 HRS core physical health file).
$^{*}p$ value < 0.05, †< 0.01, and ‡< 0.0001.
Ref. = reference.
[a]No sleep problem + no sleep med use = participants who reported no sleep problems and no use of sleep medications.
[b]No sleep problem + sleep med use = participants who reported no sleep problems but use of sleep medications.
[c]Sleep problem + no sleep med use = participants who reported sleep problems and no use of sleep medications.
[d]Sleep problem + sleep med use = participants who reported sleep problems and use of sleep medications.
[e]Full model: adjusted for age, gender, education, marital status, race, self-reported health, alcohol, number of comorbidities, limitations in IADL, limitations in ADL, limitations in mobility, self-rated eyesight, and incontinence.

Table 5: Association between sleep problems, sleep medication use, and recurrent falls in community-dwelling older adults in the US, 2010.

Variables	Single fallers Adjusted OR (95% CI)	Recurrent fallers Adjusted OR[e] (95% CI)
Sleep problems		
Yes	0.97 (0.83–1.12)	1.26† (1.12–1.42)
No	Ref.	Ref.
Sleep medication use		
Yes	1.05 (0.89–1.23)	1.21* (1.04–1.42)
No	Ref.	Ref.
Sleep problems + sleep medication use		
No sleep problem + no sleep med use[a]	Ref.	Ref.
No sleep problem + sleep med use[b]	1.24 (0.99–1.55)	1.25 (1.00–1.58)
Sleep problem + no sleep med use[c]	1.03 (0.86–1.23)	1.27† (1.10–1.47)
Sleep problem + sleep med use[d]	0.93 (0.75–1.16)	1.40† (1.17–1.68)

Data source: 2010 HRS dataset (RAND HRS data file and 2010 HRS core physical health file).
$^{*}p$ value < 0.05, †< 0.01.
Ref. = reference.
[a]No sleep problem + no sleep med use = participants who reported no sleep problems and no use of sleep medications.
[b]No sleep problem + sleep med use = participants who reported no sleep problems but use of sleep medications.
[c]Sleep problem + no sleep med use = participants who reported sleep problems and no use of sleep medications.
[d]Sleep problem + sleep med use = participants who reported sleep problems and use of sleep medications.
[e]Full model: adjusted for age, gender, education, marital status, race, self-reported health, alcohol, number of comorbidities, limitations in IADL, limitations in ADL, limitations in mobility, self-rated eyesight, and incontinence.

medications despite continued sleep problems. No significant differences in sleep quality between older adults who take benzodiazepine-receptor agonists and those who take placebos have been reported [11], and there is lack of evidence of significant treatment effect of using sedative hypnotics on a long-term basis [27].

Older adults with reported sleep problems had a significant increase in the risk of falls after adjusting for covariates (OR = 1.13; 95% CI = 1.01–1.25). The possible mechanisms could be that poor sleep may cause daytime sleepiness, cognitive dysfunction, and slower response time which could result in falls [5, 14]. Although the risk attenuated after considering covariates, the risk was still observed. However, older adults who used sleep medications or other treatments for sleep were not at increased risk of falls after adjusting for covariates. A study by Ensrud and colleagues which

TABLE 6: Associations between type of sleep problems and falls in community-dwelling older adults in the US, 2010.

Variables	Unadjusted odds ratios (95% CI)	Adjusted odds ratios[a] (95% CI)
Trouble falling asleep		
Yes	1.75‡ (1.54–1.98)	1.22† (1.07–1.40)
No	Ref.	Ref.
Trouble with waking up during the night		
Yes	1.35‡ (1.22–1.50)	1.07 (0.96–1.20)
No	Ref.	Ref.
Trouble with waking up too early and not being able to fall asleep again		
Yes	1.50‡ (1.31–1.71)	1.12 (0.98–1.30)
No	Ref.	Ref.
Trouble feeling rested when waking up in the morning		
Yes	1.54‡ (1.34–1.78)	0.98 (0.84–1.14)
No	Ref.	Ref.

Note. Data source: 2010 HRS dataset (RAND HRS data file and 2010 HRS core physical health file).
p value < 0.05, † < 0.01, and ‡ < 0.0001.
Ref. = reference.
[a]Full model: adjusted for age, sex, education, marital status, race, self-reported health, alcohol, number of comorbidities, limitations in instrumental activities of daily living (IADL), limitations in activities of daily living (ADL), limitations in mobility, self-rated eyesight, incontinence, and sleep medication use.

followed community-dwelling older women on hypnotics for one year for incidence of falls found that women taking benzodiazepines (multivariate odds ratio, MOR = 1.34; 95% CI = 1.09–1.63), antidepressants (MOR = 1.54; 95% CI = 1.14–2.07), and antiepileptics (MOR = 2.56; 95% CI = 1.49–4.41) were more likely to experience falls at least once [28]. Sedative hypnotics could increase falls by the effect on postural instability, psychomotor impairment, and cognitive dysfunction [29]. Furthermore, the risk of falls associated with these medications could be increased because of age-related changes in physiology resulting in altered pharmacokinetics and pharmacodynamics in older adults [29]. Therefore, the lack of significance in the finding could again be due to a short time frame of documented sleep medication use relative to the time frame for reported falls and lack of definition of sleep medication and treatments for the respondents in the survey.

Additionally, there was increased risk of falls among older adults who had sleep problems and who used sleep medications. However, after adjusting for covariates, older adults with no sleep problems and who used sleep medications had the highest risk of falls compared to other groups. This finding suggests that sleep medications did not have a protective effect on falls when considering sleep problems in the association. A study by Avidan and colleagues assessed the risk of falls in the same four groups with cross-tabulation of insomnia and use of sedative hypnotics: (1) insomnia, hypnotic use, (2) insomnia, no hypnotic use, (3) no insomnia, hypnotic use, and (4) no insomnia, no hypnotic use [14]. However, the results are inconsistent with the current study. Avidan and colleagues found that insomniacs who did not take hypnotics (OR = 1.55; 95% CI = 1.41–1.71) and insomniacs who took hypnotics had a significant increase in the risk of falls (OR = 1.32; 95% CI = 1.02–1.70) [14]. Insomnia without hypnotics had the highest risk of falls compared to any other groups and hypnotic use had a protective effect on falls in older adults, suggesting that the condition of insomnia might have been better treated with the medication resulting in fewer falls [14]. Although the study by Avidan and colleagues and the current study have conflicting results, the presence of sleep problems such as insomnia was found as a key risk factor for falls.

The risk of injurious falls associated with sleep problems and sleep medication use was also assessed with a multinominal logistic regression model. The effect of sleep problems and sleep medication use on the risk of injurious falls showed that the group with no sleep problems and sleep medication use had the highest risk of injurious falls compared to those with sleep problems and no sleep medication use and to those with sleep problems and sleep medication use compared to the reference group. This pattern was similar to the risk of falls generally. A prospective cohort study also found a significant increased risk of injurious falls related to the use of sedative or hypnotics (RR = 1.50; 95% CI = 1.03–2.19) [30], but other studies did not find sleep problems to be related to falls that required medical attention for an injury [31, 32]. Moreover, the risk of recurrent falls was studied. The risk of recurrent falls was seen in older adults with sleep problems and no sleep medication use and in those with sleep problems and sleep medication use but it was not seen in those with no sleep problems and sleep medication use. This could be due to the low sample size in that group. None of sleep problems and sleep medication use was associated with risk of single fall and this could be related to differences in physical performance [33] and risk factors of falls [34] between single fallers and recurrent fallers.

In this study, the risk of falls by type of reported sleep problem among older adults was also assessed. Each sleep problem had a significant increase in the unadjusted risk of falls; however, only "trouble falling asleep" significantly increased the risk of falls after adjusting for covariates including the use of sleep medications. We do not know when falls occurred in these older adults, but since they had trouble falling asleep even though they took medications or treatment for sleep, we can assume that they could have walked around during the night in a hyperarousal state which can increase the risk of falls. A study by Brassington and colleagues evaluated the same aspects of sleep disturbance in older adults as in the current study except for one type of sleep problem, which was "trouble feeling rested when waking up in the morning," and found that difficulty in falling asleep at night (OR = 1.53; 95% CI 1.04–2.24), waking up during the night (OR = 1.91; 95% CI = 1.44–2.54), and waking up too early in the morning and not being able to fall asleep again (OR = 1.64; 95% CI = 1.11–2.42) were significantly associated with the occurrence of falls after adjusting for covariates including a use of prescription medication [5]. The number of covariates that were adjusted for was fewer than in the current study and therefore may not have adjusted for the effect of confounders such as ADLs, IADLs, and mobility. In contrast, Teo and colleagues evaluated the same categories of nighttime sleep problems and used the same scale as Brassington and colleagues and reported conflicting findings [16]. Teo and colleagues did not find a significant increase in the risk of falls in the same nighttime sleep problems after adjusting for the covariates [16]. While results from our study add to the finding from previous studies, further prospective research in community-dwelling older adults is needed to accurately quantify the risk of falls by type of sleep problem.

Some strengths of this study may be noted. Since the HRS study had representative sample of older adults, national estimates were obtained. Also, several risk factors such as ADL and IADL were controlled as covariates in this study. However, as with any study, this study has limitations. First, since information was self-reported, there could be misclassification bias or recall bias. Second, because this is a cross-sectional study based on self-reported information, causal relationships cannot be explored in this study. Third, falls and medications or other treatments to help sleep were not clearly defined in the HRS survey. Variations in the definition of falls could result in misclassification bias. Fourth, unlike other questions where respondents were asked to provide information on their current sleep issues and sleep medication use, the questions on assessing falls were asked based on their experience during the last two years. The differences in the time interval may result in lack of temporal relationship between drug exposure and the outcome. Still the study results add valuable information to the current literature by shedding light on sleep problem, sleep medication use, and falls in community-dwelling older adults. Finally, information on the circumstances of falls was not collected in HRS but this information would have been useful and should be collected in future studies.

In conclusion, this study found that sleep problems, use of sleep medications, and occurrence of falls are common among community-dwelling older adults. This study adds to the literature by assessing the combined effect of sleep problems and sleep medication use on risk of falls, injurious falls, and recurrent falls in community-dwelling older adults by grouping the participants. Older adults without sleep problems and taking sleep medication had the highest risk of falls compared to other groups of those with sleep problems and taking sleep medications, those with sleep problems and not taking sleep medications, and those without sleep problems and not taking sleep medications. Healthcare professionals should consider medication-associated risk when treating sleep problems in community-dwelling older adults. Moreover, more studies are needed to examine this association in community-dwelling older adults.

Competing Interests

The authors have no competing interests to disclose.

References

[1] V. S. Stel, S. M. F. Pluijm, D. J. H. Deeg, J. H. Smit, L. M. Bouter, and P. Lips, "A classification tree for predicting recurrent falling in community-dwelling older persons," *Journal of the American Geriatrics Society*, vol. 51, no. 10, pp. 1356–1364, 2003.

[2] Panel on Prevention of Falls in Older Persons and American Geriatrics Society and British Geriatrics Society, "Summary of the Updated American Geriatrics Society/British Geriatrics Society clinical practice guideline for prevention of falls in older persons," *Journal of the American Geriatrics Society*, vol. 59, no. 1, pp. 148–157, 2011.

[3] L. Z. Rubenstein, K. R. Josephson, and A. S. Robbins, "Falls in the nursing home," *Annals of Internal Medicin*, vol. 121, no. 6, pp. 442–451, 1994.

[4] Centers for Disease Control and Prevention, WISQARS (Web-Based Injury Statistics Query and Reporting System), http://www.cdc.gov/injury/wisqars/.

[5] G. S. Brassington, A. C. King, and D. L. Bliwise, "Sleep problems as a risk factor for falls in a sample of community-dwelling adults aged 64–99 years," *Journal of the American Geriatrics Society*, vol. 48, no. 10, pp. 1234–1240, 2000.

[6] D. J. Foley, A. A. Monjan, S. L. Brown, E. M. Simonsick, R. B. Wallace, and D. G. Blazer, "Sleep complaints among elderly persons: an epidemiologic study of three communities," *Sleep*, vol. 18, no. 6, pp. 425–432, 1995.

[7] D. Foley, S. Ancoli-Israel, P. Britz, and J. Walsh, "Sleep disturbances and chronic disease in older adults: results of the 2003 National Sleep Foundation Sleep in America Survey," *Journal of Psychosomatic Research*, vol. 56, no. 5, pp. 497–502, 2004.

[8] E. L. Hill, R. G. Cumming, R. Lewis, S. Carrington, and D. G. Le Couteur, "Sleep disturbances and falls in older people," *Journals of Gerontology—Series A Biological Sciences and Medical Sciences*, vol. 62, no. 1, pp. 62–66, 2007.

[9] A. K. Helbig, A. Döring, M. Heier et al., "Association between sleep disturbances and falls among the elderly: results from the german cooperative health research in the region of augsburg-age study," *Sleep Medicine*, vol. 14, no. 12, pp. 1356–1363, 2013.

[10] K. L. Stone, S. Ancoli-Israel, T. Blackwell et al., "Actigraphy-measured sleep characteristics and risk of falls in older women," *Archives of Internal Medicine*, vol. 168, no. 16, pp. 1768–1775, 2008.

[11] J. Glass, K. L. Lanctôt, N. Herrmann, B. A. Sproule, and U. E. Busto, "Sedative hypnotics in older people with insomnia: meta-analysis of risks and benefits," *British Medical Journal*, vol. 331, no. 7526, pp. 1169–1173, 2005.

[12] J. C. Woolcott, K. J. Richardson, M. O. Wiens et al., "Meta-analysis of the impact of 9 medication classes on falls in elderly persons," *Archives of Internal Medicine*, vol. 169, no. 21, pp. 1952–1960, 2009.

[13] B. Modén, J. Merlo, H. Ohlsson, and M. Rosvall, "Psychotropic drugs and falling accidents among the elderly: a nested case control study in the whole population of Scania, Sweden," *Journal of Epidemiology and Community Health*, vol. 64, no. 5, pp. 440–446, 2010.

[14] A. Y. Avidan, B. E. Fries, M. L. James, K. L. Szafara, G. T. Wright, and R. D. Chervin, "Insomnia and hypnotic use, recorded in the minimum data set, as predictors of falls and hip fractures in Michigan nursing homes," *Journal of the American Geriatrics Society*, vol. 53, no. 6, pp. 955–962, 2005.

[15] M. A. Servais, *Overview of HRS Public Data Files for Cross-Sectional and Longitudinal Analysis*, Survey Research Center, Institute for Social Research, University of Michigan, Ann Arbor, Mich, USA, 2004.

[16] J. S. H. Teo, N. K. Briffa, A. Devine, S. S. Dhaliwal, and R. L. Prince, "Do sleep problems or urinary incontinence predict falls in elderly women?" *Australian Journal of Physiotherapy*, vol. 52, no. 1, pp. 19–24, 2006.

[17] J. M. Fabre, R. Ellis, M. Kosma, and R. H. Wood, "Falls risk factors and a compendium of falls risk screening instruments," *Journal of Geriatric Physical Therapy*, vol. 33, no. 4, pp. 184–197, 2010.

[18] R. C. van Nieuwenhuizen, N. van Dijk, F. G. van Breda et al., "Assessing the prevalence of modifiable risk factors in older patients visiting an ED due to a fall using the CAREFALL Triage Instrument," *American Journal of Emergency Medicine*, vol. 28, no. 9, pp. 994–1001, 2010.

[19] M. E. Tinetti and C. Kumar, "The patient who falls: 'it's always a trade-off'," *Journal of the American Medical Association*, vol. 303, no. 3, pp. 258–266, 2010.

[20] T.-Y. Chen and M. C. Janke, "Predictors of falls among community-dwelling older adults with cancer: results from the health and retirement study," *Supportive Care in Cancer*, vol. 22, no. 2, pp. 479–485, 2014.

[21] T. R. Gure, R. J. McCammon, C. T. Cigolle, T. M. Koelling, C. S. Blaum, and K. M. Langa, "Predictors of self-report of heart failure in a population-based survey of older adults," *Circulation: Cardiovascular Quality and Outcomes*, vol. 5, no. 3, pp. 396–402, 2012.

[22] E. A. Kerr, M. Heisler, S. L. Krein et al., "Beyond comorbidity counts: how do comorbidity type and severity influence diabetes patients' treatment priorities and self-management?" *Journal of General Internal Medicine*, vol. 22, no. 12, pp. 1635–1640, 2007.

[23] Guideline for the Prevention of Falls in Older Persons, "American Geriatrics Society, British Geriatrics Society, and American Academy of orthopaedic surgeons panel on falls prevention," *Journal of the American Geriatrics Society*, vol. 49, no. 5, pp. 664–672, 2001.

[24] J. M. Gaines, J. L. Poey, K. A. Marx, J. M. Parrish, and B. Resnick, "Health and medical services use: a matched case comparison between CCRC residents and national health and retirement study samples," *Journal of Gerontological Social Work*, vol. 54, no. 8, pp. 788–802, 2011.

[25] A. M. Tromp, S. M. F. Pluijm, J. H. Smit, D. J. H. Deeg, L. M. Bouter, and P. Lips, "Fall-risk screening test: a prospective study on predictors for falls in community-dwelling elderly," *Journal of Clinical Epidemiology*, vol. 54, no. 8, pp. 837–844, 2001.

[26] M. H. C. Bleijlevens, J. P. M. Diederiks, M. R. C. Hendriks, J. C. M. Van Haastregt, H. F. J. M. Crebolder, and J. T. Van Eijk, "Relationship between location and activity in injurious falls: An Exploratory Study," *BMC Geriatrics*, vol. 10, article 40, 2010.

[27] T. Unbehaun, K. Spiegelhalder, V. Hirscher, and D. Riemann, "Management of insomnia: update and new approaches," *Nature and Science of Sleep*, vol. 2, pp. 127–138, 2010.

[28] K. E. Ensrud, T. L. Blackwell, C. M. Mangione et al., "Central nervous system-active medications and risk for falls in older women," *Journal of the American Geriatrics Society*, vol. 50, no. 10, pp. 1629–1637, 2002.

[29] H. Allain, D. Bentué-Ferrer, E. Polard, Y. Akwa, and A. Patat, "Postural instability and consequent falls and hip fractures associated with use of hypnotics in the elderly: a comparative review," *Drugs & Aging*, vol. 22, no. 9, pp. 749–765, 2005.

[30] M. Stenbacka, B. Jansson, A. Leifman, and A. Romelsjö, "Association between use of sedatives or hypnotics, alcohol consumption, or other risk factors and a single injurious fall or multiple injurious falls: A Longitudinal General Population Study," *Alcohol*, vol. 28, no. 1, pp. 9–16, 2002.

[31] J. E. Byles, G. D. Mishra, M. A. Harris, and K. Nair, "The problems of sleep for older women: changes in health outcomes," *Age and Ageing*, vol. 32, no. 2, pp. 154–163, 2003.

[32] A. C. Grundstrom, C. E. Guse, and P. M. Layde, "Risk factors for falls and fall-related injuries in adults 85 years of age and older," *Archives of Gerontology and Geriatrics*, vol. 54, no. 3, pp. 421–428, 2012.

[33] N. D. A. Boyé, F. U. S. Mattace-Raso, E. M. M. Van Lieshout, K. A. Hartholt, E. F. Van Beeck, and T. J. M. Van der Cammen, "Physical performance and quality of life in single and recurrent fallers: data from the Improving Medication Prescribing to Reduce Risk of Falls study," *Geriatrics and Gerontology International*, vol. 15, no. 3, pp. 350–355, 2015.

[34] T.-Y. Wu, W.-C. Chie, R.-S. Yang, K.-L. Kuo, W.-K. Wong, and C.-K. Liaw, "Risk factors for single and recurrent falls: a prospective study of falls in community dwelling seniors without cognitive impairment," *Preventive Medicine*, vol. 57, no. 5, pp. 511–517, 2013.

21

Effect of Electronic Messaging on Physical Activity Participation among Older Adults

Chantrell Antoine Parker and Rebecca Ellis

Georgia State University, Atlanta, GA 30302, USA

Correspondence should be addressed to Rebecca Ellis; rellis@gsu.edu

Academic Editor: Guido Iaccarino

The purpose of this study was to determine if electronic messaging would increase min of aerobic physical activity (PA) among older adults. Participants were active older adults (n = 28; M age = 60 years, SD = 5.99, and range = 51–74 years). Using an incomplete within-subjects crossover design, participants were randomly assigned to begin the 4-week study receiving the treatment condition (a morning and evening text message) or the control condition (an evening text message). Participants self-reported min of completed aerobic PA by cell phone text. The 1-way within-subjects ANOVA showed significant group differences ($p < 0.05$). Specifically, when participants were in the treatment condition, they reported significantly greater average weekly min of aerobic PA (M = 96.88 min, SD = 62.9) compared to when they completed the control condition (M = 71.68 min, SD = 40.98). Electronic messaging delivered via cell phones was effective at increasing min of aerobic PA among older adults.

1. Introduction

Regular physical activity (PA) has many physical and mental health benefits for older adults including lowering the risk of early death, improving bone health, increasing cardiorespiratory and muscular fitness, decreasing levels of body fat, and reducing anxiety and depression [1]. To achieve these benefits, the 2008 Physical Activity Guidelines for Americans (PAG) recommend that adults should complete 150 min a week of moderate intensity aerobic PA or 75 min a week of vigorous intensity aerobic PA (or a combination of both), as well as two days a week of muscle strengthening activities [2]. PA participation progressively declines as people age, and currently only 17.1% and 15.9% of adults 55–64 years and 65 years and older, respectively, meet these guidelines; therefore, interventions to increase PA participation among older adults are warranted [3].

Meta-analytic evidence demonstrated that interventions are effective for increasing PA participation [4, 5], and specific characteristics of the intervention produced larger effects on behavior. For instance, in a review of 141 studies, Dishman and Buckworth [5] found significantly larger effect sizes for interventions that used behavior modification strategies such as reinforcement, stimulus control, or behavioral contracts (r = 0.92 weighted; r = 0.56 not weighted) and for those that were delivered using a mediated approach via indirect implementation through mailings or telecommunications (r = 0.91 weighted; r = 0.41 not weighted). Behavior modification techniques are based on the premise that the antecedents and consequences (including expected consequences) of the activity influence behavior [6]. Stimulus control involves manipulating environmental conditions, such as using prompts or reminders to decrease the problem behavior (physical inactivity) and increase the targeted behavior (PA participation [6]) and this strategy has frequently been incorporated into health behavior interventions.

In a systematic review of 19 weight loss, PA, and diet interventions that used periodic prompts, Fry and Neff [7] found that 11 studies reported positive intervention effects. The type of prompt (i.e., messages, reminders, and feedback), delivery periodicity (i.e., delivered daily, weekly, or monthly), and method of administration (i.e., sent using e-mail, telephone, and mail) were examined to determine which prompt characteristics had the greatest impact on behavior change. Of the 11 studies with positive results, 5 studies showed significant increases in PA when messages were delivered weekly by telephone and e-mail. Overall, these findings demonstrated that prompts delivered periodically are effective for promoting behavior change, and specifically can increase PA participation. Furthermore, Fry and Neff [7] acknowledge that the use of mobile technology as an alternative method for prompt delivery may be another cost-effective way to promote behavior change that warrants future research.

The use of cell phones, and specifically text messaging, to prompt PA participation is advantageous for promoting healthy behaviors because (a) there is a high penetration of mobile telephones across income and ethnic groups; (b) mobile phones are popular, portable, and convenient; and (c) information can be delivered quickly [8]. Gerber et al. [8] found that participants reported positive feedback and attitudes toward text messaging as a way to cultivate healthy behaviors. In a review of 14 health behavior change interventions that were delivered via mobile telephone short-message service (SMS) text messages, Fjeldsoe et al. [9] observed significant positive behavioral changes in 8 studies, and an additional 5 studies demonstrated positive behavior trends using SMS as a reminder to increase adherence to treatment programs.

Fanning et al. [10] conducted a recent meta-analysis of 11 studies that used mobile devices to increase PA. Specifically, interventions were delivered via SMS (eight studies), mobile software (four studies), and a personal digital assistant (PDA; two studies). The results of the meta-analysis showed that interventions delivered via mobile devices produced significant moderate effects on PA behavior ($g = 0.54$, 95% CI = 0.17 to 0.91, and $p = 0.01$). Moreover, a significant moderate effect was found for those interventions delivered with a mobile phone ($g = 0.52$, 95% CI = 0.11 to 0.94, and $p = 0.01$). However, of the 11 studies reviewed, only 2 reported samples with an average age of at least 60 years [11, 12].

King et al. [11] compared an intervention group that received a programmed alert on their PDA twice a day to a control group that received standard health educational written materials about PA. They found significantly larger increases in PA among older-aged adults when the intervention was delivered via a handheld computer (i.e., PDA). Nguyen et al. [12] compared a mobile self-monitored group to a mobile coached group that sent daily text message updates on exercise and symptoms of COPD. In return, both groups received a weekly thank-you standard text message. However, the mobile self-monitored group did not receive personalized feedback regarding exercise and symptoms of COPD. Although both groups increased PA, the mobile self-monitored group showed significant improvements in total steps per day compared to the mobile coached group. Therefore, using cell phones as a way to merge communication technologies with intervention strategies to increase PA participation in adults warrants more research in general and specifically among older adults.

To date, a limited number of research studies have examined the use of mobile technology to promote PA among adults aged 50 years and older [13–15]. Now that many older adults own and use a mobile phone, the purpose of this study was to determine if electronic prompts delivered via cell phones would increase min of aerobic PA among adults aged 50 years and older. It was hypothesized that participants would report significantly greater average weekly min of aerobic PA during the intervention condition than when they were in the control condition.

2. Methods

2.1. Participants. Participants were recruited from a certified personal training studio within the Metro-Atlanta area. Study participants met the following inclusion criteria: (1) 50 years of age or older, (2) worked with a personal trainer for at least six consecutive months, (3) currently working with a personal trainer at least twice a week for strength training, but did not meet the PAG for weekly aerobic PA, and (4) able to send and receive e-mail and/or text messages from a cell phone during a 4-week period. Thirty volunteers signed the university IRB approved informed consent form and were given information about the study. Volunteers were between 51 and 74 years of age.

2.2. Design and Procedures. This study used an incomplete within-subjects crossover design with counterbalancing of conditions to control for carryover effects between the treatment and control conditions. At the beginning of the 4-week period, the Principal Investigator (PI; the first author) met face to face with each volunteer for about 15 min. During the meeting, the PI explained and received a signature on the informed consent form. Participants also completed the personal history questionnaire. Participants were then randomly assigned to the treatment condition (Group 1) or the control condition (Group 2). During the first two weeks of the study, Group 1 (treatment condition) participants received a morning and evening text message to prompt aerobic PA three days a week. The morning prompt stated "Don't forget to do cardio today" and the evening prompt stated "Did you do your cardio today?" Prompting aerobic PA three days a week was chosen to supplement the two days a week of strength training participants were completing with their personal trainers. Although the participants were not currently meeting the PAG of 150 min a week of aerobic PA, the objective of the research was to test the efficacy of the intervention for increasing weekly min of aerobic PA, not necessarily to achieve 150 min or more. Participants in Group 2 (control condition) received only the evening text message (i.e., "Did you do your cardio today?") three days a week for two weeks.

All participants completed the electronic PA participation form by cell phone e-mail or text message on the days the text messages were received. Participants were informed that with a "*yes*" response to the evening message, they should report the type of aerobic PA, duration in min, and intensity (moderate or vigorous). With a "*no*" response to the evening message, participants were asked to report the reason for not performing aerobic PA (e.g., barriers). At the end of the first two weeks, participants crossed over to the other condition (i.e., Group 1 completed the control condition and Group 2 completed the treatment condition) and the procedures were executed exactly the same as described during the first two weeks.

2.3. Measures

2.3.1. Personal History Questionnaire. Participants reported age, gender, marital status, race/ethnicity, education, and income. Marital status was categorized as married and other (e.g., domestic partner, single, widowed, and divorced); race/ethnicity was categorized as White and other (e.g., Hispanic or Latino); education was categorized as high school or less, some college or associate's degree, and bachelor's degree or more; and income was categorized as low (<$1306 per month), medium ($1307–$1836 per month), high (≥$25,000 per year), and not reported.

2.3.2. Electronic Physical Activity Participation Form. The electronic PA participation form was used to record the participants' responses to the evening text message during the treatment and control conditions (i.e., "Did you do your cardio today? If yes, what did you do and if no, why not?"). Participants who reported "*yes*" to the completion of aerobic PA provided the type performed (walk, bike, swim, etc.), duration in min, and intensity (moderate or vigorous). Participants who reported "*no*" to the completion of aerobic PA reported barriers that prevented them from engaging in aerobic PA (e.g., no time, work, bad weather, etc.).

2.4. Analyses. Tests of outliers and normality were conducted. Participant demographic characteristics were described using frequencies, means, and standard deviations. If outliers were identified and removed from the sample, ANOVA and Chi-square were used to compare group differences between the outliers and remaining sample across demographic variables (e.g., age, gender, marital status, race, education level, and income level). ANOVA and Chi-square were also used to examine group differences across demographic variables between the participants who began the study in Group 1 (treatment condition) and those who began the study in Group 2 (control condition). Self-reported weekly min of aerobic PA and barriers to aerobic PA were summarized using frequencies. Weekly min of aerobic PA were categorized as 0–29 min, 30–59 min, 60–89 min, 90–119 min, 120–149 min, and 150 min or more. Finally, a 1-way within-subjects ANOVA was used to determine significant differences in average weekly min of aerobic PA by condition. SPSS version 18.0 was used to perform all data analyses denoting a statistically significant value of alpha levels at $p < 0.05$.

3. Results

Thirty older adults volunteered to participate in the study; however, two were identified as multivariate outliers and removed from the analyses. There were no significant group differences between the outliers and the remaining sample across demographic characteristics except on income level. One of the participants removed as an outlier reported a significantly lower income level (e.g., $1306 or less monthly versus $25,000 or more annually) than the other study participants, χ^2 $(2, N = 30) = 14.63$, $p = 0.001$; however, it should be noted this was the only volunteer in the sample who reported low income. The final sample included 28 male and female older adults (M age = 60 years, SD = 5.99, Range = 51–74 years; see Table 1). There were no significant group differences between the participants initially randomized into Group 1 (treatment condition) and those who began the study in Group 2 (control condition) across demographic characteristics.

The weekly min of aerobic PA for Group 1 and Group 2 were summarized using frequencies (see Table 2). The 1-way within-subjects ANOVA showed significant differences between conditions on total min of aerobic PA, Wilks' Lambda = 0.82, $F(1, 27) = 5.76$, $p = 0.024$, $\eta p^2 = 0.18$, and observed power = 0.64. Specifically, while participants were in the treatment condition they reported significantly greater average weekly min of aerobic PA (M = 96.88 min, SD = 62.90) compared to when they were in the control condition (M = 71.68 min, SD = 40.98; see Figure 1).

There were seven common barriers reported among participants that prevented them from engaging in aerobic PA (see Figure 2). The most commonly reported barriers during the treatment condition were (a) did not make time (31%) and (b) work (31%) and the most commonly reported barriers to aerobic PA during the control condition were (a) did not make time (28%), (b) work (26%), and (c) not feeling well (e.g., sick/injury; 18%).

4. Discussion

The purpose of this study was to determine if electronic prompts on cell phones would increase aerobic PA participation among adults aged 50 years and older. Average weekly min of aerobic PA were significantly greater during the treatment condition than during the control condition. Although future studies are warranted, current findings are consistent with previous research in that prompts effectively increase PA behavior and demonstrate the promise of using cell phone technology to deliver prompts to older adults. The clinical implications of these findings suggest that this is a feasible and effective intervention strategy for promoting aerobic PA among those 50 years and older who are members and regular users of fitness facilities because this intervention strategy was tested in a real-world setting.

As hypothesized, participants reported significantly greater average weekly min of aerobic PA during the treatment condition when they received the electronic reminder in the morning than during the control condition when the morning reminder was not delivered, and this treatment effect ($p = 0.024$; $\eta p^2 = 0.18$) was found despite a small sample size and reduced statistical power (0.64). These results are consistent with previous research that demonstrated the effectiveness of prompt interventions with mediated delivery [5, 7–10]. A recent meta-analysis by Fanning et al. [10] found a significant moderate effect for physical activity interventions that were specifically delivered via mobile phones; however, few of the studies reviewed included older adults. Therefore, the findings from this study extend the literature by providing evidence that electronic prompts delivered via cell phones can also be a successful strategy for increasing PA levels among adults aged 50 years and older.

TABLE 1: Demographics for Group 1 and Group 2 participants.

Characteristic	Group 1 (*n* = 13) M (SD)		Group 2 (*n* = 15) M (SD)		Total (*n* = 28) M (SD)	
Age	58.23 (6.59)		61.60 (5.15)		60.04 (5.99)	
Gender						
Male	*n* = 2	15.4%	*n* = 3	20.0%	*n* = 5	17.9%
Female	*n* = 11	84.6%	*n* = 12	80.0%	*n* = 23	82.1%
Marital status						
Married	*n* = 7	53.8%	*n* = 13	86.7%	*n* = 20	71.4%
Other	*n* = 6	46.2%	*n* = 2	13.3%	*n* = 8	28.6%
Race						
White	*n* = 12	92.3%	*n* = 15	100%	*n* = 27	96.4%
Other	*n* = 1	7.7%			*n* = 1	3.6%
Education level						
High school or less	*n* = 2	15.4%	*n* = 1	6.7%	*n* = 1	3.6%
Some college or associate's degree	*n* = 11	84.6%	*n* = 4	26.7%	*n* = 6	21.4%
Bachelor's degree or more			*n* = 10	66.7%	*n* = 21	75.0%
Income level						
$25,000 or more annually	*n* = 12	92.3%	*n* = 10	66.7%	*n* = 22	78.6%
Did not report	*n* = 1	7.7%	*n* = 5	33.3%	*n* = 6	21.4%
History of disease*						
Cardiovascular	*n* = 3	23.1%	*n* = 2	13.3%	*n* = 5	17.9%
Cancer	*n* = 0	0.0%	*n* = 3	20.0%	*n* = 3	10.7%
Thyroid	*n* = 0	0.0%	*n* = 3	20.0%	*n* = 3	10.7%
Bone	*n* = 1	7.7%	*n* = 1	6.7%	*n* = 2	7.1%
Spine	*n* = 2	15.4%	*n* = 0	0.0%	*n* = 2	7.1%
Other	*n* = 3	23.1%	*n* = 2	13.3%	*n* = 5	17.9%
No disease reported	*n* = 6	46.2%	*n* = 5	33.3%	*n* = 11	39.3%

Note. Group 1 = treatment condition first. Group 2 = control condition first. *Frequencies may not equal total sample sizes or 100% because 3 participants reported 2 illnesses.

TABLE 2: Weekly min of aerobic physical activity for Group 1 and Group 2 participants.

Categories	0–29 min		30–59 min		60–89 min		90–119 min		120–149 min		≥150 min	
Week 1												
Group 1 (TX)	*n* = 2	15.4%	*n* = 3	23.1%	*n* = 1	7.7%	*n* = 1	7.7%	*n* = 4	30.8%	*n* = 2	15.4%
Group 2	*n* = 1	6.7%	*n* = 5	33.3%	*n* = 3	20.0%	*n* = 3	20.0%	*n* = 1	6.7%	*n* = 2	13.3%
Week 2												
Group 1 (TX)	*n* = 2	15.4%	*n* = 2	15.4%	*n* = 2	15.4%	*n* = 2	15.4%	*n* = 1	7.7%	*n* = 4	30.8%
Group 2	*n* = 4	26.7%	*n* = 1	6.7%	*n* = 3	20.0%	*n* = 2	13.3%	*n* = 4	26.7%	*n* = 1	6.7%
Week 3												
Group 1	*n* = 2	15.4%	*n* = 3	23.1%	*n* = 2	15.4%	*n* = 6	46.2%	*n* = 0	0.0%	*n* = 0	0.0%
Group 2 (TX)	*n* = 5	33.3%	*n* = 1	6.7%	*n* = 3	20.0%	*n* = 0	0.0%	*n* = 3	20.0%	*n* = 3	20.0%
Week 4												
Group 1	*n* = 3	23.1%	*n* = 4	30.8%	*n* = 3	23.1%	*n* = 1	7.7%	*n* = 1	7.7%	*n* = 1	7.7%
Group 2 (TX)	*n* = 1	6.7%	*n* = 3	20.0%	*n* = 1	6.7%	*n* = 1	6.7%	*n* = 7	46.7%	*n* = 2	13.3%

Note. TX = treatment condition. Group 1 (*n* = 13) = treatment condition first. Group 2 (*n* = 15) = control condition first.

In addition to examining the use of electronic messaging via cell phones to increase PA participation among older adults, common barriers to aerobic PA participation were recorded. The most common barriers during both conditions were "did not make time" and "work," which are consistent with previous research [16]. However, fewer barriers were reported while participants were in the treatment intervention ($n = 32$) than in the control ($n = 39$), suggesting that

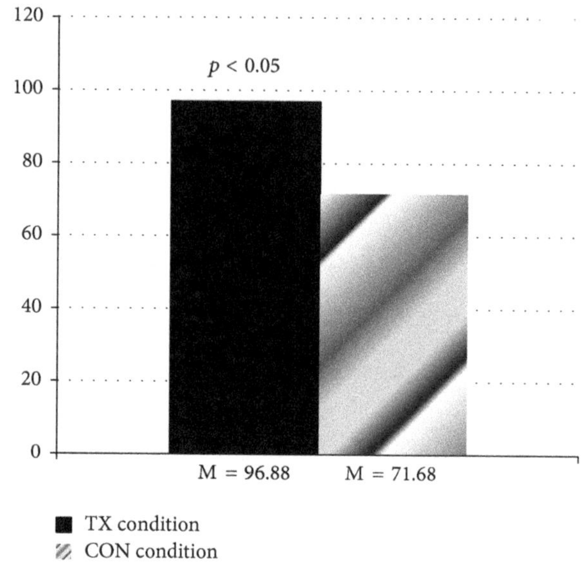

Figure 1: Average weekly min of aerobic physical activity. TX = treatment condition. CON = control condition.

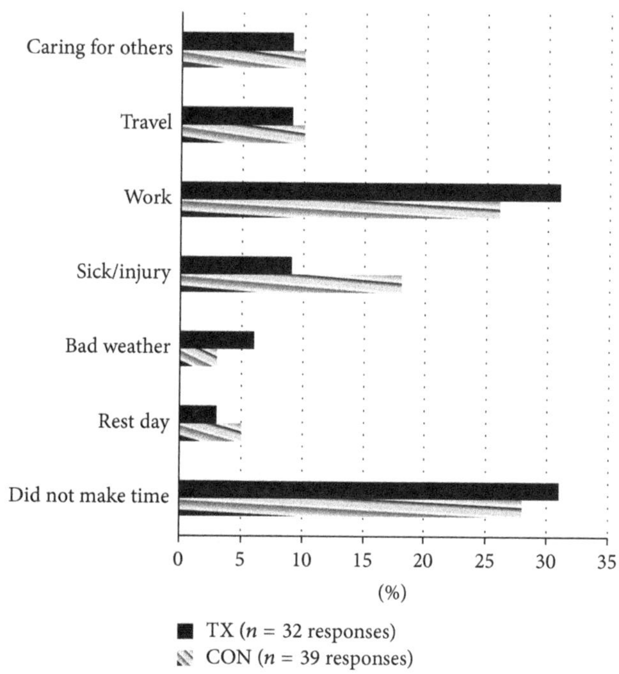

Figure 2: Barriers to aerobic physical activity. TX = treatment condition. CON = control condition.

the electronic prompts may have assisted with barrier removal. These findings show promise for using electronic prompts delivered via cell phones to increase PA participation as well as to assist with barrier removal.

Although the results of this study suggest that use of electronic prompts delivered via cell phones to promote aerobic PA among older adults is effective, it is not without limitations. First, the generalizability of the findings is limited to a small sample of mostly White, wealthy, well-educated women with access to cell phones who were already physically active (e.g., working with a personal trainer for strength training) and relatively healthy; however, it should be noted that the study sample was representative of the facility population from which volunteers were recruited. Moreover, the study sample was similar to samples included in previous studies that used mobile devices to prompt PA among older adults [11, 12]. These studies also included small samples of mostly White women that held at least a bachelor's degree and earned more than $50,000 a year with an average age of 60 years or more. Second, within a crossover design, although participants were randomized into Group 1 and Group 2, contamination between the groups did occur in participants that partnered together during personal training sessions. Specifically, a husband and wife pair began the study in opposite groups, and the husband in Group 1 asked his wife in Group 2 to walk with him. This contamination may have resulted in increased PA among the control participants.

Finally, the duration of the intervention and the frequency of the electronic prompt delivery may be considered inadequate despite the demonstration of positive results. However, this intervention should be viewed in the context of previous research that shares similar characteristics and also demonstrated the effectiveness of prompts for changing behavior. For instance, interventions that were less than six weeks were included in the Fry and Neff [7] review (see [17, 18]), and the frequency of electronic prompt delivery in this study is within a range of frequencies (e.g., daily, once a week, and once a month) found in studies included in the Fry and Neff [7] and Fjeldsoe et al. [9] reviews (see [11, 12, 17, 19, 20]). In addition, it should be noted that during the treatment condition participants were averaging about 32 min of aerobic PA per bout (6 bouts during 2-week condition) versus 24 min of aerobic PA during the control condition. These values suggest that if the treatment had been delivered 5 times per week, participants were on track to meet the 150 weekly min of aerobic activity. Although longer interventions are necessary to determine the effectiveness of electronic prompts for the maintenance of aerobic PA in older adults, the evidence is promising for the effects of this strategy for promoting adoption and short-term aerobic PA.

5. Conclusions

Few studies have examined electronic prompts on cell phones to increase PA participation among older adults [13–15], and few have been tested in real-world settings. The results of this study are consistent with previous research and indicate that electronic prompts can increase aerobic PA among older adults and may assist with barrier removal. Future research interventions using mobile technology are needed to confirm the study findings using a randomized between-subjects design with a larger sample size of older adults across different income levels, educational backgrounds, ethnicities, and health status. Future research interventions should also test the use of the video components (i.e., FaceTime and Skype) of mobile technology for prompt delivery. In summary, the use of electronic prompts on cell phones may be a feasible, cost-effective, and convenient method to increase aerobic PA among older adults. Physicians, physical therapists, and personal trainers may want to consider integrating mobile technology into their practice by using cell phones to deliver reminder, informational, and even instructional prompts to patients and clients.

Competing Interests

There is no financial conflict of interests to report. It should be noted that Chantrell Antoine Parker was an employee at BodyFitz when this research was conducted.

Acknowledgments

The authors would like to thank Mr. Daniel FitzSimons, owner of BodyFitz, for allowing them to conduct this research study at his personal training studio.

References

[1] US Department of Health and Human Services, National Institute on Aging, 2011, http://nihseniorhealth.gov/exerciseforolderadults/toc.html.

[2] U.S. Department of Health and Human Services, "*Physical activity guidelines for Americans*," 2008, http://www.health.gov/paguidelines/guidelines/summary.aspx.

[3] Centers for Disease Control and Prevention, "Adult participation in aerobic and muscle strengthening physical activities: United States, 2011," *Morbidity and Mortality Weekly Report (MMWR)*, vol. 62, no. 17, pp. 326–330, 2013.

[4] V. S. Conn, A. R. Hafdahl, and D. R. Mehr, "Interventions to increase physical activity among healthy adults: meta-analysis of outcomes," *American Journal of Public Health*, vol. 101, no. 4, pp. 751–758, 2011.

[5] R. K. Dishman and J. Buckworth, "Increasing physical activity: a quantitative synthesis," *Medicine & Science in Sports & Exercise*, vol. 28, no. 6, pp. 706–719, 1996.

[6] J. M. Williams, Ed., *Applied Sport Psychology: Personal Growth to Peak Performance*, Mayfield Publishing Company, Mountain View, Calif, USA, 2001.

[7] J. P. Fry and R. A. Neff, "Periodic prompts and reminders in health promotion and health behavior interventions: systematic review," *Journal of Medical Internet Research*, vol. 11, no. 2, pp. e16–e52, 2009.

[8] B. S. Gerber, M. R. Stolley, A. L. Thompson, L. K. Sharp, and M. L. Fitzgibbon, "Mobile phone text messaging to promote healthy behaviors and weight loss maintenance: a feasibility study," *Health Informatics Journal*, vol. 15, no. 1, pp. 17–25, 2009.

[9] B. S. Fjeldsoe, A. L. Marshall, and Y. D. Miller, "Behavior change interventions delivered by mobile telephone short-message service," *American Journal of Preventive Medicine*, vol. 36, no. 2, pp. 165–173, 2009.

[10] J. Fanning, S. P. Mullen, and E. Mcauley, "Increasing physical activity with mobile devices: a meta-analysis," *Journal of Medical Internet Research*, vol. 14, no. 6, pp. e161–e177, 2012.

[11] A. C. King, D. K. Ahn, B. M. Oliveira, A. A. Atienza, C. M. Castro, and C. D. Gardner, "Promoting physical activity through hand-held computer technology," *American Journal of Preventive Medicine*, vol. 34, no. 2, pp. 138–142, 2008.

[12] H. Q. Nguyen, D. P. Gill, S. Wolpin, B. G. Steele, and J. O. Benditt, "Pilot study of a cell phone-based exercise persistence intervention post-rehabilitation for COPD," *International Journal of Chronic Obstructive Pulmonary Disease*, vol. 4, pp. 301–313, 2009.

[13] D. Bossen, C. Veenhof, K. E. Van Beek, P. M. Spreeuwenberg, J. Dekker, and D. H. De Bakker, "Effectiveness of a web-based physical activity intervention in patients with knee and/or hip osteoarthritis: randomized controlled trial," *Journal of Medical Internet Research*, vol. 15, no. 11, article e257, 2013.

[14] B. H. Kim and K. Glanz, "Text messaging to motivate walking in older african americans: a randomized controlled trial," *American Journal of Preventive Medicine*, vol. 44, no. 1, pp. 71–75, 2013.

[15] M. Tabak, H. Op den Akker, and H. Hermens, "Motivational cues as real-time feedback for changing daily activity behavior of patients with COPD," *Patient Education and Counseling*, vol. 94, no. 3, pp. 372–378, 2014.

[16] J. Salmon, D. Crawford, N. Owen, A. Bauman, and J. F. Sallis, "Physical activity and sedentary behavior: a population-based study of barriers, enjoyment, and preference," *Health Psychology*, vol. 22, no. 2, pp. 178–188, 2003.

[17] A. Prestwich, M. Perugini, and R. Hurling, "Can implementation intentions and text messages promote brisk walking? A randomized trial," *Health Psychology*, vol. 29, no. 1, pp. 40–49, 2010.

[18] R. Sirriyeh, R. Lawton, and J. Ward, "Physical activity and adolescents: an exploratory randomized controlled trial investigating the influence of affective and instrumental text messages," *British Journal of Health Psychology*, vol. 15, no. 4, pp. 825–840, 2010.

[19] P. P. Cheung, B. C. Chow, and G. Parfitt, "Using environmental stimuli in physical activity intervention for school teachers: a pilot study," *International Electronic Journal of Health Education*, vol. 11, pp. 47–56, 2008.

[20] R. Hurling, M. Catt, M. De Boni et al., "Using internet and mobile phone technology to deliver an automated physical activity program: randomized controlled trial," *Journal of Medical Internet Research*, vol. 9, no. 2, article e7, 2007.

22

Successful Aging: A Psychosocial Resources Model for Very Old Adults

G. Kevin Randall,[1] Peter Martin,[2] Mary Ann Johnson,[3] and Leonard W. Poon[4]

[1] *CC Wheeler Institute, Bradley University, 05 Bradley Hall, 1501 W. Bradley Avenue, Peoria, IL 61625, USA*
[2] *Gerontology Program, Iowa State University, 1096 LeBaron Hall, Ames, IA 50011-1120, USA*
[3] *Department of Foods & Nutrition, The University of Georgia, 143 Barrow Hall, 115 DW Brooks Dr, Athens, GA 30602, USA*
[4] *Institute of Gerontology, College of Public Health, The University of Georgia, 255 E. Hancock Avenue, Athens, GA 30602-5775, USA*

Correspondence should be addressed to G. Kevin Randall, krandall@bradley.edu

Academic Editor: Roger A. Fielding

Objectives. Using data from the first two phases of the Georgia Centenarian Study, we proposed a latent factor structure for the Duke OARS domains: Economic Resources, Mental Health, Activities of Daily Living, Physical Health, and Social Resources. *Methods.* Exploratory and confirmatory factor analyses were conducted on two waves of the Georgia Centenarian Study to test a latent variable measurement model of the five resources; nested model testing was employed to assess the final measurement model for equivalency of factor structure over time. *Results.* The specified measurement model fit the data well at Time 1. However, at Time 2, Social Resources only had one indicator load significantly and substantively. Supplemental analyses demonstrated that a model without Social Resources adequately fit the data. Factorial invariance over time was confirmed for the remaining four latent variables. *Discussion.* This study's findings allow researchers and clinicians to reduce the number of OARS questions asked of participants. This has practical implications because increased difficulties with hearing, vision, and fatigue in older adults may require extended time or multiple interviewer sessions to complete the battery of OARS questions.

1. Introduction

Aging is often conceptualized as a developmental challenge to maintain balance between the gains and losses of resources necessary for adaptation to age-related change, with losses increasing over the lifespan [1, 2]. Yet, Von Faber and colleagues [3] reminded us that, "Successful aging as an optimal state implicates more than physical well-being and fits the World Health Organization's definition of health as a state of complete physical, mental, and social well-being and not merely the absence of disease or infirmity." These resources-material, social, or personal characteristics essential for successful aging-hold a prominent position in studies of older adults [4–6]. Consequently, the need for a valid, reliable, and efficient resource measure, designed for use in clinical and community settings with older adults, arose. In response, Fillenbaum [7] and associates developed the *Multidimensional Functional Assessment of Older Adults: The Duke Older Americans Resources and Services Procedures* (OARS hereafter). Since development of the OARS, advances in statistical methodology, computer technology, and software programs have made factor analytic procedures commonplace, enabling researchers to suggest less complex and shorter versions of measurement scales and to model measurement error in empirical studies. To date, we know of no studies that investigated the underlying, latent factor structure of the five OARS resources with data from older adults—the purpose of the present study.

Studies on multiple resources and successful aging among older adults have grown tremendously [8–11], spawning psychometric concerns regarding how and what to assess [12]. Researchers have demonstrated the need to expand investigations of multidimensional resources in older populations [13, 14]. This body of work was motivated not only by the increased prevalence of older adults but also by a growing concern among those assessing and caring for frail older adults. The OARS was developed by a multidisciplinary team who recognized that older adults' personal well-being encompasses many aspects or multiple functions [7]. Because older adults often present with chronic disabilities or ailments [15, 16], the developers of the OARS designed an assessment tool that focused primarily on adaptation and the maintenance of personal well-being in five resources: Social Resources, Economic Resources, Mental Health, Physical Health, and self-care capacity or functional health (including both instrumental activities of daily living (IADL) and activities of daily living (ADLs)). This instrument has received widespread use by a diverse group of geriatric practitioners, researchers, and service group providers such as epidemiologists characterizing particular populations, clinicians assessing patient status, resource allocators providing services, and program evaluators investigating the impacts of interventions [12, 17–19].

In addition, because clinical work and empirical research may be tiring and confusing for older participants, a reduced version of the five OARS resources as modeled by five latent variables would prove helpful in reducing the time required to assess older adults' resources. However, few studies have specified the OARS resources as latent variables [20–22]. Further, to date, no study was found that developed a measurement model for all five OARS resources.

The purpose of this study was to specify and test the latent factor structure of the five OARS resources administered to participants in their 60s, 80s, and 100s. We hypothesized that (a) the resource model proposed by Fillenbaum [7] can be obtained using data from old and very old individuals and (b) a reduced short version of the OARS will yield a satisfactory latent variable solution.

2. Methods

2.1. Procedure and Participants. Participants were selected through the assistance of the University of Georgia Survey Research Center, the Office of the Governor of Georgia, the media, and local older adult service organizations [23–25]. Selection criteria for the final sample of community-dwelling individuals included a score of 23 or higher on the Mini-Mental Status Examination (MMSE; [26]) or a score of 2 or lower on the Global Deterioration Scale [27].

The data collection at phase one included 321 older adults (217 women, 104 men), classified as sexagenarians (n = 91), octogenarians (n = 93), and centenarians (n = 137). At time two, 201 participants provided data for this longitudinal study: 70 sexagenarians, 63 octogenarians, and 68 centenarians. Those in their 60s and 80s were followed up within 60 months; due to mortality attrition, centenarians were followed up within 20 months. Almost one-third of the sample was African American (27.7% and 30.8% at Time 1 and Time 2, resp.). The majority of the sample was female (67.6%), well-educated (at least graduated from high school), and rated their health as excellent or good (Table 1).

Table 1: Sample demographic characteristics.

Variables	Time 1		Time 2		χ^2
	n	%	n	%	
Sex					1.59
Male	104	32.4	60	29.9	
Female	217	67.6	141	70.1	
Race					2.61
Black	89	27.7	62	30.8	
White	232	72.3	139	69.2	
Age group					18.86***
60s	91	28.3	70	34.8	
80s	93	29.0	63	31.3	
100s	137	42.7	68	33.8	
Education					6.19
0-8 years	90	28.2	55	28.8	
High school	84	26.3	42	22.0	
Business/trade school	23	7.2	14	7.3	
College	75	23.6	44	23.0	
Graduate school	47	14.7	36	18.8	
Self-rated health					4.7
Excellent	67	21.1	39	20.2	
Good	159	50.2	93	48.2	
Fair	79	24.9	52	26.9	
Poor	12	3.8	9	4.7	

Because of rounding, percentages may not add to 100.
***$P < .001$.

As noted earlier, in this sample of old and very old adults, mortality attrition resulted in a reduction of participants, particularly among the centenarians, from 321 at time 1 to 201 at time 2. Table 2 examines the differences for the OARS manifest variables and two measures of cognitive status. Overall, the sample at time 2 showed significantly higher scores relative to time 1.

2.2. Measures. Because the purpose of this study was to develop a latent variable model for the five OARS resources, in this section we provide a brief overview of the measures based upon Fillenbaum's [7] work. Details of our final latent variables and corresponding indicators are presented in Section 3. In addition, the appendix lists each resource and its indicators and associated questions, based on our final results.

2.2.1. Economic Resources. Six questions were asked; examples included "How well does the amount of money you have take care of your needs—very well, fairly well, or poorly?" and "Please tell me how well you think you are now doing financially as compared to other people your age—better, about the same, or worse?" These items were scaled from 0: poorly or worse to 2: very well or better.

2.2.2. Mental Health. Satisfaction (six items), sleep disturbance (two items), lethargy (6 items), and paranoid (three

Table 2: Differences between participants at Time 1 and participants at Time 1 and Time 2.

Variables	Time 1 Only		Time 1 and Time 2		t
	M	SD	M	SD	
Mini-Mental (MMSE)	25.30	2.72	26.31	3.01	−3.03**
Short Portable (SPMSQ)	8.63	1.58	9.04	1.38	−2.41*
Economic Resources	4.73	1.48	4.82	1.47	.48
Mental Health	5.12	1.33	5.27	1.24	.97
IADLs	4.81	1.30	5.25	1.19	3.02**
Physical Health	3.73	1.70	4.24	1.58	2.73**
Social Resources	4.49	1.55	4.57	1.47	.42

*$P < .05$. **$P < .01$.

items) comprised the four dimensions of Mental Health [7]. Examples of questions included (a) satisfaction: "In general, do you find life exciting, pretty routine, or dull?" scaled so that 0: dull, 1: pretty routine, and 2: exciting; (b) sleep disturbance: "Do you wake up fresh and rested most mornings?" scaled so that 0: no, 1: yes; (c) lethargy: "Have you had periods of days, weeks, or months when you couldn't take care of things because you couldn't "get going?" scaled so that 0: no, 1: yes; (d) paranoid: "Does it seem that no one understands you?" scaled so that 0: no, 1: yes.

2.2.3. ADLs. Two commonly used dimensions, instrumental activities of daily living (IADL; seven items) and physical activities of daily living (PADLs; six items), comprised the self-care capacity assessment. An example of an IADL question included "Can you do your housework?" scaled so that 2: without help (can clean floors, etc.); 1: with some help (can prepare some things but unable to cook full meals yourself) or 0: are you completely unable to prepare any meals? A PADL question was "Can you dress and undress yourself" scaled so that 2: without help (able to pick out clothes, dress and undress yourself) 1: with some help, or 0: are you completely unable to dress and undress yourself?

2.2.4. Physical Health. Three questions assessing subjective self-rated health were included. For example, participants responded to "How would you rate your overall health at the present time—excellent, good, fair, or poor?" scaled so that 0: poor and 3: excellent.

2.2.5. Social Resources. Social Resources were measured using seven questions. An example of a question focusing on the interaction aspect of social support was "How many people do you know well enough to visit with in their homes?" Participants chose from a scale of 0: none to 3: five or more. An assessment of dependability of social support included two questions. These questions were answered 1: yes and 0: no. For example, one question was "Do you have someone you can trust and confide in?" A third assessment of the affective domain of social support also included two questions, scaled 1: yes and 0: no. For example, one question was "Do you see your relatives and friends as often as you want to or not?"

2.3. Data Analysis. The analyses conducted to confirm a measurement model included the following steps for each resource: (a) specifying and testing Fillenbaum's subscales; (b) adapting Fillenbaum's recommendations when modeling difficulties were encountered; (c) employing exploratory factor analyses (i.e., principal axis factoring retaining three factors with oblique rotation) to assess relationships within the data and to posit possible indicators for latent constructs; (d) testing the measurement model by confirmatory factor analyses. We developed at least three indicators for each resource and then tested the latent variable measurement model via confirmatory factor analysis. Table 3 provides assessment of measurement model fit, standardized loadings, and the uniqueness or R^2 for each indicator. All variables were scaled so that higher scores indicated higher levels of the resource. In the appendix, we provide a nontechnical summary of our results, listing the recommended questions for each indicator of the five OARS resources.

We used full-information maximum likelihood (FIML) to estimate our models [28, 29]. For our latent variable analyses we used *M*plus 6.11 [30] and employed FIML with the estimator MLR (maximum likelihood parameter estimates with standard errors and a mean-adjusted chi-square test statistic that are robust to nonnormality).

Exploratory factor analyses were conducted using SPSS 18.0, whereas confirmatory factor analyses and structural equation modeling were conducted with *M*plus [30]. Overall model fit was assessed by employing the Satorra-Bentler chi-square test statistic. This type of chi-square test statistic provided maximum likelihood parameter estimates with standard errors and a mean-adjusted chisquare test statistic that is robust to nonnormality of measures. Because the chisquare goodness of fit test and its corresponding probability value are sensitive to sample size, often making it difficult to accurately assess model fit when limited to this single statistic [31, 32], other measures of model fit were reported including the Comparative Fit Index (CFI) [33], the Tucker-Lewis coefficient (also called the NNFI) (TLI) [34], Browne and Cudeck's [35] root mean squared error of approximation (RMSEA), and the standardized root mean squared residual (SRMR). It has been suggested that values close to .95 for TLI and CFI, .08 for SRMR, and .06 for RMSEA are necessary before concluding that a relatively good fit between the observed data and the hypothesized model exists [36, 37].

TABLE 3: OARS resources latent variable measurement model results.

Construct/indicators	Loadings (λ)[a]	Uniqueness (R^2)	Loadings (λ)[a]	Uniqueness (R^2)
	T1*		T2**	
Economic Resources				
Sufficient Income	.81[b]	.66	.96[b]	.93
Overall Income	.70	.49	.61	.37
Meet Payments	.63	.40	.30	.09
Mental Health				
Exciting	.60[b]	.36	.53[b]	.28
Overall Mental Health	.53	.29	.49	.24
Life Satisfaction	.50	.25	.69	.47
IADLS				
Getting Out	.89[b]	.80	.94[b]	.88
Housework	.88	.78	.94	.88
Medicine	.65	.42	.77	.59
Physical Health				
Low Troubles	.70[b]	.49	.86[b]	.73
Overall Physical Health	.66	.44	.49	.24
Comparative Health	.46	.21	.48	.23
Social Resources				
Phone Talk	.64[b]	.41	.94[b]	.89
Visit Network Number	.47	.22	.08	.01
Visits With Others	.42	.17	.29	.08

[a] Parameter estimates are from the standardized solution. [b] These indicator loadings were fixed to 1.0 (unstandardized) for model identification; all estimated loadings $P < .01$; except Time 2 Social Resources.
*T1 Fit Indices: MLR χ^2 ($N = 321$; df = 80) = 144; CFI = .94; TLI = .92; RMSEA = .05; SRMR = .05.
**T2 Fit Indices: MLR χ^2 ($N = 201$; df = 80) = 136; CFI = .93; TLI = .90; RMSEA = .06; SRMR = .07.

3. Results

Economic Resources included six items. We conducted an exploratory factor analysis (principal axis factoring) with an oblique rotation and extracted three factors, accounting for 76 percent of the variance. Based upon these results, we constructed three indicators. First, we summed the three dichotomous items tapping the sufficiency of the respondent's economic resources to meet emergencies and provide extras currently and in the future (Cronbach's alpha = .81). This indicator, *Sufficient Income*, was recorded so that the scores ranged from 0 to 2. (Because we summed these indicators to create a manifest variable in other analyses, we recorded the indicators for equal weighting.) Second, two items loaded on a second factor, both asking the respondents how well they were doing financially. These two items were then averaged to create a second indicator, *Overall Income*, and assessed how well the respondents felt they were doing relative to their overall financial well-being (Cronbach's alpha = .59). Finally, the last item, *Meet Payments*, assessed the participant's expenses, was recorded to 0–2, and used as a third indicator. This item tapped the respondents, ability to meet payments. The three indicators loaded significantly and substantively on the latent variable, Economic Resources, at Time 1 and Time 2 (Table 3).

Inspection of the *Mental Health* assessment revealed that five items had 90% or more respondents scoring alike, five had 80% or more of respondents scoring alike, and three had 70% or more of respondents scoring alike. Thus, we did not use these items and specified a latent variable with three single-item indicators: (a) "In general, do you find life exciting, pretty routine, or dull?" (b) "How would you rate your mental or emotional health at the present time?" and (c) "Taking everything into consideration how would you describe your satisfaction with life in general at the present time?" These three indicators, *Exciting*, *Overall Mental Health*, and *Life Satisfaction*, loaded significantly and substantively on the latent variable Mental Health at Time 1 and Time 2 (Table 3).

Activities of Daily Living (IADL) consisted of instrumental activities of daily living (seven items) and physical activities of daily living (six items). Because descriptive statistics demonstrated that for those in their 60s and 80s few difficulties with physical activities of daily living were encountered, we did not include this subscale but created three indicators for IADL based upon an exploratory factor analysis of the seven items of IADL. The first indicator, labeled *Getting Out*, included items assessing (a) "Can you use the phone?" (b) "Can you get to places out of walking distance?" and (c) "Can you go shopping for groceries or clothes?" Cronbach's alpha for these three items was .76. The second indicator, *Housework*, was comprised of three items (Cronbach's alpha = .88) assessing: (a) "Can you prepare your own meals?" (b) "Can you do your own housework?" and (c) "Can you handle your own money?" The third indicator, *Medicine*, was a single item, "Can you take your own medicine?" The three indicators loaded significantly and substantively on the latent variable IADL at Time 1 and Time 2 (Table 3).

Physical Health consisted of three single-item indicators assessing subjective health perceptions. First, for the indicator *Low Troubles*, respondents were asked, "How much do your health troubles stand in the way of your doing the things you want to do?" Second, the question for the indicator *Overall Health* asked "How would you rate your overall health at the present time?" A third question for the indicator *Comparative Health* asked, "Is your health now better, about the same, or worse than it was five years ago?" These three indicators loaded significantly and substantively on the latent variable Physical Health at Time 1 and Time 2 (Table 3).

Social Resources included seven items. Because three dichotomous items did not provide much variance (over 90% of respondents scored "yes"), we did not use them. We then conducted an exploratory factor analysis on the remaining questions. Four items were used in our initial latent variable: (a) "How many times did you talk to friends, relatives, or others on the phone in the past week?" (b) "How many people do you know well enough to visit in their homes?" (c) "How many times in the past week did you spend some time with someone who does not live with you?" and (d) "Do you find yourself feeling lonely?" (recorded so that high scores reflected low loneliness). Thus, a latent variable was specified with *Phone Talk* as the first indicator, with *Visit Network Number* as a second indicator, *Visits With Others* as a third indicator, and *Loneliness* as a fourth.

Based on the previous exploratory factor analyses, we specified and tested a measurement model using confirmatory factor analysis and comprised of the five factors and their respective indicators as previously discussed. However, in the first test of the measurement model, loneliness did not significantly load on the latent variable for Social Resources at Time 1 ($t = 1.62$); this item was dropped and not used as an indicator in further analyses. Next, we conducted a similar analysis and these indicators loaded on the latent factor, Social Resources, significantly and substantively at Time 1 (see Table 3 for the results). However, at Time 2 the second and third indicators did not load significantly or substantively, although the overall measurement model fit to the data was adequate. This indicates that the construct might have changed over time, and the results for Time 2 Social Resources need to be stated with caution (Table 3).

The five latent variables were significantly correlated with one another at each measurement occasion with a few exceptions at Time 2 (Table 4). For example, at Time 2 Social Resources was only significantly associated with IADL; also, Physical Health was not significantly associated with either Mental Health or Social Resources at Time 2. Also, power issues may have influenced the results as the sample size was $N = 321$ at time 1 and $N = 201$ at Time 2, resulting in a lack of findings that may have existed. For example, consider the correlation between Social Resources and Mental Health at Time 2: $r = .25, P > .05$. However, at Time 1, with the larger sample size, two correlations close to the same magnitude as that between Social Resources and Mental Health at Time 2—the correlation between Economic Resources and IADL ($r = .25, P \leq .01$) and the correlations between Economic

Table 4: Correlation Matrix of OARS Resources Latent Variables (Time1 below the diagonal; Time 2 above the diagonal).

	1	2	3	4	5
1. Economic Resources	—	.26**	.43**	.27**	.08
2. Physical Health	.46**	—	.15	.58**	.14
3. Mental Health	.60**	.83**	—	.38**	.25
4. IADLS	.21**	.56**	.42**	—	.45**
5. Social Resources	.27**	.34**	.35**	.50**	—

** $P < .01$.

Resources and Social Resources ($r = .27, P \leq .01$)—are significant, indicating a likely reduction in power at Time 2. Table 5 presents the final correlations and descriptive statistics for all indicators of the OARS measurement model.

Finally, we attempted a nested model test for factorial invariance over time by constraining the loadings of each indicator at Time 1 equal to the same indicator at Time 2. Also, the residual for each indicator at Time 1 was correlated with its counterpart at Time 2. This constrained or nested model did not fit the data well: MLR χ^2 (354, $N = 201$) = 527.03, $P = .001$, CFI = .91, TLI = .89, RMSEA = .05, and SRMR = .07. However, despite increasing the number of iterations and specifying starting values, we were not able to get the unconstrained or base model to converge. This measurement model included the Social Resources latent construct at Time 2 that did not have significant loadings for its estimated indicators. Thus, the overall poor model fit may be due to a poor measurement model for Social Resources.

As a follow-up, we decided to fit a measurement model without the Social Resources latent variable. The unconstrained or base model, including the four latent variable resource constructs (without Social Resources at Time 1 and Time 2), specified with correlated residuals across time, fit the data well: MLR χ^2 (211, $N = 201$) = 289.09, $P = .001$, CFI = .95, TLI = .94, RMSEA = .04, and SRMR = .06. Next, we added across time constraints to the factor loadings for each corresponding indicator and ran the model. This constrained or nested model with eight more degrees of freedom fit the data well also: MLR χ^2 (219, $N = 201$) = 300.18, $P = .001$, CFI = .95, TLI = .94, RMSEA = .04, and SRMR = .07. Finally, we performed a nested model chi-square difference test following the specifications provided by B. Muthén and L. Muthén [30] for the MLR chi-square. In this case, the chi-square difference was 11.06 with eight degrees of freedom, $P = .20$. Thus, no significant difference was found between these two models and it is reasonable to assume factorial invariance over time.

4. Discussion

The focus of this study was a widely used integral part of the *Multidimensional Functional Assessment of Older Adults: The Duke Older Americans Resources and Services Procedures* [7]. To date, few studies have specified one or more of the five OARS resources as latent variables [20–22] and we found no studies with older adults, especially centenarians, specifying

TABLE 5: Correlation matrix of indicators for OARS measurement model (Time 1 below the diagonal; Time 2 above the diagonal).

Variables	1	2	3	4	5	6	7	8	9	10	11	12	13	14	15	16		
(1) Age Group	—	−.18**	.02	−.08	−.22**	−.23**	−.13	−.72**	−.71**	−.47**	−.27**	−.10	−.09	−.40**	−.18**	−.03		
(2) Sufficient Income	−.05	—	.58**	.28**	.17**	.18**	.32**	.27**	.25**	.12	.19**	.30**	.04	.14	−.02	.16		
(3) Overall Income	.07	.56**	—	.22**	.07	.14	.21*	.02	.04	−.01	.02	.16*	.04	.08	.10	.09		
(4) Meet Payments	−.04	.55**	.41**	—	.09	.06	.14	.12	.10	.06	.21**	.10	.13	−.02	−.06	−.01		
(5) Exciting	−.24**	.22**	.27**	.20**	—	.29**	.35**	.23**	.17	.22**	.05	.13	−.09	.14*	.06	.20**		
(6) Overall Mental Health	−.08	.28**	.31**	.16**	.27**	—	.33**	.16**	.21**	.07	.00	.33**	.01	.07	.13*	.03		
(7) Life Satisfaction	−.10	.22**	.24**	.24**	.38**	.23**	—	.19*	.26**	.20*	.09	.18**	−.02	.16**	.04	.17**		
(8) Getting Out	−.69**	.17**	.11	.18**	.33**	.13**	.20**	—	.88**	.73**	.46**	.32**	.17*	.40**	.13	.02		
(9) House Work	−.63**	.04	.07	.16**	.29**	.11	.14**	.79**	—	.72**	.48**	.27**	.16*	.40**	.07	.07		
(10) Medicine	−.38**	.19**	.00	.02	.21**	.03	.07	.55**	.61**	—	.38**	.27**	.14	.31**	.07	.05		
(11) Low Troubles	−.26**	.19**	.25**	.21**	.32**	.26**	.28**	.41**	.35**	.30**	—	.40**	.41**	.09	−.14*	.00		
(12) Overall Physical Health	−.16**	.30**	.29**	.22**	.33**	.48**	.20**	.28**	.24**	.17**	.45**	—	.33**	.16*	.03	.08		
(13) Comparative Health	−.28**	.08	.12	.11	.25**	.17**	.13**	.29**	.27**	.19**	.35**	.28**	—	.10	−.13	−.03		
(14) Phone Talk	.23**	.04	.18**	.03	.16**	.08	.11	.35**	.30**	.20**	.15*	.20**	.01	—	.07	.27**		
(15) Visit Network Number	−.21**	.03	.07	.09	.11**	.05	.04	.32**	.21**	.19	.10	.13	.09	.24**	—	.19		
(16) Visits With Others	−.03	.14**	.05	−.01	.10	.09	.11	.10	.00	.08	.11	.09	−.01	.31**	.25**	—		
Means	Time 1	$N = 321$	1.14	1.52	1.44	1.78	1.41	2.06	1.75	1.63	1.58	1.83	1.29	1.89	.86	2.41	2.86	2.16
	Time 2	$N = 201$	.99	1.52	1.42	1.72	1.42	1.97	1.77	1.55	1.47	1.77	1.17	1.83	.78	2.41	2.87	2.08
SD	Time 1	$N = 321$	.78	.78	.52	.50	.57	.70	.47	.46	.59	.40	.76	.77	.62	.85	.49	.77
	Time 2	$N = 201$	.83	.78	.77	.58	.57	.72	.49	.55	.67	.51	.78	.80	.61	.89	.48	.88

$^*P \leq .05$. $^{**}P \leq .01$.

all five OARS resources as latent variables. Thus, empirical and clinical attention to multidimensional assessments of older adults and their successful aging, especially those in their 80s and 100s, and the continued popularity of the OARS instrument as a standardized scale motivated this study development of a measurement model of psychosocial resources essential to successful aging for very old adults.

Five latent variables with three indicators each, corresponding to the five OARS resources, were specified; the combined measurement model fit the data adequately using a sample of older adults in their 60s, 80s, and 100s. Three results from the measurement analyses are noteworthy. First, because of advances in SEM programs and techniques allowing specification of measurement error and latent factor modeling, a comprehensive measurement model of the five OARS resources would prove useful to researchers and those assessing and caring for older adults. With the exception of Social Resources at Time 2, researchers employing the OARS may confidently specify the measurement model tested in this study. The measurement model tested in this study fit the data well at Time 1 and Time 2. Factor loadings (except those of Social Resources at Time 2) were significant and substantive, providing adequate evidence of an acceptable latent variable measurement model for the five OARS resources.

Second, supplementary analyses of factorial invariance over time, conducted without Social Resources at Time 2, revealed that in this sample, the four latent variables (i.e., Economic Resources, IADL, Physical Health, and Mental Health) fit the data well and did not change significantly over time. It is noted that for the younger participants (i.e., those in their 60s and 80s), five years elapsed between measurement occasions, whereas, for the centenarians, 20 months. Researchers interested in developmental questions of change over time are encouraged to employ the measurement model verified by this study and to extend this work by carefully considering the time intervals necessary for proximal and distal influences to unfold among older adults.

Third, Social Resources tended to have the lowest loadings per indicator. In this sample, relative to the other indicators, talking on the phone is the main indicator tapping the respondent's Social Resources. Burholt and colleagues [38] investigated OARS Social Resources in a population-based study of older adults living independently in six Western European countries and argued that the items demonstrated a breadth of conceptual assessment. It is our contention that such is the case with the three single-item indicators for the latent variable Social Resources. These indicators may assess a breadth of structure and at times the items may not be related. These three items may better serve as a checklist of social resources structure. Expecting relatively high factor loadings for such a construct may be unfounded (see [39], for a discussion regarding why checklist assessments often exhibit low internal consistency). Thus, other valid and reliable assessments of social support might be examined to augment or supplant the items included in the OARS assessment. Finally, empirical work investigating the relationship between measures of social support and loneliness has demonstrated discriminant validity; despite the strong association these measures tap different constructs [40, 41]. This is consistent with the finding of this study; the loneliness item did not load significantly on the Social Resources latent variable and was not included in the final measurement model.

4.1. Limitations and Direction for Future Research. Several limitations, however, exist that affect the generalization of this study's results. First, the participants were Southeastern older adults in reasonably good health, mentally competent, and community-dwelling. Second, the younger age groups (those in their 60s and those in their 80s) were randomly selected by race and gender to approximate older adults in Georgia. However, in contrast, centenarians were selected using convenience sampling through state and local agencies. Also, the sexagenarians and octogenarians were assessed in testing locations; centenarians completed their assessments at home. In addition, for the two younger age groups, measurement occasions were five years apart, but for the centenarians the measurement occasions were approximately 20 months apart. With only two waves of data, longitudinal results are to be interpreted with caution. Future research will want to employ other valid assessments of similar assessments of the five resources for comparison, particularly with larger, more homogeneous samples. This would provide opportunity to compare the relationships between the revised OARS latent resources based on our results and other known measures. Also, using a more homogenous sample of older adults might mitigate some of the methodological difficulties inherent in our heterogeneous sample that includes three age groups of old (60s and 80s) and very old adults (100s).

Finally, the items used for Social Resources in this study could be improved in future research. All the latent variables except Social Resources were fairly consistent across measurement occasions. In fact, for the models tested without the Social Resources latent variable, the overall measurement model fit the data well and factorial invariance of the latent variables over time was substantiated. Future research is encouraged to consider other measures of Social Resources (see [42], for 12 different measures assessing social support).

This study employed data from the Georgia Centenarian Study and used the popular Duke OARS [7] to develop a measurement model consisting of latent variables for Economic Resources, Instrumental Activities of Daily Living, Physical Health, Mental Health, and Social Resources. The model was specified and affirmed using longitudinal (two waves) data from a sample of sexagenarians, octogenarians, and centenarians, further substantiating the robustness of these latent variables in research with older adults. The results of this study allow reduction of the numerous items used in assessing the five OARS resources. This has valuable and practical implications because increased difficulties with hearing, vision, and fatigue in older adults may require extended time or multiple interviewer sessions to complete the extensive battery of questions in the OARS. Thus, researchers conducting etiological investigations, health professionals conducting intake and out-patient assessments, and other practitioners wishing to employ the OARS with older populations and the resources essential to successful aging will benefit from using this reduced version.

Appendices

A. OARS Economic Resources

A.1. Sufficient Income

Are your assets and financial resources sufficient to meet emergencies?

1 Yes

0 No

Do you usually have enough to buy those little "extras," that is, those small luxuries?

1 Yes

0 No

At the present time do you feel that you will have enough for your needs in the future?

1 Yes

0 No

A.2. Overall Income

Please tell me how well you think you are now doing financially as compared to other people your age—better, about the same, or worse?

3 Better

2 About the same

1 Worse

How well does the amount of money you have take care of your needs—very well, fairly well, or poorly?

3 Very well

2 Fairly well

1 Poorly

A.3. Meet Payments

Are your expenses so heavy that you cannot meet the payments, or can you barely meet the payments, or are your payments no problem to you?

0 Subject cannot meet payments

1 Subject can barely meet payments

2 Payments are no problem

B. OARS Mental Health

B.1. Exciting

In general, do you find life exciting, pretty routine, or dull?

2 Exciting

1 Pretty routine

0 Dull

B.2. Overall Mental Health

How would you rate your mental or emotional health at the present time—excellent, good, fair, or poor?

3 Excellent

2 Good

1 Fair

0 Poor

B.3. Life Satisfaction

Taking everything into consideration how would you describe your satisfaction with life in general at the present time—good, fair, or poor?

2 Good

1 Fair

0 Poor

C. OARS IADL

C.1. Getting Out

Can you use the telephone...

2 without help, including looking up numbers and dialing?

1 with some help (can answer phone or dial operator in an emergency, but need a special phone or help in getting the number or dialing)?

0 are you completely unable to use the telephone?

Can you get to places out of walking distance...

2 without help (drive your own car, or travel alone on buses, or taxis)?

1 with some help (need someone to help you or go with you when traveling)?

0 are you unable to travel unless emergency arrangements are made for a specialized vehicle like an ambulance?

Can you go shopping for groceries or clothes (assuming subject has trans)...

2 without help (taking care of all shopping needs yourself, assuming you had transportation)?

1 with some help (need someone to go with you on all shopping trips)?

0 are you completely unable to do any shopping?

C.2. Housework

Can you prepare your own meals...

2 without help (plan and cook full meals yourself)?

1 with some help (can prepare some things but unable to cook full meals yourself)?

0 are you completely unable to prepare any meals?

Can you do housework...

2 without help (can clean floors, etc.)?

1 with some help (can do light housework but need help with heavy work)?

0 are you completely unable to do any housework?

Can you handle your own money...

2 without help (write checks, pay bills, etc.)?

1 with some help (manage day-to-day buying but need help with managing your checkbook and paying your bills)?

0 are you completely unable to handle money?

C.3. Medicine

Can you take your own medicine...

2 without help (in the right dose at the right time)?

1 with some help (able to take medicine if someone prepares it for you and/or reminds you to take it)?

0 are you completely unable to take your medicines?

D. OARS Physical Health

D.1. Low Troubles

How much do your health troubles stand in the way of your doing the things you want to do—not at all, a little (some), or a great deal?

2 Not at all

1 A little (some)

0 A great deal

D.2. Overall Health

How would you rate your overall health at the present time—excellent, good, fair, or poor?

3 Excellent

2 Good

1 Fair

0 Poor

D.3. Comparative Health

Is your health now better, about the same, or worse than it was five years ago?

2 Better

1 About the same

0 Worse

E. OARS Social Resources

E.1. Visit Network Number

How many people do you know well enough to visit with in their homes?

3 Five or more

2 Three to four

1 One or two

0 None

E.2. Phone Talk

About how many times did you talk to someone—friends, relatives, or others—on the telephone in the past week (either you called them or they called you?) (if subject has no phone, question still applies).

3 Once a day or more

2 2–6 times

1 Once

0 Not at all

E.3. Visits with Others

How many times during the past week did you spend some time with someone who does not live with you, that is, you went to see them or they came to visit you, or you went out to do things together?

3 Once a day or more

2 2–6 times

1 Once

0 Not at all

Acknowledgment

This research was supported in part by NIH grant RO1-43435 and PO1 AG17533-01A1.

References

[1] P. B. Baltes, "On the incomplete architecture of human ontogeny: selection, optimization, and compensation as foundation of developmental theory," *American Psychologist*, vol. 52, no. 4, pp. 366–380, 1997.

[2] P. B. Baltes and M. M. Baltes, *Successful Aging: Perspectives from the Behavioral Sciences*, Cambridge University Press, Cambridge, UK, 1990.

[3] M. Von Faber, A. Bootsma-Van Der Wiel, E. Van Exel et al., "Successful aging in the oldest old," *Archives of Internal Medicine*, vol. 161, no. 22, pp. 2694–2700, 2001.

[4] S. E. Hobfoll, "Social and psychological resources and adaptation," *Review of General Psychology*, vol. 6, no. 4, pp. 307–324, 2002.

[5] L. W. Poon, P. Martin, A. Bishop et al., "Understanding centenarians' psychosocial dynamics and their contributions to health and quality of life," *Current Gerontology and Geriatrics Research*, vol. 2010, Article ID 680657, 13 pages, 2010.

[6] P. Martin, "Individual and social resources predicting well-being and functioning in the later years: conceptual models, research, and practice," *Ageing International*, vol. 27, no. 2, pp. 3–29, 2002.

[7] G. G. Fillenbaum, *Multidimensional Functional Assessment of Older Adults: The Duke Older Americans Resources and Services Procedures*, Lawrence Erlbaum Associates, Hillsdale, NJ, USA, 1988.

[8] H. B. Bosworth and K. W. Schaie, "The relationship of social environment, social networks, and health outcomes in the Seattle longitudinal study: two analytical approaches," *Journals of Gerontology*, vol. 52, no. 5, pp. P197–P205, 1997.

[9] M. Martin, M. Grünendahl, and P. Martin, "Age differences in stress, social resources, and well-being in middle and older age," *Journals of Gerontology*, vol. 56, no. 4, pp. P214–P222, 2001.

[10] M. Pinquart and S. Sörensen, "Influences of socioeconomic status, social network, and competence on subjective well-being in later life: a meta-analysis," *Psychology and Aging*, vol. 15, no. 2, pp. 187–224, 2000.

[11] R. A. Pruchno, M. Wilson-Genderson, M. Rose, and F. Cartwright, "Successful aging: early influences and contemporary characteristics," *Gerontologist*, vol. 50, no. 6, pp. 821–833, 2010.

[12] D. G. Blazer, "Psychiatry and the oldest old," *American Journal of Psychiatry*, vol. 157, no. 12, pp. 1915–1924, 2000.

[13] C. McCamish-Svensson, G. Samuelsson, and B. Hagberg, "Correlated and prevalence of loneliness from young old to oldest old: results from a Swedish cohort," *Hallym International Journal of Aging*, vol. 3, pp. 1–24, 2001.

[14] R. M. Suzman, D. P. Willis, and K. G. Manton, *The Oldest Old*, Oxford University Press, New York, NY, USA, 1992.

[15] A. J. Selim, G. Fincke, D. R. Berlowitz et al., "Comprehensive health status assessment of centenarians: results from the 1999 large health survey of veteran enrollees," *Journals of Gerontology*, vol. 60, no. 4, pp. 515–519, 2005.

[16] M. L. Stek, J. Gussekloo, A. T. F. Beekman, W. Van Tilburg, and R. G. J. Westendorp, "Prevalence, correlates and recognition of depression in the oldest old: the Leiden 85-plus study," *Journal of Affective Disorders*, vol. 78, no. 3, pp. 193–200, 2004.

[17] C. Bailey, J. Corner, J. Addington-Hall, D. Kumar, M. Nelson, and J. Haviland, "Treatment decisions in older patients with colorectal cancer: the role of age and multidimensional function," *European Journal of Cancer Care*, vol. 12, no. 3, pp. 257–262, 2003.

[18] P. Krach, S. DeVaney, C. DeTurk, and M. H. Zink, "Functional status of the oldest-old in a home setting," *Journal of Advanced Nursing*, vol. 24, no. 3, pp. 456–464, 1996.

[19] M. C. Tierney, J. Charles, G. Naglie, S. Jaglal, A. Kiss, and R. H. Fisher, "Risk factors for harm in cognitively impaired seniors who live alone: a prospective study," *Journal of the American Geriatrics Society*, vol. 52, no. 9, pp. 1435–1441, 2004.

[20] A. J. Bishop, P. Martin, and L. Poon, "Happiness and congruence in older adulthood: a structural model of life satisfaction," *Aging and Mental Health*, vol. 10, no. 5, pp. 445–453, 2006.

[21] B. S. Fees, P. Martin, and L. W. Poon, "A model of loneliness in older adults," *Journals of Gerontology*, vol. 54, no. 4, pp. P231–P239, 1999.

[22] P. Martin, B. Hagberg, and L. W. Poon, "Predictors of loneliness in centenarians: a parallel study," *Journal of Cross-Cultural Gerontology*, vol. 12, no. 3, pp. 203–224, 1997.

[23] P. A. Holtsberg, L. W. Poon, C. A. Noble, and P. Martin, "Mini-Mental State Exam status of community-dwelling cognitively intact centenarians," *International Psychogeriatrics*, vol. 7, no. 3, pp. 417–427, 1995.

[24] P. Martin, M. V. Long, and L. W. Poon, "Age changes and differences in personality traits and states of the old and very old," *Journals of Gerontology*, vol. 57, no. 2, pp. P144–P152, 2002.

[25] L. W. Poon, G. M. Clayton, P. Martin et al., "The georgia centenarian study," in *in The Georgia Centenarian Study: A Special Issue of the International Journal of Aging and Human Development*, L. W. Poon, Ed., vol. 34, pp. 1–18, Baywood Publishing, Amityville, NY, USA, 1992.

[26] M. F. Folstein, S. E. Folstein, and P. R. McHugh, "'Mini mental state'. A practical method for grading the cognitive state of patients for the clinician," *Journal of Psychiatric Research*, vol. 12, no. 3, pp. 189–198, 1975.

[27] B. Reisberg, S. H. Ferris, M. J. De Leon, and T. Crook, "The global deterioration scale for assessment of primary degenerative dementia," *American Journal of Psychiatry*, vol. 139, no. 9, pp. 1136–1139, 1982.

[28] A. C. Acock, "Working with missing values," *Journal of Marriage and Family*, vol. 67, no. 4, pp. 1012–1028, 2005.

[29] P. D. Allison, "Missing data techniques for structural equation modeling," *Journal of Abnormal Psychology*, vol. 112, no. 4, pp. 545–557, 2003.

[30] B. Muthén and L. Muthén, *Mplus User's Guide*, Muthén & Muthén, Los Angeles, Calif, USA, 3rd edition, 2004.

[31] B. M. Byrne, *Structural Equation Modeling with LISREL, PRELIS, and SIMPLIS: Basic Concepts, Applications, and Programming*, Lawrence Erlbaum Associates, Hillsdale, NJ, USA, 1998.

[32] J. B. Ullman and P. M. Bentler, "Structural equation modeling," in *Handbook of Psychology: Research Methods in Psychology*, J. A. Schinka and W. F. Velicer, Eds., vol. 2, pp. 607–634, John Wiley & Sons, New York, NY, USA, 2003.

[33] P. M. Bentler, "Comparative fit indexes in structural models," *Psychological Bulletin*, vol. 107, no. 2, pp. 238–246, 1990.

[34] P. M. Bentler and D. G. Bonett, "Significance tests and goodness of fit in the analysis of covariance structures," *Psychological Bulletin*, vol. 88, no. 3, pp. 588–606, 1980.

[35] M. W. Browne and R. Cudeck, "Single sample cross-validation indices for covariance structures," *Multivariate Behavioral Research*, vol. 24, pp. 445–455, 1989.

[36] L. T. Hu and P. M. Bentler, "Cutoff criteria for fit indexes in covariance structure analysis: conventional criteria versus new alternatives," *Structural Equation Modeling*, vol. 6, no. 1, pp. 1–55, 1999.

[37] R. C. MacCallum and J. T. Austin, "Applications of structural equation modeling in psychological research," *Annual Review of Psychology*, vol. 51, pp. 201–226, 2000.

[38] V. Burholt, G. Windle, D. Ferring et al., "Reliability and validity of the Older Americans Resources and Services (OARS) social resources scale in six European countries," *Journals of Gerontology*, vol. 62, pp. S371–S379, 2007.

[39] T. B. Herbert and S. Cohen, "Measurement issues in research on psychosocial stress," in *Psychosocial Stress: Perspectives on Structure, Theory, Life-Course, and Methods*, H. B. Kaplan, Ed., pp. 295–332, Academic Press, San Diego, Calif, USA, 1996.

[40] D. W. Russell, "UCLA Loneliness Scale (Version 3): reliability, validity, and factor structure," *Journal of Personality Assessment*, vol. 66, no. 1, pp. 20–40, 1996.

23

Robotic Seals as Therapeutic Tools in an Aged Care Facility

Melanie Birks,[1] Marie Bodak,[2] Joanna Barlas,[3] June Harwood,[4] and Mary Pether[5]

[1] *Nursing, Midwifery, and Nutrition, Centre for Nursing and Midwifery Research, College of Healthcare Sciences, James Cook University, Townsville, QLD, Australia*
[2] *Nursing, Midwifery, and Nutrition, College of Healthcare Sciences, James Cook University, Townsville, QLD, Australia*
[3] *Clinical Psychology, College of Healthcare Sciences, James Cook University, Singapore Campus, Singapore*
[4] *Aged Care Services Australia Group, Launceston, TAS, Australia*
[5] *Regis Aged Care, Townsville, QLD, Australia*

Correspondence should be addressed to Melanie Birks; melanie.birks@jcu.edu.au

Academic Editor: F. R. Ferraro

Robots, including robotic seals, have been used as an alternative to therapies such as animal assisted therapy in the promotion of health and social wellbeing of older people in aged care facilities. There is limited research available that evaluates the effectiveness of robot therapies in these settings. The aim of this study was to identify, explore, and describe the impact of the use of Paro robotic seals in an aged care facility in a regional Australian city. A qualitative, descriptive, exploratory design was employed. Data were gathered through interviews with the three recreational therapists employed at the facility who were also asked to maintain logs of their interactions with the Paro and residents. Data were transcribed and thematically analysed. Three major themes were identified from the analyses of these data: "a therapeutic tool that's not for everybody," "every interaction is powerful," and "keeping the momentum." Findings support the use of Paro as a therapeutic tool, revealing improvement in emotional state, reduction of challenging behaviours, and improvement in social interactions of residents. The potential benefits justify the investment in Paro, with clear evidence that these tools can have a positive impact that warrants further exploration.

1. Introduction

Residential aged care facilities provide an important service in promoting the health and social wellbeing of elderly individuals. Over 230,000 individuals currently reside in aged care facilities in Australia, with approximately 52% having a diagnosis of dementia [1]. Recreational therapy is a significant component of the health care regime for aged care residents and is effective in promoting the physical, social, and psychological wellbeing of all older adults residing in aged care facilities.

Animal assisted therapy is perhaps the best known form of recreational therapy in the aged care setting. Animal assisted therapy began in the USA in the 1960s and, despite the recognised benefits of this form of therapy for use with the elderly, there is minimal research on its effectiveness [2]. The limited amount of recent work that has been done in this area emanates from Italy. These studies suggest that animal assisted therapy reduces depressive symptoms and agitation and results in an overall positive experience for the resident [2–4]. Animal assisted therapy is not without its problems, however, which has seen these programs fall out of favour because of limited availability of appropriate animals and issues of hygiene and safety [5]. As a result, robots, and particularly pet robots, have arisen as a viable alternative.

Much of the recent research in the area of robots in healthcare has arisen from Canada [6–8], New Zealand [9–11], Europe [12–16], and Australia [17]. While some of this work explores robots generally [7, 10], most examines the use of robots with the elderly in broad terms [9, 13, 14, 16, 17], with some focus on dementia [6, 11, 12, 15] and disability [8].

A number of systematic [12, 17] and other structured [6, 13] reviews of the literature form much of the current work. These reviews raise issues in respect of worth of earlier research, arguing for greater emphasis on rigour and overall quality. Some studies, for example, simply compare one type of robot or system with another [10, 11], with limited consideration for the absolute value of robots in a given setting. In another study, Wolbring and Yumakulov [8] delivered an online survey, with no ability of the respondents to actually view the capabilities of the robot.

The Paro robotic seal is a socially responsive robot that has been in use since 2003 [18]. This high technology therapeutic tool reacts to the individual in response to the way in which it is treated. Paro has been shown to effect connections with elderly individuals who may be socially, cognitively, or emotionally isolated [19]. Research into seal robots provides an example of the conflict of interests evident in this field of research. Takanori Shibata, the inventor of the Paro robotic seal, has undertaken various studies into the use and value of his product. One example is the administration of a questionnaire sent with the robot when purchased [20], with a subsequent study comparing video recordings of elderly persons with dementia interacting with Paro versus a stuffed toy lion [21].

Other independent researches support the value of Paro. One group of researchers in the USA [22, 23] used observations and video recordings of participants interacting with Paro [23] or combined these with interviews with therapists to identify the positive potential that Paro has when used with people living with dementia [22]. Researchers from New Zealand [24] similarly used video and interviews with a broad range of residents and staff at an aged care facility to identify primarily social benefits. Ahn et al. [9], also from New Zealand, used interview, observation, and nonrandomised and randomised trials to add physical benefits to the list of positive outcomes. Studies from Europe mostly relied on quantitative methods [25, 26] to further demonstrate the potential value of Paro in dementia care in particular.

Most of the existing literature examining the effects of Paro describes studies conducted with residents of care facilities in almost all cases focusing on the care of persons with dementia. The research presented in this paper aims to contribute to the existing body of knowledge by exploring the experiences of therapists using Paro as a therapeutic tool with a more diverse group of residents in an aged care facility in regional Australia.

2. Materials and Methods

This study employed a qualitative descriptive, exploratory design. The setting was an aged care facility in a regional Australian city. This 127-bed facility was operated by a Nongovernment Organisation (NGO) and employed 125–130 staff. The research team was contacted by the facility when the robotic seals were purchased with an invitation to assist with research to evaluate their effectiveness. The research team attended an event to launch the use of the robotic seals (named "George" and "Sally" by the residents) in the facility and at this time explained the purpose of the research and the study design to the staff, residents, family, and friends in attendance. The original intention was to recruit from this broader pool of stakeholders. The three recreational (diversional) therapists employed at the facility were those most involved with the use of the robotic seals, however, and it was these staff who participated in the study.

Prior to implementing the robotic seals project, the therapists participated in a number of short training sessions (tool boxes) led by the facility manager, who had worked previously with the Paro robotic seals. These workshops aimed to develop foundational understanding of how these robotic seals could be used as a therapeutic tool to benefit the day-to-day experiences of the residents. Following approval by the university's Human Research Ethics Committee, the therapists were asked to maintain a journal of their interactions with residents when using Paro. Paro was employed daily as a diversional therapy with selected residents in either an individual or group activity. Each session was 30–40 minutes in duration. During these sessions, residents were encouraged to interactively engage with Paro including stroking, cuddling, and speaking to the robotic seal.

After the seals had been in use for a period of approximately four months, semistructured interviews were conducted with the participants for approximately one hour each. While a group interview was planned, one therapist was unavailable and so was interviewed separately from the other two. Two members of the research team undertook an inductive thematic analysis of the data obtained from the verbatim interview transcripts and therapists' journals. This analysis was checked by a third researcher and the results are presented in Section 3.

3. Results

The findings of this study present an overview of the impact of Paro robotic seals on residents, from the perspective of the recreational therapists. The following discussion present an integrated analysis of the interviews and participant journals. The major themes derived from the analysis were as follows: *a therapeutic tool that's not for everybody*; *every interaction is powerful*; and *keeping the momentum*.

3.1. A Therapeutic Tool That's Not for Everybody. This theme encompasses the diversity of reactions to the Paro seals. In the case of residents, participants noticed a range of initial reactions from outright dismissal through curiosity to excitement. Those residents who dismissed the robots were noted by the participants to be more negative in their use of language. Amongst those who were curious, some apprehension was observed, which was overcome with encouragement from the participants.

> *There have been a couple of residents that have been a little bit wary of George and Sally. I've gone back to those residents, and some of them have actually come forward and stroked George or Sally. The others have dismissed me straight away; don't want to have anything to do with it. [Participant 1]*

> *I believe over 50 per cent are really interested to know more about this and then we get those who think it's a load of rubbish. [Participant 3]*

These varying initial reactions were thought to be driven by normal individual differences and differences relating to mental and physical health status. The participants in this study acknowledged and respected individual preferences for one activity over another. There was a sense that these healthcare workers viewed the robots as another optional activity that could form part of a therapeutic toolbox to draw on when working with elderly residents.

> *...it is a therapeutic tool, but still I don't think it's for everybody. [Participant 1]*

Participants observed that Paro elicited more of a response from residents with dementia, even those with more advanced-stage dementia. There was a suggestion that some residents with dementia appeared to lack understanding that it was not real.

> *I think the [residents with] dementia react better. They smile a lot more, or they frown, or their eyes sparkle. [Participant 1]*

> *I think the interaction particularly with somebody with dementia who's like third stage was just wonderful. [Participant 3]*

In contrast, those who were more immediately dismissive of Paro were described by the participants as more cognitively able or *"mentally with-it."* Differing reactions not only were dependent on whether or not the resident had dementia but seemed to relate to physical, cognitive, and emotional impairment more widely. According to the participants, those with depression and disabilities or those under palliative care, for example, were observed to respond positively to Paro.

> *...one lady that there's nothing wrong [with cognitively], but physically she can't move or do anything. And her eyes just sparkle when I walk in and I put George or Sally on the bed table, because she can touch and stroke [him] and all that. [Participant 1]*

A diversity of reactions from residents' caregivers (family members and staff) to the Paro seals was also described. Participants in this study commented that the response from family members was primarily positive; they expressed interest in understanding the purpose of the Paros and shared views about the anticipated reactions from their relatives.

> *...they've actually asked questions about where they came from and why we have them here, and most families have been very positive. [Participant 1]*

One of the participants observed the Paro facilitates an expression of affection between a resident who could not speak and her husband.

> *...you could see the look on her face and his face and the touching which would - she touched his hand and they both touched Paro so it was a really wonderful experience. [Participant 3]*

Some negativity was observed, however, such as when derogatory comments were made about staff members using Paro:

> *...somebody said to me, a family member said "oh, I've seen somebody carrying that around, they're like a complete idiot". [Participant 3]*

The participants also observed staff expressing negative views about Paro. These included apparent concerns about the use of Paro infantilizing the residents by dismissing Paro as *"that toy."* Negative reactions from other caregivers appeared to be driven by lack of understanding about the use of Paro. Some staff believed it was *"a waste of money"* and the participants in this study thought that these staff did not *"realize its benefits to the residents."* One participant also reported that some staff expressed seemingly paranoid views about Paro being used as a recording device, perhaps with the intention of monitoring their behaviour at work.

> *They walk away and the hands up "I'm not talking - I'm not talking while that's around and while it's turned off". Then you're in the nurses' station, "is that turned off?" [Participant 3]*

3.2. Every Interaction Is Powerful. A number of therapeutic benefits for residents were observed by participants. Three subthemes were developed in this category. These subthemes encapsulated the emotional, behavioural, and social benefits of the Paro seals.

One common theme related to the emotional benefits. In one example, a participant reported that during a 15- to 20-minute one-on-one session some residents *"came out of their shells"* and seemingly had more *"spark"* in them.

> *On entering the room I noticed her looking forlorn, distant and looking into space... she spotted George (Paro) in my arms and her whole body language changed immediately by showing exuberance, verve in her movements and in her face. She immediately held out her arms to hold George. [Participant 3 log entry]*

In some cases, participants reported that they witnessed an emotional bond developed between the resident and the robot. The Paro became something towards which they could express affection, talk, and welcome back like an old friend.

> *He invited me into his room. As soon as he viewed George his eyes opened wide and a huge smile appeared on his face. With his focus on George, he placed his water on the bed side table and opened out his arms ready to take hold of him and commenced talking to George as if he was continuing his conversation from the last visit with Sally. He commenced with, "What have you been*

doing with yourself? " Conversation flowed as he held George. [Participant 3 log entry]

Participants also suggested that the emotional benefits extended to providing happiness and comfort at the end of life. This phenomenon was just one example of the powerful effect that these simple therapeutic tools can have.

> *I used it on a palliative care resident and that was - it was a wonderful experience because she was able to verbalise how she was feeling [through] the tactile - feeling, the sensory part... "Yes dear, yes, I am feeling..." she looked at Paro "yes dear, I'm feeling like this"... I think that...she could see that she was thinking about her thoughts and she wanted to pass it on to somebody. [Participant 3]*

> *George came in, he jumped - generated conversation. Even only a small bit of conversation but at least he was able to verbalise. I think in the last legs of his life, he was happy. [Participant 3]*

Behavioural benefits followed as a result of interacting with the robotic seals. The participants in this study were very excited by the positive influence the interaction with the Paro was having for the residents. They used adjectives such as beautiful, pleasing, sparkling eyes, giggling, and a powerful experience. Significantly, these positive effects extended to residents who had been exhibiting disruptive, loud behaviour as they became more relaxed, contented, and settled for a period of time.

> *At the end of the activity I [noticed] that [this resident's] manner [had] changed from the interaction with George from one of vagueness and a far-away look to having energy in his approach and showing calmness and love. [Participant 3 log entry]*

> *I heard [the resident] yelling out, "Help, Help, Help!" As soon as he saw me he stopped yelling and beckoned for me to come to him with George. He spent the rest of the time... touching and observing [the] movements of George. After leaving, I listened and he did not commence his usual yelling for help. Also I returned 20 minutes later to listen for yelling and did not hear [the resident] verbalizing." [Participant 3 log entry]*

In addition to emotional and behavioural benefits, the participants described social benefits to the use of Paro. While there was clearly a positive impact from the use of Paro directly, some of the indirect benefits noted by participants included a deepening of relationships between therapists and the residents.

> *There was one lady...she's a loner and she stays in her room at all times. Having...Sally placed in her arms, it just reminded her of her baby. She just opened up and her face just lit up...it was a just powerful moment and...it was just beautiful just to be there to experience it... I believe that she changed there and then on the spot. So even today, even though we've got a good rapport, I think it's even closer.... [Participant 3]*

One therapist used Paro to foster social connection by encouraging a group of residents to work together to create lyrics about Paro to a familiar old tune.

> *They were all excited. It was a noisy atmosphere and everyone was talking at the same time, laughing, giggling and elbowing each other trying to come up some rhyming words. Some residents [came] up with funny words and some [were] not suitable, but it sounded very funny and they all laughed... Residents were using their brains it stimulation them. It was also good social interaction and a good laugh. Until next time, I am planning to record the song on CD when completed. [It's a] good sense of achievement for the residents. [Participant 2 log entry]*

Social and relationship benefits were noted to extend from other residents and carers to the family members, in one example prompting recall of memories.

> *Both mother and daughter had a good laugh at the way her mother was talking to George; [the] daughter [said] "it reminds me [of] when I was little, she spoke to us like that, it's funny it makes me laugh". [Participant 2 log entry]*

The participants in this study also observed that family members recognised the value of Paro and appreciated the positive impact that the robotic seals had for their loved one. In one case, the daughter of a resident, concerned that her mother would be distressed that she could not make her regular visit, specifically asked a participant that her mother be given some time with Paro.

> *I took George this morning to see a resident, her daughter came to me the other day and said... "I won't be visiting mum ... on Thursday, could you please take George or Sally up to her?" [Participant 1]*

3.3. Keeping the Momentum. This final theme reflects the participants' initial sense of responsibility towards ensuring the success of Paro as a therapeutic tool. Despite indicating that they had come into the trial project without any preconceived ideas, participants appeared hopeful rather than sceptical about the use of Paro. This attitude likely helped them to wholly embrace the possibilities of Paro. Therapists incorporated the robotic seals into their daily activities with residents and sought to educate and reduce scepticism amongst others as part of their role.

> *But you do that... as an educator – I suppose that's part of me inside is making sure that people understand why we do it and we need to continue to keep the momentum happening. [Participant 3]*

Therapists were keen to share the benefits of Paro and in particular to *"include the nurses as well."* They encouraged cynical staff members to observe Paro being used, understanding the power of witnessing the change in residents' behaviour.

> *They came in and they observed him and they couldn't believe what he was doing, like singing all these songs - they've never ever heard this cranky man in their life sing, smile so much. They've never seen his teeth and here he is smiling and his face is lit up... Watch, observe and I said, he's your client, now you know what he can do... when he's cranky, you now can put a smile on his face. So that... Paro made him come out of his shell [and made] the staff more aware of what was actually happening.... [Participant 3]*

The advocacy for the use of Paro shown by the participants in this study was likely related to their own experiences of witnessing the benefits, which included a seemingly vicarious sharing of residents' emotions.

> *It's just the reaction... They're in the moment on the spot... it just gives you joy, you can see their faces. [Participant 2]*

> *I went and had a bit of a cry.... [Participant 3]*

These participants clearly saw the enduring value of Paro beyond the initial trial period. Their suggestions comprised using Paro to assist with care planning, activities of daily living (ADLs), and wound care and to reduce incidences of challenging behaviour. The consensus appeared to be that use of Paro required regularity and momentum to effect maximum benefits.

> *I'd like to see them used daily, and different areas. If money wasn't an issue, or staffing wasn't an issue, it'd be lovely to be able to have them in each area. [Participant 1]*

4. Discussion

The findings of this study present an interesting overview of the impact of Paro on residents in an aged care facility from the perspective of the therapists who employed these robotic seals in their practice. These findings add to the existing contemporary literature about robot seals and their use with the elderly. Furthermore, this study expands knowledge from a qualitative perspective as well as in respect of what is known about the use of robot seals with the elderly beyond that of dementia care. These participants reported mixed reactions from residents, family, and staff. Giusti and Marti [27] suggest that a number of factors determine how an individual may interact with Paro, including the context and their personal history. Recognition of these factors, combined with the findings evident in this study, highlights the importance of care planning that respects and accommodates individual differences, preferences, and needs.

The potential impact of personal history explains the use of a seal form of the robot. While participants reported confusion for residents in some instances, the use of an animal with which the residents are unlikely to be familiar removes the potential impact of any existing preconceptions or experiences. A baby harp seal is an endearing and relatively innocuous creature to which an individual can direct their affection [19]. Physical and cognitive status are further factors that influence the reaction of those who come into contact with the robot and this can be seen from the findings described in this paper. In particular, participants noted that residents with dementia were likely to perceive Paro as a living thing, reflecting the results of Giusti and Marti [27].

The findings in this paper indicate that participants perceived a degree of negativity amongst some residents, their relatives, and other staff. This finding is in contrast with the work of both Heerink et al. [15] and Robinson et al. [11], who found that Paro was received favourably by these groups. Lack of understanding of the value and capability of the robotic seal no doubt contributed to the negative reaction from some who came into contact with it. Indeed, members of the research team themselves were initially unsure of the value or significance of these therapeutic tools when they were first encountered. As was also found by Bemelmans [26], sceptics of Paro can become enthusiasts once the positive effects are seen.

Some of the negativity towards the Paro might result from a perception that the use of robots with cognitively impaired individuals is humiliating and demeaning. This might particularly be the case when those who witness the resident interacting with the robotic seal lack an understanding of its therapeutic capability, such as untrained carers [14]. While recent work has discussed the ethical implications of using seals in the care of the elderly [13, 14, 19], no such specific concerns were evident in this study. Nonetheless, these findings highlight the importance of education for those people who work directly and indirectly with Paro to avoid ethical issues arising.

Past research identified therapeutic benefits emotionally [22, 26], physically [9], behaviourally [28], and socially [9, 21, 23, 24]. The research reported in this paper adds support to these findings for the use of Paro in improving mood, reducing challenging behaviour, and facilitating social interactions. As a result of its qualitative design, the current study also brought to light some of the processes involved in these therapeutic improvements in specific contexts. Participants reported positive responses to Paro that involved physical touch, verbal communication, and expressed affection, similar to those observed between pet owners and their pets [29]. It is hypothesised that such benefits could improve the quality of life and reduce the distress of residents. By doing so, they have the potential to reduce the worry and distress of family members and the stress and potential for burnout in residential staff.

Reduced loneliness has been identified previously as a benefit of Paro [9, 23] and the observations of participants in this study suggested two main processes in this respect: the establishment of a direct relationship with the robotic seal and its use in facilitating better social connections with others. Isolated and withdrawn residents talked to Paro in a conversational manner and end-of-life residents verbalised their internal world, in both contexts seemingly reducing a sense of being alone. This finding highlights distinctions between the loss of ability to communicate, the loss of desire to communicate, and the loss of opportunities to communicate.

Chang et al. [22] described Paro as a "*good social mediator*" (p. 102) and participants in this study provided descriptive examples of such processes occurring between groups of residents, residents and staff, and residents and family members. These findings suggest that staff members can use the robotic seal as a rapport-building tool with otherwise socially and verbally withdrawn residents. In groups, it can be used as an external and nonthreatening focal point for group activities. With family members, Paro can be used for both day-to-day conversation and reminiscence, in line with Sung et al. [28].

Calo et al. [19] have previously written about the ethics and value of replacing human relationships with robot relationships and the issue of using a robotic seal as a replacement social relationship was raised in this research. It was beyond the scope of this research to consider whether the relationship between human and Paro is best understood as an attachment relationship as occurs with pets [30] or where Paro is a transitional object as proposed by Taggart et al. [31].

It was clear to the research team that the participants in this study were very excited at the results of their work with the residents and Paro. They expressed a desire to teach others about the benefits of using Paro in the hope of motivating them to employ it as a therapeutic tool. Beyond the social and behavioural benefits described by the participants, there is clear potential for Paro to be used effectively in assisting residents with activities of daily living such as at meal times, in preparation for showering, and at night when they are unable to sleep. Although Bemelmans et al. [26] found no significant benefit of using Paro in care activities, that finding was confounded by the limited number of care activities examined and an associate learning curve in the use of the robot for this purpose. Those authors did, however, find that Paro had a significant therapeutic impact. Previous work has shown that Paro can alter the psychosocial environment [25] and function as a social catalyst [24] thereby establishing a context where elderly residents are more likely to be receptive to care interventions. The findings of the study described in this paper confirm the positive impact of Paro detailed in early work and suggest that there is even greater scope for its use in the support of residents in aged care facilities.

4.1. Recommendations and Limitations. A number of recommendations arise from this study. In respect of practice, it is clear that if robotic seals are to be introduced into the practice environment, it is necessary for those who will be involved in their use to be adequately prepared. The gradual introduction of Paro into the clinical or residential setting, with increasing visibility and accessibility, may maximise the potential for success. Sharkey [14] believes that therapeutic benefits of robots are the result of skilled use. Thus, the carer must be adequately trained before they are deployed in any setting. Given the positive effect of Paro suggested by this and earlier work, the expansion of its use to include other caregivers, in particular nurses, may broaden its potential therapeutic reach.

Future research is recommended that validates the findings of this study and explores issues that arise from this work. Perspectives of other caregivers, particularly those who express negativity towards the robotic seal, may identify barriers to its use. Studies on the value of Paro in improving caregiver wellbeing and reducing staff burnout are also warranted. Longitudinal work would also confirm the long-term therapeutic value of Paro found by Jøranson et al. [25] and support Sabanovic et al.'s [23] assertion that the benefits are not simply due to a novelty effect. It is acknowledged that the positive impact observed by the participants may be attributable in part to their presence and not confined to the therapeutic value of Paro, consistent with the assertions of Jøranson et al. [25]. A comparative trial using standard therapeutic measures as an intervention, such as what was used by those authors, may highlight the unique value of Paro in the provision of care.

The major limitation of this study relates to the small sample size and its focus on a single facility. Nonetheless, the findings reinforce those of earlier studies and provide greater understanding of the potential value of Paro and other social responsive robots to those who work in facilities such as the one described in this paper.

5. Conclusions

Ensuring a safe, therapeutic, and respectful environment for the elderly members of our society is a key concern for people working in residential aged care facilities. Both professional caregivers and significant others work with limited resources in managing the often complex physical, cognitive, social, and emotional needs of the elderly. Any and all tools that can aid in promoting the wellbeing of aged residents should not be dismissed until potential has been fully assessed. This paper has presented the findings of a study into the use of the Paro robotic seal by recreational therapists in an aged care facility. While it is clear that not all those who come in contact with these robotic devices will see their value, there is evidence that these tools can have a positive impact that warrants further exploration. The potential benefits clearly justify the investment.

Competing Interests

The authors declare that there is no conflict of interests regarding the publication of this paper.

References

[1] Department of Social Services, *2013-14 Report on the Operation of the Aged Care Act 1997*, Department of Social Services, Canberra, Australia, 1997.

[2] L. F. Menna, M. Fontanella, A. Santaniello et al., "Evaluation of social relationships in elderly by animal-assisted activity," *International Psychogeriatrics*, vol. 24, no. 6, pp. 1019–1020, 2012.

[3] V. Bernabei, D. De Ronchi, T. La Ferla et al., "Animal-assisted interventions for elderly patients affected by dementia or psychiatric disorders: a review," *Journal of Psychiatric Research*, vol. 47, no. 6, pp. 762–773, 2013.

[4] F. Moretti, D. De Ronchi, V. Bernabei et al., "Pet therapy in elderly patients with mental illness," *Psychogeriatrics*, vol. 11, no. 2, pp. 125–129, 2011.

[5] W. D. Stiehl, J. Lieberman, C. Breazeal, L. Basel, L. Lalla, and M. Wolf, "Design of a therapeutic robotic companion for relational, affective touch," in *Proceedings of the 14th IEEE Workshop on Robot and Human Interactive Communication (RO-MAN '05)*, pp. 408–415, August 2005.

[6] E. Mordoch, A. Osterreicher, L. Guse, K. Roger, and G. Thompson, "Use of social commitment robots in the care of elderly people with dementia: a literature review," *Maturitas*, vol. 74, no. 1, pp. 14–20, 2013.

[7] K. Pangka, Y. Hui, and A. Yan, "Robots in medicine," *University of Western Ontario Medical Journal*, vol. 82, no. 2, pp. 29–30, 2013.

[8] G. Wolbring and S. Yumakulov, "Social robots: views of staff of a disability service organization," *International Journal of Social Robotics*, vol. 6, no. 3, pp. 457–468, 2014.

[9] H. S. Ahn, E. Broadbent, I. Han Kuo et al., "Long-term study of a healthcare robot system for senior people in rest homes, hospitals, and a dementia unit," in *Proceedings of the IEEE/RSJ International Conference on Intelligent Robots and Systems Workshop on Assistive Robotics for Individuals with Disabilities: HRI Issues and Beyond*, Chicago, Ill, USA, September 2014.

[10] J. A. Mann, B. A. Macdonald, I.-H. Kuo, X. Li, and E. Broadbent, "People respond better to robots than computer tablets delivering healthcare instructions," *Computers in Human Behavior*, vol. 43, pp. 112–117, 2015.

[11] H. Robinson, B. A. MacDonald, N. M. Kerse, and E. Broadbent, "Suitability of healthcare robots for a dementia unit and suggested improvements," *Journal of the American Medical Directors Association*, vol. 14, no. 1, pp. 34–40, 2013.

[12] R. Bemelmans, G. J. Gelderblom, P. Jonker, and L. de Witte, "Socially assistive robots in elderly care: a systematic review into effects and effectiveness," *Journal of the American Medical Directors Association*, vol. 13, no. 2, pp. 114–120.e1, 2012.

[13] S. Frennert and B. Östlund, "Review: seven matters of concern of social robots and older people," *International Journal of Social Robotics*, vol. 6, no. 2, pp. 299–310, 2014.

[14] A. Sharkey, "Robots and human dignity: a consideration of the effects of robot care on the dignity of older people," *Ethics and Information Technology*, vol. 16, no. 1, pp. 63–75, 2014.

[15] M. Heerink, J. Albo-Canals, M. Valenti-Soler et al., "Exploring requirements and alternative pet robots for robot assisted therapy with older adults with dementia," in *Social Robotics*, vol. 8239 of *Lecture Notes in Computer Science*, pp. 104–115, Springer, 2013.

[16] E. Torta, F. Werner, D. O. Johnson et al., "Evaluation of a small socially-assistive humanoid robot in intelligent homes for the care of the elderly," *Journal of Intelligent and Robotic Systems: Theory and Applications*, vol. 76, no. 1, pp. 57–71, 2014.

[17] R. Kachouie, S. Sedighadeli, R. Khosla, and M.-T. Chu, "Socially assistive robots in elderly care: a mixed-method systematic literature review," *International Journal of Human-Computer Interaction*, vol. 30, no. 5, pp. 369–393, 2014.

[18] PARO Robots US, *PARO Therapeutic Robot*, 2014, http://www.parorobots.com/.

[19] C. J. Calo, N. Hunt-Bull, L. Lewis, and T. Metzler, "Ethical implications of using the paro robot, with a focus on dementia patient care," in *Proceedings of the AAAI Workshop on Human-Robot Interaction in Elder Care*, WS-2011-2012, San Francisco, Calif, USA, 2011.

[20] T. Shibata, Y. Kawaguchi, and K. Wada, "Investigation on people living with seal robot at home," *International Journal of Social Robotics*, vol. 4, no. 1, pp. 53–63, 2012.

[21] K. Takayanagi, T. Kirita, and T. Shibata, "Comparison of verbal and emotional responses of elderly people with mild/moderate dementia and those with severe dementia in responses to seal robot, PARO," *Frontiers in Aging Neuroscience*, vol. 6, article 257, 2014.

[22] W.-L. Chang, S. Šabanović, and L. Huber, "Use of seal-like robot PARO in sensory group therapy for older adults with dementia," in *Proceedings of the 8th ACM/IEEE International Conference on Human-Robot Interaction (HRI '13)*, pp. 101–102, IEEE Press, Tokyo, Japan, March 2013.

[23] S. Sabanovic, C. C. Bennett, W.-L. Chang, and L. Huber, "PARO robot affects diverse interaction modalities in group sensory therapy for older adults with dementia," in *Proceedings of the IEEE 13th International Conference on Rehabilitation Robotics (ICORR '13)*, Seattle, Wash, USA, June 2013.

[24] H. Robinson, E. Broadbent, and B. MacDonald, "Group sessions with Paro in a nursing home: structure, observations and interviews," *Australasian Journal on Ageing*, vol. 35, no. 2, pp. 106–112, 2016.

[25] N. Jøranson, I. Pedersen, A. M. M. Rokstad, and C. Ihlebæk, "Effects on symptoms of agitation and depression in persons with dementia participating in robot-assisted activity: a cluster-randomized controlled trial," *Journal of the American Medical Directors Association*, vol. 16, no. 10, pp. 867–873, 2015.

[26] R. Bemelmans, G. J. Gelderblom, P. Jonker, and L. de Witte, "Effectiveness of robot paro in intramural psychogeriatric care: A Multicenter Quasi-Experimental Study," *Journal of the American Medical Directors Association*, vol. 16, no. 11, pp. 946–950, 2015.

[27] L. Giusti and P. Marti, "Interpretative dynamics in human robot interaction," in *Proceedings of the 15th IEEE International Symposium on Robot and Human Interactive Communication (RO-MAN '06)*, pp. 111–116, IEEE, Hatfield, UK, September 2006.

[28] H.-C. Sung, S.-M. Chang, M.-Y. Chin, and W.-L. Lee, "Robot-assisted therapy for improving social interactions and activity participation among institutionalized older adults: a pilot study," *Asia-Pacific Psychiatry*, vol. 7, no. 1, pp. 1–6, 2015.

[29] E. Prato-Previde, G. Fallani, and P. Valsecchi, "Gender differences in owners interacting with pet dogs: an observational study," *Ethology*, vol. 112, no. 1, pp. 64–73, 2006.

[30] S. Zilcha-Mano, M. Mikulincer, and P. R. Shaver, "An attachment perspective on human-pet relationships: conceptualization and assessment of pet attachment orientations," *Journal of Research in Personality*, vol. 45, no. 4, pp. 345–357, 2011.

[31] W. Taggart, S. Turkle, and C. D. Kidd, "An interactive robot in a nursing home: preliminary remarks," in *Toward Social Mechanisms of Android Science*, Workshop Paper, Cognitive Science Society, Stresa, Italy, 2005.

24

Weekly Physical Activity Levels of Older Adults Regularly Using a Fitness Facility

Michael J. Turner,[1] Emily E. Schmitt,[2] and Tricia Hubbard-Turner[3,4]

[1] *Laboratory of Systems Physiology, University of North Carolina at Charlotte, Charlotte, NC 28223, USA*
[2] *Biology of Physical Activity Laboratory, Texas A&M University, College Station, TX 77843, USA*
[3] *Biodynamics Research Laboratory, Department of Kinesiology, University of North Carolina at Charlotte, Charlotte, NC 28223, USA*
[4] *Center for Biomedical Engineering & Science, University of North Carolina at Charlotte, Charlotte, NC 28223, USA*

Correspondence should be addressed to Michael J. Turner; miturner@uncc.edu

Academic Editor: Enrica Menditto

The aim of this paper was to determine if weekly physical activity levels were greater in an independent-living older adult population that was regularly participating in structured fitness activities. Also, lifetime exercise history and sex differences were investigated in an effort to understand how they relate to current weekly step activity. Total weekly step counts, measured with a pedometer, were assessed in two older adult groups; the first consisted of members of a local senior center who regularly used the fitness facility (74.5 ± 6.0 yrs; mean ± SD) while the second group consisted of members who did not use the fitness facility (74.8 ± 6.0 yrs). Participants also completed the Lifetime Physical Activity Questionnaire (LPAQ). No significant difference was found in the total number of weekly steps between groups ($p = 0.88$) or sexes ($p = 0.27$). The LPAQ suggested a significant decline in activity with aging ($p = 0.01$) but no difference between groups ($p = 0.54$) or sexes ($p = 0.80$). A relationship was observed between current step activity and MET expenditure over the past year ($p = 0.008$, $r^2 = 0.153$) and from ages 35 to 50 years ($p = 0.037$, $r^2 = 0.097$). The lack of difference in weekly physical activity level between our groups suggests that independent-living older adults will seek out and perform their desired activity, in either a scheduled exercise program or other leisure-time activities. Also, the best predictor of current physical activity level in independent-living older adults was the activity performed over the past year.

1. Introduction

Maintaining aerobic capacity and increasing muscular strength are known to lead to improvements in overall function in the aging population. An increase or maintenance of regular physical activity levels with aging would likely aid in the improvement in the functional capacity of the older adult. After 16 weeks of an exercise program focusing on improving aerobic capacity, muscular strength, and muscular endurance, Fahlman et al. [1] reported improvements in older adults on measures of aerobic fitness and functional ability. Nakamura et al. [2] demonstrated similar results in which participation in physical activity (walking, recreational activities, and resistance training) at least three times a week over a twelve-week period led to improvements in body composition. Importantly, participation in a regular structured exercise program has been found to improve health and well-being [1–3] and lead to an increase in the amount of physical activity performed outside of the exercise class on nonstructured exercise days [4]. Therefore, participation in regular structured exercise programming would likely benefit the aging population.

In addition, past research has shown that those who participate in exercise during youth and adolescent years have increased exercise levels in adulthood and lower body mass index levels [5, 6]. Those who report moderate to vigorous physical activity in midlife have been observed to possess better mobility later in life [6]. However, research is limited in this area; therefore identifying possible relationships between past exercise and current fitness levels remains an important goal for gerontological studies. In the current study a sample of both males and females were studied, ranging in age from 65 to 95 years. The use of a Lifetime Physical Activity Questionnaire [7] allowed for a look at physical activity across the lifespan to provide evidence as to whether past exercise can be used as a predictor of future levels of physical activity in later adulthood.

The purpose of this study was to assess total weekly steps taken in two older adult groups who frequent a local senior center using a pedometer. The first group consisted of members of a senior center who used the fitness facility at least two times a week (FIT). The second group consisted of members who have never used a fitness facility (NFIT). We hypothesized that those who participate in using the exercise facility at a senior center would have a greater total number of steps than those who did not use the fitness facility. Also, we hypothesized that those who regularly participated in exercise earlier in life would perform a greater number of total steps compared to those less active earlier in life. Finally, based on the past literature [6, 8–11] we hypothesized that males would exhibit a greater number of weekly steps compared to the female participants.

2. Methods

2.1. Participants. Eighteen males and 27 females ranging in age from 65 to 95 years were recruited from the Charlotte-Mecklenburg Senior Center in Charlotte, North Carolina. This study consisted of mostly European American participants ($n = 42$), two African Americans ($n = 2$), and one Asian ($n = 1$). Volunteers were recruited from advertising for interested individuals who regularly frequented the facility. This study was approved by the Institutional Review Board of the University of North Carolina at Charlotte.

2.2. Study Design. Participants were placed into one of two groups. The first group consisted of 13 males and 16 females who were members of the senior center and regularly used the fitness facility at least two times a week (FIT). The second group was composed of 5 males and 11 females who were members of the senior center but never used a fitness center, either in the senior center or elsewhere (NFIT).

The potential benefits and risks of participating in this study were fully explained to each participant. Participants were required to complete a medical history form and provide written informed consent before receiving a pedometer to measure daily steps for one full week. Subjects were also instructed about completing the Lifetime Physical Activity Questionnaire (LPAQ) [7] throughout the one-week period during which daily steps were measured. Height (cm) and body mass (kg) were recorded at the start of the study period, with body mass also recorded on the last day of the study period to monitor any changes. Subject's body mass (kg) was measured on a standard scale (J.A. King and Company, Inc., Greensboro, NC). From the height and initial mass measurements, body mass index (BMI) was calculated in kg/m^2.

2.3. Measurement of Physical Activity Levels

2.3.1. Pedometers. All volunteers were provided with a Digi-Walker SW-200 pedometer (New Lifestyles, Inc., Lees Summit, Missouri) at the beginning of the study period. Subjects were instructed on the proper way to wear the pedometer (on the waistband or belt close to the hip joint) and were reminded to wear the device at all times except when bathing, showering, swimming, or sleeping at night. Participants were asked to put on the pedometer first thing in the morning and remove the pedometer from the belt or waistline, complete the provided daily step log, and zero the pedometer before going to bed for seven consecutive days. Daily step totals were added together and the calculated sum equaled the weekly total for each participant. All subjects were asked to maintain their typical daily routine and leisure activities for the duration of the study.

2.3.2. Lifetime Physical Activity Questionnaire (LPAQ). Each subject was given a LPAQ [7] on the first day of the study. They were instructed on how to complete the questionnaire and were asked to fill it out and return it at the end of the study period with the pedometer. When the participant returned the LPAQ [7], the completed questionnaire was reviewed with the principal investigator. Intensity was determined by asking each participant how intensely they were working while performing a certain activity. Intensity was measured in multiples of metabolic equivalents (MET, 3.5 mL/kg/min) with intensity levels being assigned using the *Compendium of Physical Activities* [12].

The data from the LPAQ [7] were scored by calculating the minutes per year a person was performing a certain activity multiplied by the MET levels assigned to that activity. Total MET expenditure was determined for each age period (15–21 years, 22–34 years, 35–50 years, 51–65 years, and the past year) and for total lifetime.

2.4. Statistical Analyses. All descriptive data were analyzed using a one-way analysis of variance between groups. A two-way analysis of variance by group and sex was used to determine any differences in the total number of weekly steps taken between groups (FIT versus NFIT) and between males and females. Group changes in body mass during the study period were compared using a two-way analysis of variance with repeated measures. Any relationships between the LPAQ [7] MET levels for each age period and current weekly step count were determined by performing linear squares regression analyses for all participants and for each group. Also, linear regression analyses were performed for all participants and for each group between pre body mass and BMI versus total weekly steps. The LPAQ [7] MET levels for each age period were compared by two-way analysis of variance with repeated measures between groups (group × age) and sexes (sex × age). All statistical conclusions were based on an alpha level of 0.05 and performed using JMP Statistical Analysis software (SAS Institute, Cary, NC).

3. Results

3.1. Subject Characteristics. A total of 29 people in the FIT group (female $n = 16$, male $n = 13$) and a total of 16 people in the NFIT group (female $n = 11$, male $n = 5$) participated in the study. There was no difference in age between the two

TABLE 1: Mean (±SD) descriptive characteristics of fitness and nonfitness participants.

	Fitness	Nonfitness
Age (yr)		
All	74.5 ± 6.0	74.8 ± 6.0
Female	73.8 ± 6.2	73.6 ± 5.4
Male	75.4 ± 5.9	77.4 ± 7.3
Height (cm)		
All	168.7 ± 9.7	165.4 ± 8.1
Female	161.5 ± 5.6	161.5 ± 5.6
Male	177.5 ± 4.6	173.2 ± 7.1
Pre mass (kg)		
All	73.3 ± 14.3	75.5 ± 9.4
Female	63.6 ± 7.1	74.5 ± 10.3
Male	85.1 ± 11.6	77.7 ± 7.7
Post mass (kg)		
All	73.5 ± 14.4	75.4 ± 9.4
Female	63.7 ± 7.1	74.2 ± 10.2
Male	85.5 ± 11.6	77.9 ± 7.6
BMI (kg/m^2)*		
All	25.6 ± 3.3	27.7 ± 3.9
Female	24.3 ± 2.3	28.5 ± 3.8
Male	27.0 ± 3.8	26.1 ± 3.9

*Denoting significant difference between groups ($p = 0.05$).

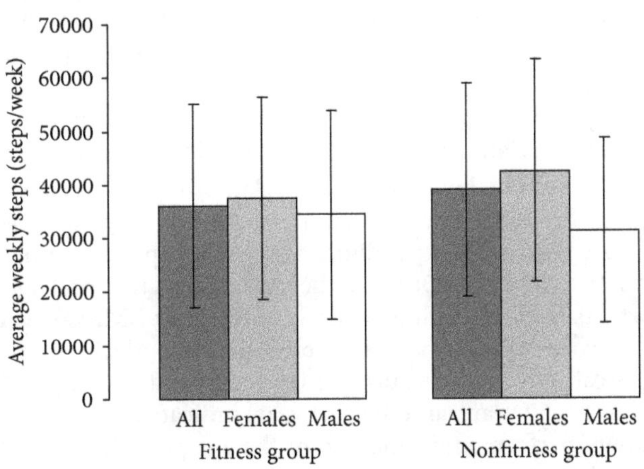

FIGURE 1: Mean (±SD) of average weekly steps for the participants in the fitness and nonfitness group.

groups ($p = 0.88$). A summary of the descriptive data can be found in Table 1. Also, there was no difference in height between groups ($p = 0.22$). There was no difference between groups for pre body mass ($p = 0.58$), post body mass ($p = 0.60$), or across time ($p = 0.55$). However, BMI was found to be different between groups ($p = 0.05$), with FIT exhibiting a greater BMI than the NFIT group.

3.2. Total Number of Weekly Steps. Analysis of total number of weekly steps between FIT and NFIT exhibited no significant difference ($p = 0.88$; Figure 1). No difference in total number of weekly steps was observed between males and females ($p = 0.27$). Also, no interaction was observed for total weekly steps for sex and group ($p = 0.53$).

TABLE 2: Correlation table (r^2 values) of total weekly steps and LPAQ MET levels for all subjects and each group.

	Past year	51–65 yrs	35–50 yrs	22–34 yrs	15–21 yrs
All	0.153*	0.040	0.097*	0.034	0.010
Fitness	0.150*	0.030	0.098	0.017	0.037
Nonfitness	0.254*	0.057	0.095	0.132	0.030

*Denoting significant relationship with total weekly steps ($p < 0.05$).

3.3. Lifetime Physical Activity Questionnaire MET Levels. A two-way analysis of variance for group and age with Lifetime Physical Activity Questionnaire (LPAQ) [7] MET levels found no difference between groups ($p = 0.54$) but a significant decrease in activity level with age ($p = 0.01$). There was no significant interaction effect ($p = 0.37$).

A two-way analysis of variance for sex and age with the LPAQ [7] found no difference between sexes ($p = 0.80$), a significant decrease with age ($p = 0.01$), and a significant interaction ($p = 0.003$). The sex by age interaction effect suggests that male activity decline begins after 22–34 years while female activity declines after 35–50 years.

3.4. Comparing Total Weekly Steps and LPAQ MET Levels. Linear least squares regression was performed between total weekly steps and the different age periods with the LPAQ METs per year [7]. Total weekly steps were significantly related for all subjects to the past year MET levels ($p = 0.008$; $r^2 = 0.153$) and 35–50 yr age period ($p = 0.037$; $r^2 = 0.097$). There were no other relationships between total weekly steps and the remaining age periods. All r^2 values are displayed in Table 2.

For FIT participants, total weekly steps were significantly related with past year MET expenditure ($p = 0.038$; $r^2 = 0.150$). For NFIT participants, total weekly steps were significantly related to past year MET expenditures ($p = 0.047$; $r^2 = 0.254$). There were no other relationships between total weekly steps and the remaining age periods within each group. All r^2 values are displayed in Table 2.

3.5. Comparing Pre Body Mass and BMI with Total Weekly Steps. Linear least squares regression values between pre body mass and total weekly steps for all participants were not significantly related ($p = 0.78$; $r^2 = 0.002$). For the FIT group, pre body mass and total weekly steps were not significantly correlated ($p = 0.93$; $r^2 = 0.0003$). With all NFIT participants pre body mass was not related with total weekly steps ($p = 0.39$; $r^2 = 0.053$).

There was no significant relationship between BMI and total weekly steps for all participants ($p = 0.63$; $r^2 = 0.006$). For FIT, BMI was not related with total weekly steps ($p = 0.95$; $r^2 = 0.0002$). Additionally, BMI was not related to total weekly steps for the NFIT group ($p = 0.38$; $r^2 = 0.055$).

4. Discussion

We found no difference in total number of weekly steps between older adults who regularly participate in the exercise facility at a senior center and those who do not use an exercise facility. Depending on the age period, the current study found a relationship between current steps per week and past activity levels over the past year and from the age period of 35–50 years. Additionally, both groups (i.e., FIT and NFIT) were analyzed by sex to determine any sex-related differences in regular physical activity level. No sex-related differences in physical activity level were observed in this study.

Our first hypothesis was not supported by the findings, which indicate no significant difference in the total number of weekly steps taken between those who regularly use and those who do not use an exercise facility (Figure 1). To our knowledge this is the first study to compare weekly step counts in two groups of older adults who do and do not participate in structured exercise. The findings of the current study may be a result of the observations of Whaley and Ebbeck [13] who interviewed older adults at a senior center to find perceived constraints to participating in structured exercise. Nine females and eight males were interviewed to better understand perceived barriers to exercise class participation. The authors reported that older adults might choose to not participate in structured exercise because they are frequently active elsewhere. The researchers found that some older adults would rather walk around the neighborhood, swim, or ride bikes [13]. They also discovered that older adults claimed that they were too busy to exercise or exercise conflicted with other appointments. Some found structured exercise to be inconvenient [13].

Several studies have outlined how important it is for older adults to participate in structured exercise in order to meet exercise guidelines. Rejeski et al. [14] examined the influence of a physical activity intervention program on satisfaction with self-efficacy along with physical function for older adults who ranged in age from 70 to 89 years. The researchers found that older adults who participated in physical activity (aerobic, strength, balance, and flexibility) had better profiles for satisfaction with physical function and self-efficacy for the 400-meter walk compared to those in a successful aging program. In addition, Tudor-Locke et al. [4] found that older adults who participated in structured exercise experienced an increase in physical activity on the exercise program days relative to other days of the week. The researchers found that walking for exercise was the most prevalent form of exercise outside of a structured exercise class [4].

A previous study assessing physical activity levels of older adults using a pedometer recruited 415 participants [15]. Strath et al. [15] wanted to examine walking volume in older adults by examining personal characteristics associated with walking behavior. These authors showed that race and ethnicity significantly influenced one's average steps per day. They noted that African American older adults took approximately 750 fewer steps per day than European American of the same age [15]. The demographics of our FIT and NFIT groups did not differ significantly in this study and consisted of 42 European Americans, two African Americans, and one Asian participant(s). The current study did not recruit a wide range of ethnic diversity, which could be why there was no statistically significant difference between races.

The current study also found that body mass and BMI did not relate to weekly step count in an older adult population. Body mass and total weekly step counts were not significantly related for all study participants ($p = 0.78$). Scott et al. [16] investigated the effects of pedometer use as a means of encouraging and assessing ambulatory activity in a group of older adults. This study was part of a larger cohort study (Tasmanian Older Adult Cohort Study) to look at the progression of osteoarthritis and osteoporosis in older adults aged 50 to 79 years. These authors [16] observed a negative relationship between body fatness and daily step activity ($p < 0.001$, $r = -0.54$). Although we observed no relationship of step activity and BMI for any of the groups, past studies [16, 17] suggesting body fatness or BMI influencing step activity recruited significantly larger and more heterogeneous sample sizes compared to the current study. These studies incorporated younger adults and individuals with a larger variance in body composition compared to the current study population. Therefore, lack of a relationship in weekly step counts and BMI could be attributed to the lack of a large number of overweight or obese subjects in our groups. Strath et al. [15] reported that older adults considered overweight took about 2,000 steps less than those in the normal weight category while those in the obese category took about 2,500 fewer steps than those in the normal weight category. With only 11.1% of the males and 6.6% of the females in the current study being classified as obese with respect to their BMI, we expect that the high number of normal BMI subjects could be influencing our lack of relationship between BMI and total weekly steps.

The second hypothesis of a relationship between past activity levels and current steps per week was only supported by past year MET expenditure and MET expenditure from ages 35 to 50 years. Other studies have found that past sport participation in childhood can lead to lower BMI values in adult women [5]. Also, results from Patel et al. [6] who studied physical activity levels during three age periods in life (20–40 years, 40–60 years, and the past year) indicated that physical activity performed during two of the age periods (ages 20–40 and 40–60 years) was associated with better mobility and slower onset of chronic disease states in older adulthood determined by functional assessments.

The current study observed a significant decrease in activity level with an increase in age. This is in line with past studies [6, 8, 18, 19]. Norman et al. [19] conducted a study that examined recalled physical activity at 15, 30, and 50 years of age in a large sample of older Swedish men. It was concluded that a decrease in physical activity over time was due to a reduction in leisure-time activities [19]. Patel et al. [6] reported that physical activity levels in older adults over the past year were significantly lower than levels reported for midlife. The Centers for Disease Control and Prevention (CDC) has reported the prevalence of leisure-time physical activity declined for the US population from the years 1994 to 2004 [18]. The largest decline was in the older adult population (men aged 50–59 years and women aged 60–69 years) [18]. In addition,

Armstrong et al. [8] showed that men and women generally had declining levels of activity across the lifespan.

Friedman et al. [20] argue that activity levels are somewhat stable from childhood into middle and late adulthood. Friedman et al. [20] continued the Terman Life-Cycle Study, which was started in 1922 by Lewis Terman. The original Life-Cycle Study was composed of 1528 mostly middle class European American boys and girls. Subjects' activity levels were followed throughout their lives with assessments every 5 to 10 years. Data were reviewed for subjects born between the years 1904–1915. The researchers concluded that, after studying significant associations across almost six decades, active children grow into active, energetic adults. Friedman et al. [20] also argued that it is not important to know whether individuals are more active than others, but it is more beneficial to understand past activity levels from the last decade in order to understand current activity levels. Our findings are in agreement with this statement by Friedman et al. [20] with the relationship of current activity levels matching past year's MET expenditures.

Lastly, the current study observed no sex differences in total weekly steps between males and females whether they were in the FIT or NFIT group. This finding does not agree with most research. Past research generally indicates that men are more active than women [6, 8–11]. Lee [10] found that women were significantly less active than men in duration of exercise. The study also noted that 26% of older adult males and 12% of older adult females engaged in the recommended amount of physical activity (30 minutes a day, 5 days a week) [10]. In addition, Yasunaga et al. [11] measured physical activity levels in older adults and concluded that older adult men accumulated more step counts than their female counterparts. Armstrong et al. [8] found that walking was greater in older adult males compared to older adult females. However, recent reviews of physical activity by Friedman et al. [20] and Strath et al. [15] reported little difference between sexes in older adult populations. Friedman et al. [20] found patterns of physical activity across the lifespan to be about the same for males and females. Strath et al. [15] found no significant differences between males and females in any race or ethnic category when investigating steps per day in an older adult population.

4.1. Study Limitations. Limitations of this study include the sample population. This research was conducted at a senior center where the majority of individuals were very independent and mostly of high socioeconomic status. Also, the population was all healthy individuals who did not exhibit a wide range of BMI values, with only 11.1% of males and 6.6% of females being categorized as obese. The CDC national averages for BMI in the older adult population show that 32.2% of men and 30.5% of women over the age of 65 years are obese [19]. Additionally, there were few males in the NFIT group. The pedometer was used for the daily assessment of physical activity in our older adult population. Recently Colbert et al. [21] compared the validity values of physical activity measures in older adults using three different activity models. The authors discovered that more expensive devices did not rank physical activity any better than the pedometer, and the pedometer was the most cost-effective method for ranking physical activity level in older adults [21].

Another limitation of this study was the Lifetime Physical Activity Questionnaire (LPAQ) [7]. This questionnaire was used to assess physical and leisure-time activities throughout the lifespan. The decades in which the questionnaire asked about were past activity amounts categorized into different age periods (15–21 years, 22–34 years, 35–50 years, 51–65 years, and the past year). Certain activities and ages may have been missed with this survey tool. For example, an individual who filled out this survey who was 72 years of age was not asked about the age period of 66–71 years. This creates age gaps that could miss pertinent information in regard to lifetime physical activity. Also, with any questionnaire recall can be a problem. Asking an older adult to recall activities they did decades earlier can certainly be a difficult task, especially with regard to intensity levels.

5. Conclusions

In conclusion, no difference was observed in the total number of weekly steps taken by older adults who regularly participate at an exercise facility and those who do not use an exercise facility. This finding suggests that independent-living older adults will seek out and perform weekly physical activity, whether in a scheduled exercise program or with other leisure-time activities. To our knowledge the current study is the first to compare weekly step counts in two groups of older adults who do and do not participate in structured exercise. In addition, using questionnaire recall with the LPAQ [7] we observed that physical activity declined with age (3, 5, 15, and 17) [6, 8, 19]. Using the LPAQ [7] we only observed a relationship between current steps per week and MET expenditure over the past year and from ages 35 to 50 years. Also, the current study observed no sex differences in weekly step count between males and females, for all participants or in the FIT or NFIT group.

Competing Interests

The authors have no conflict of interests to declare.

Acknowledgments

The authors would like to thank the participants from the Charlotte-Mecklenburg Senior Centers.

References

[1] M. M. Fahlman, R. Topp, N. McNevin, A. L. Morgan, and D. J. Boardley, "Structured exercise in older adults with limited functional ability," *Journal of Gerontological Nursing*, vol. 33, no. 6, pp. 32–39, 2007.

[2] Y. Nakamura, K. Tanaka, N. Yabushita, T. Sakai, and R. Shigematsu, "Effects of exercise frequency on functional fitness in older adult women," *Archives of Gerontology and Geriatrics*, vol. 44, no. 2, pp. 163–173, 2007.

[3] K. R. Fox, A. Stathi, J. McKenna, and M. G. Davis, "Physical activity and mental well-being in older people participating

in the Better Ageing Project," *European Journal of Applied Physiology*, vol. 100, no. 5, pp. 591–602, 2007.

[4] C. Tudor-Locke, G. R. Jones, A. M. Myers, D. H. Paterson, and N. A. Ecclestone, "Contribution of structured exercise class participation and informal walking for exercise to daily physical activity in community-dwelling older adults," *Research Quarterly for Exercise and Sport*, vol. 73, no. 3, pp. 350–356, 2002.

[5] C. M. Alfano, R. C. Klesges, D. M. Murray, B. M. Beech, and B. S. McClanahan, "History of sport participation in relation to obesity and related health behaviors in women," *Preventive Medicine*, vol. 34, no. 1, pp. 82–89, 2002.

[6] K. V. Patel, A. K. Coppin, T. M. Manini et al., "Midlife Physical Activity and Mobility in Older Age. The InCHIANTI Study," *American Journal of Preventive Medicine*, vol. 31, no. 3, pp. 217–224, 2006.

[7] L. Chasan-Taber, J. B. Erickson, J. W. McBride, P. C. Nasca, S. Chasan-Taber, and P. S. Freedson, "Reproducibility of a self-administered lifetime physical activity questionnaire among female college alumnae," *American Journal of Epidemiology*, vol. 155, no. 3, pp. 282–289, 2002.

[8] T. Armstrong, A. Bauman, and J. Davies, *Physical Activity Patterns of Australian Adults: Results of the 1999 National Physical Activity Survey*, Australian Institute of Health and Welfare, Canberra, Australia, 2000.

[9] A. M. Kavanagh and R. Bentley, "Walking: a gender issue?" *Australian Journal of Social Issues*, vol. 43, no. 1, pp. 45–64, 2008.

[10] Y.-S. Lee, "Gender differences in physical activity and walking among older adults," *Journal of Women and Aging*, vol. 17, no. 1-2, pp. 55–70, 2005.

[11] A. Yasunaga, F. Togo, E. Watanabe et al., "Sex, age, season, and habitual physical activity of older Japanese: the Nakanojo Study," *Journal of Aging and Physical Activity*, vol. 16, no. 1, pp. 3–13, 2008.

[12] B. E. Ainsworth, W. L. Haskell, M. C. Whitt et al., "Compendium of physical activities: an update of activity codes and MET intensities," *Medicine and Science in Sports and Exercise*, vol. 32, no. 9, pp. S498–S504, 2000.

[13] D. E. Whaley and V. Ebbeck, "Older adults' constraints to participation in structured: exercise classes," *Journal of Aging and Physical Activity*, vol. 5, no. 3, pp. 190–212, 1997.

[14] W. J. Rejeski, A. C. King, J. A. Katula et al., "Physical activity in prefrail older adults: confidence and satisfaction related to physical function," *Journals of Gerontology: Psychological Sciences and Social Sciences*, vol. 63, no. 1, pp. P19–P26, 2008.

[15] S. J. Strath, A. M. Swartz, and S. E. Cashin, "Ambulatory physical activity profiles of older adults," *Journal of Aging and Physical Activity*, vol. 17, no. 1, pp. 46–56, 2009.

[16] D. Scott, L. Blizzard, J. Fell, and G. Jones, "Ambulatory activity, body composition, and lower-limb muscle strength in older adults," *Medicine and Science in Sports and Exercise*, vol. 41, no. 2, pp. 383–389, 2009.

[17] C. Tudor-Locke, D. R. Bassett Jr., W. J. Rutherford et al., "BMI-referenced cut points for pedometer-determined steps per day in adults," *Journal of Physical Activity and Health*, vol. 5, no. 1, pp. S126–S139, 2008.

[18] Centers for Disease Control and Prevention, "Trends in leisure-time physical inactivity by age, sex, and race/ethnicity—United States, 1994–2004," *Morbidity and Mortality Weekly Report*, vol. 54, no. 39, pp. 991–994, 2005.

[19] A. Norman, R. Bellocco, F. Vaida, and A. Wolk, "Age and temporal trends of total physical activity in Swedish men," *Medicine and Science in Sports and Exercise*, vol. 35, no. 4, pp. 617–622, 2003.

[20] H. S. Friedman, L. R. Martin, J. S. Tucker, M. H. Criqui, M. L. Kern, and C. A. Reynolds, "Stability of physical activity across the lifespan," *Journal of Health Psychology*, vol. 13, no. 8, pp. 1092–1104, 2008.

[21] L. H. Colbert, C. E. Matthews, T. C. Havighurst, K. Kim, and D. A. Schoeller, "Comparative validity of physical activity measures in older adults," *Medicine and Science in Sports and Exercise*, vol. 43, no. 5, pp. 867–876, 2011.

25

Recruiting and Engaging Older Men in Evidence-Based Health Promotion Programs: Perspectives on Barriers and Strategies

Chelsie Anderson, Laura R. Seff, Anamika Batra, Chintan Bhatt, and Richard C. Palmer

Florida International University, Miami, FL 33199, USA

Correspondence should be addressed to Richard C. Palmer; richard.palmer@fiu.edu

Academic Editor: Elke Bromberg

Evidence-based health promotion programs are effective at reducing health risks and healthcare costs among older adults, but few men participate in the programs. This mixed methods study aimed to gain insight into the barriers to recruiting and engaging older men in evidence-based health promotion programs offered by the Healthy Aging Regional Collaborative of South Florida (HARC). Fourteen program coordinators participated in a focus group to identify barriers and strategies to improve male participation, and 49 instructors participated in a survey to triangulate the findings. Themes among barriers to male participation included women outnumbering men in the implementation sites and programs, conflict between male gender roles and the programs, and preference for other activities. Themes among strategies included public support of programs by male community leaders, program advertisements featuring males, and adapting program content. Survey results supported themes identified in the focus group. Nearly 78% of the survey respondents agreed that the perception of exercise programs as feminine was a barrier and over 90% of the survey respondents believed program advertisements featuring men would increase male participation. Findings indicate that health promotion programs and recruiting strategies need to be tailored to the unique needs and preferences of older men to improve participation.

1. Introduction

The number of adults aged 65 and older in the United States is projected to increase to 71 million by 2030 [1]. Eighty percent of older adults have at least one chronic disease and 50% have at least two chronic diseases [1]. Treatment of chronic conditions for older adults accounts for 66% of the healthcare budget in the United States [2]. Impairment and disability are also common and costly among older adults [3]. The chronic disease burden, disability, and healthcare costs associated with an aging population have made the health status of older adults a top priority for the Centers for Disease Control and Prevention (CDC), the Administration on Aging (AoA), and Medicare.

To ensure that limited resources for improving the health status of older adults are used effectively and efficiently, policymakers, funders, and members of the aging networks are increasingly calling for the use of evidence-based health promotion (EBHP) programs. Research supports the effectiveness of EBHP programs in improving health behaviors and health outcomes among older adults of different ethnicities and in different communities [4–9]. Researchers have also demonstrated that EBHP programs reduce healthcare utilization and healthcare costs [6, 7, 10].

Federal law now requires health promotion and disease prevention programs to be evidence-based in order to be eligible for Older Americans Act Title IIID funding [11]. In 2014, 43 programs that underwent the Older Americans Act Title IIID submission process met the highest-level criteria for evidence-based programs and include programs such as the Stanford Self-Management programs, EnhanceFitness, and Matter of Balance [12]. Evidence-based programs are supported as being effective; however, members of the intended population must participate in the programs in order to benefit from them.

A variety of factors may influence an older individual's willingness to participate in health promotion programs. Cultural beliefs, attitudes about health promotion, gender roles, age-related issues, and mistrust of research have been reported as reasons why older Korean Americans do not participate in health promotion programs [13]. Fatalism, underestimation of risk, poor self-efficacy, and stigma associated with programs for older people were identified as barriers to participation in fall prevention programs [14]. Research with participants, nonparticipants, and administrators of a health promotion program designed to reduce cardiovascular disease in older adults suggests that time constraints, transportation, lack of information about the programs, and lack of comfort are barriers to participation [15, 16]. Focus groups conducted at a senior wellness center revealed that social support, interpersonal engagement, and programs tailored to individual needs, interests, and limitations facilitate participation in community-based health promotion programs [17]. A study of older adults who declined to join or joined an exercise program revealed that those who joined were socially inclined and desired accountability while those who declined to join reported already getting enough exercise, lack of motivation, and lack of affiliation with people in the program [18].

A significant issue related to older adult participation in EBHP programs is that men are often underrepresented [4, 8, 19–21]. Given that males also suffer higher rates of most illnesses than females and have higher healthcare costs than females from the age of 60 to approximately the age of 90, efforts are needed to ensure that older men participate in EBHP programs [22]. While it is clear from the literature that men and women differ in the frequency of many health behaviors that may contribute to gender disparities in healthcare costs, the reasons why men are less likely than women to engage in health behaviors such as participating in EBHP programs are poorly understood [23].

Research suggests that a one-size-fits-all approach to male health promotion will not be successful because men are a heterogeneous group with varying health information needs and preferences [24, 25]. There is a lack of research addressing the participation of older men in health promotion programs. The present study aimed to address this gap by examining program coordinator and instructor perspectives on low male participation in EBHP programs offered by the Healthy Aging Regional Collaborative of South Florida (HARC). Males represented 44% of the population aged 60 and older in counties where HARC offered programs, but males represented only 19% of HARC participants [26]. As program implementers, HARC coordinators and instructors are responsible for recruiting and engaging participants and thus were selected to participate in this study to identify barriers to recruiting and engaging older male participants and to identify strategies to increase male participation.

2. Method

2.1. Setting. The Health Foundation of South Florida established the Healthy Aging Regional Collaborative (HARC) in 2008 to disseminate evidence-based health promotion programs in Broward, Miami-Dade, and Monroe counties. Programs were selected to address physical inactivity, fall prevention, and chronic conditions among older adults. The HARC programs included EnhanceFitness (EF), Chronic Disease Self-Management (CDSMP), Tomando Control de su Salud (TCS), Diabetes Self-Management (DSMP), Manejo Personal de la Diabetes (MDP), Matter of Balance (MOB), and Asunto de Equilibrio (ADE). HARC member agencies implemented one or more of the evidence-based programs listed to meet the needs of the older adults they served. This study was approved by the Institutional Review Board at Florida International University.

2.2. Participants. Program coordinators and instructors of HARC programs were included in this study to learn why older men were not participating in HARC programs. Program coordinators and instructors were chosen as study participants because they have extensive experience working with program participants and are knowledgeable about the feasibility of potential strategies to increase participation. Each HARC agency selected a program coordinator or multiple program coordinators to manage the implementation of one or more evidence-based programs. Twenty program coordinators representing the 14 HARC member agencies in 2013 were invited by email to participate in a focus group. The 14 program coordinators who participated in the focus group (70% participation rate) represented 11 of the 14 member agencies.

The agencies represented in the focus group included area agencies on aging, nonprofits, healthcare organizations, recreation organizations, and social service agencies. All of the coordinators had managed the HARC programs for multiple years at the time of the study. Program coordinators were responsible for recruiting program participants, so they have knowledge about individuals who participated and individuals who were informed about the programs but decided not to participate.

Program instructors were selected by the HARC agencies and participated in instructor training according to program requirements. HARC program instructors had professional experience in a wide range of fields and facilitated the programs on a part-time or volunteer basis. Program instructors interacted closely with the participants in each program session and were likely to develop a sense of the barriers to participation based on observations and feedback from participants. The 269 program instructors who taught one or more HARC workshops between 2008 and 2013 were invited by email to participate in an online survey. Instructors who were also program coordinators were excluded from the survey. Instructors were sent two reminder emails in an effort to improve the response rate. Forty-nine instructors responded to the survey (18% response rate). Thirty-nine of the respondents (80%) were female and 10 were male (20%). Respondents and nonrespondents did not differ in gender.

2.3. Data Collection. This mixed methods study used a focus group to elicit information from HARC program coordinators about the most important barriers and strategies for male participation in HARC programs and to develop a survey about male participation that was subsequently administered to HARC instructors to triangulate findings. The focus group was moderated by a member of the HARC local evaluation team and lasted approximately two hours.

To identify barriers to male participation, the moderator first asked coordinators to provide reasons why more men do not participate in HARC programs and why it is difficult to recruit male participants. The moderator then asked the coordinators to identify strategies that might be effective in increasing male interest and participation in HARC programs. The moderator followed up the initial questions with probes to collect additional information. The moderator documented the ideas reported on an interactive whiteboard grid so that all participants could see the responses as they were given and clarify or expand upon the responses if desired. A note taker from the HARC local evaluation team typed comments from the discussion in an electronic document during the session.

After completing the analysis of the focus group comments, a questionnaire was developed in order to examine instructor perspectives on male participation and to triangulate findings. Major themes from the focus group discussion, interesting but infrequent coordinator comments from the focus group, and participation barriers described in the literature were developed into survey items to examine whether HARC instructors agreed that the factors mentioned by coordinators and existing research were barriers to participation for HARC program participants and whether the suggested strategies were likely to be successful with HARC program participants. HARC instructors received an email inviting them to participate in an online survey. The email included an explanation of the purpose of the study, instructions for accessing the survey questionnaire, a statement explaining that participation was voluntary, and a description of the confidentiality of responses. If participants did not complete the survey within two weeks of receiving the first email, they received two reminder emails spaced one week apart.

The questionnaire was administered using Qualtrics online software and included items that assessed barriers to participation and strategies to increase participation. Items regarding barriers required respondents to rate their level of agreement with several possible explanations for nonparticipation by older males and several statements about their perceptions of male program participants. Items regarding strategies required respondents to indicate the likelihood that each of several potential strategies would be successful in increasing male participation in HARC programs. Open-ended questions asked respondents to describe any barriers to male participation in HARC programs and to list any strategies to increase male participation in HARC programs.

2.4. Data Analysis. The focus group data were analyzed by two members of the HARC local evaluation team who collaboratively organized statements from the SMART Board grids and the discussion document into common topics and summarized the data. Descriptive statistics were calculated for the fixed-choice survey questions. In the analysis, ratings of "strongly disagree" and "disagree" were collapsed and ratings of "agree" and "strongly agree" were collapsed. Similarly, ratings of "very unlikely" and "unlikely" were collapsed and ratings of "likely" and "very likely" were collapsed.

Thematic analysis was used to examine the responses to the open-ended survey questions. Thematic analysis involves familiarizing oneself with the dataset, generating codes, combining the codes into themes, and reviewing and refining the themes [27]. The responses to the open-ended survey questions were downloaded from Qualtrics. A member of the evaluation team assigned open codes to words, phrases, or sentences. A second member of the evaluation team validated the codes and then worked collaboratively with the first coder to group the codes into themes.

3. Results

3.1. Focus Group. When asked to provide reasons why it is difficult to recruit men in HARC programs, coordinators expressed that older men may not be comfortable in activities where most participants are women and that attention to health in general is not consistent with male gender roles. Coordinators also reported that health promotion programs are not a part of the senior male culture, there are fewer men at senior sites where coordinators recruit participants, social programs are not appealing to men, and there are too many women instructors. Coordinators also believed that men view EnhanceFitness (EF) as an aerobics class and would prefer other physical activities.

When asked to provide a list of strategies to increase male interest and participation in HARC programs, coordinators suggested getting male community leaders to support the programs, producing advertisements showing men, encouraging women to bring men to the workshops, and providing meaningful incentives. Coordinators also suggested encouraging instructors to do less dancing in EF and hiring more male instructors.

3.2. Survey

3.2.1. Agreement with Barriers to Male Participation and Men's Beliefs. When asked in the online survey whether older men's viewing exercise programs as aerobics classes for females was a barrier to participation, nearly 78% of the instructors agreed (Table 1). Similarly, nearly 74% of the instructors agreed that machismo or cultural beliefs prevent older men from participating and that older males think personal problems should not be discussed. More than 80% of the instructors disagreed with statements that older males are uncomfortable with female instructors and that older males think they will not be respected if they participate in health promotion programs.

When asked in the online survey to rate their level of agreement with statements regarding men's beliefs and participation, almost 96% of the respondents agreed that men are more likely to participate if they see other men in the group and 87% agreed that men are more likely to participate if they come with their spouse or partner (Table 2).

TABLE 1: Agreement with statements explaining why older males do not participate in HARC programs.

Statement	Agree	Disagree
Older males view exercise programs as aerobics classes for females.	77.6%	22.4%
Machismo or cultural beliefs prevent older men from participating in health promotion programs.	73.5%	26.5%
Older males think personal problems should not be discussed.	73.5%	26.5%
There are too many women in health promotion classes.	49.0%	51.0%
Older males feel that there is a negative stigma associated with participating in health promotion programs for older adults.	42.9%	57.1%
Older males believe that they will be perceived as old if they participate in a health promotion program.	30.6%	69.4%
Older males think that they will not be respected if they participate in a health promotion program.	22.5%	77.5%
Older males are not comfortable with female instructors.	18.4%	81.6%

Note. For all statements, the sample size was $n = 49$.

TABLE 2: Agreement with statements regarding men's beliefs and participation.

Statement	Agree	Disagree
Men are more likely to participate if they see other men in the group.	95.7%	4.3%
Men are more likely to participate with their spouse/partner.	87.2%	12.8%
Men view group exercise as a female activity.	76.6%	23.4%
Men are reluctant to attend organized health promotion activities.	66.0%	34.0%
Men believe they have little control over what happens to them in the aging process.	57.4%	42.6%
Male participants are not actively engaged in workshops.	57.4%	42.6%
Men think that seeking health advice makes them seem weak or dependent.	55.3%	44.7%
Men will stop coming to classes if they are the only male in the class.	55.3%	44.7%
Men feel awkward or embarrassed in an exercise or health education class.	51.1%	48.9%
Male participants think the material covered in the workshops is "silly" or too "touchy-feely."	44.7%	55.3%
Male participants are likely to lose interest during a workshop session.	44.7%	55.3%
Men prefer male instructors to female instructors.	25.5%	74.5%

Note. For all statements, the sample size was $n = 47$.

Over 74% of the respondents disagreed that men prefer male instructors.

3.2.2. Descriptions of Barriers to Male Participation. Four themes emerged from open-ended items that asked instructors to describe barriers to male participation. Instructors expressed that more women attend health promotion classes, so men feel outnumbered by women if they do attend. Male gender roles became another apparent theme. One respondent said, "traditionally, females attend to the family's health issues," and another said, "older males like to feel independent, self-sufficient, and knowledgeable. I think they believe attending one of the classes will indicate the opposite." Respondents also expressed that men are often not comfortable seeking help or engaging in conversations about health issues.

Another common theme was that men prefer to do other activities rather than attending workshops. Instructors explained that men prefer physical activities and competition. One respondent said, "sitting in a classroom is not something that older males look forward to," and another said, "older men are more about doing and fixing than talking." Regarding the EnhanceFitness (EF) program in particular, a common theme was that males would prefer other types of fitness activities. Respondents explained that men feel EF is not vigorous enough and emphasizes dancing too much.

A final theme that emerged was negative perceptions of health promotion programs. One respondent said, "the biggest barrier seems to be the attitude of older men towards the healthcare profession. They are less inclined to visit doctors and are not as proactive about their health as women." One instructor shared that a man described the health promotion classes as "long-winded with a lot of common sense stuff."

3.2.3. Likelihood That Strategies Will Succeed in Increasing Male Participation. When presented with a list of strategies and asked to rate the likelihood that each strategy would increase male participation, all of the strategies were rated as likely to succeed by the majority of instructors. Over 90% of the instructors rated advertisements showing men engaging in health promotion and including pictures of single older males in promotional materials as likely to succeed (Table 3).

3.2.4. Strategies Suggested to Increase Male Participation. Three main themes emerged from the open-ended question regarding strategies to improve male participation in health promotion programs. The most common theme among strategies suggested by respondents involved advertising and

TABLE 3: Likelihood of strategies successfully increasing male participation in HARC programs.

Strategy	Likely	Unlikely
Produce advertisements that show men engaging in health promotion programs.	95.7%	4.3%
Have pictures of single older males in program brochures, flyers, and posters (not just couples).	91.3%	8.7%
Get male community leaders to publicly support the program (e.g., church leaders, politicians, and community leaders as advocates).	89.1%	10.9%
Air public service announcements aimed at men.	89.1%	10.9%
Get well known public figures to endorse male participation.	87.0%	13.0%
Encourage women who register for classes to bring men.	82.6%	17.4%
Provide meaningful incentives (e.g., gift card to a store where men typically shop).	78.3%	21.7%
Go to barbershops.	63.0%	37.0%
Hire more male instructors.	60.9%	39.1%

Note. For all strategies, the sample size was $n = 46$.

support for the HARC programs. Instructors suggested using local sports franchises and retired athletes to endorse the programs. They also suggested having male instructors and doctors promote the programs. Social media, television, and newspapers were suggested as important mediums for advertising older men participating in health promotion programs. Targeting advertisements where men congregate and actually offering programs where men congregate were also suggested to increase male participation.

The second theme discovered among suggested strategies was normalizing male participation in health promotion programs. The strategies to normalize male participation are closely linked with strategies to improve advertising and support for the programs. Including men in class advertisements and having recognized men in the community endorse male participation were suggested as strategies to "make attendance more acceptable or normal for older men." Instructors also mentioned that offering men-only programs may help.

Another common theme that emerged deals with the content and perceptions of the EF program. Instructors suggested that the male participation in EF would be improved by using exercises that resemble circuit training, incorporating sports moves that both men and women could enjoy, and reducing the amount of dancing.

4. Discussion

People who engage in healthy lifestyle behaviors have a reduced risk for chronic disease morbidity and mortality [28]. Evidence-based health promotion programs have the potential to help participants adopt health behaviors to improve their wellbeing, but participation by males is suboptimal. Maximizing male participation in health promotion is an important goal for public health, because men are more likely than women to engage in most health risk behaviors, die at higher rates than women from the leading causes of death, and have shorter life spans than women [23, 29].

The current study enrolled HARC program coordinators and instructors who provided their perspectives on the barriers to recruiting older males in EBHP programs and suggested potential strategies to increase male participation. Coordinators and instructors are responsible for recruiting and engaging participants in EBHP, so their combined perspectives are valuable in understanding and improving male participation. The findings from the focus group and survey revealed that male gender roles, men's views of health promotion programs, preferences for other activities, and the low numbers of males in the classes are barriers to engaging males in health promotion programs. The findings from the survey supported most of the ideas reported in the focus group. Survey respondents did not, however, support the idea that women instructors are a barrier to male participation.

The findings from this study are in line with previous research which has reported that gender is associated with different health beliefs and behavior [30, 31]. From the perspective of the constructionist theory of gender, men and women think and act as they do because of socially constructed concepts about masculinity and femininity in their culture [32, 33]. The male gender role includes being independent, strong, and self-reliant and does not tend to include seeking care [23]. Applying this theory, men may avoid attending health promotion programs if participation in the program does not align with their concepts of masculinity.

Coordinators and instructors reported that men hold negative views of health promotion programs and the healthcare profession. This finding may reflect men's view of help-seeking in general. Researchers have reported that men with traditional beliefs about male gender roles have more negative attitudes about seeking help and are less willing to seek help [34]. Machismo, defined as strong masculine pride, has also been reported to affect help-seeking among Latino men and South Florida has a large Latino population [35]. Latino men who participated in a study of gender beliefs and prostate cancer screening indicated that machismo impedes preventive healthcare and screening [36]. The present study builds upon previous research by indicating that machismo acts as a barrier to male participation in EBHP programs as well.

A qualitative study of older British men's health needs indicates that although masculine culture has a strong influence on the way men think about health, men still wanted more health services and information, were open to discussing their healthcare needs, and were dissatisfied with masculine stereotypes in advertising and health information for men [25]. These findings emphasize the importance of acknowledging the influence of masculinity reported in the current study while remaining sensitive to the multitude of other factors, such as culture, socioeconomic status, ethnicity, and sexual orientation, which may influence men's needs and preferences related to health promotion programs.

Coordinators and instructors indicated that older men prefer alternatives to the current discussion-based activities provided in HARC programs. Previous research on masculinity and health beliefs supports the notion that men do not discuss health issues unless they are serious and solvable and that men are averse to disclosing vulnerability [37]. Gast and Peak reported that men are willing to discuss health concerns but that male-friendly health education programs are needed because men may not feel comfortable with the way services are currently delivered [38]. Men's Sheds represent a novel approach to enhancing the health of men in Australia by providing a male-friendly space and should be investigated for use with older men in the United States [39]. The Men's Shed is a large shed that allows men to come together to socialize and partake in meaningful activities such as woodwork or metalwork which help to provide a sense of connection and purpose that support health [39]. The Australian Men's Sheds do not ensure the provision of specific health information or skills needed by older adult men, but lessons learned from work with Men's Sheds about the activities and environments used to reach men could be applied to health promotion programs and recruiting strategies.

Coordinators and instructors expressed that females' outnumbering males was a barrier to participation. Carroll et al. found that homogenous group composition was important for creating a safe dynamic and supported the engagement of men in community-based health and physical activity promotion programs [40]. Saunders et al. also found that men were more likely to participate in male-only church-based programs and appreciated the opportunity to develop relationships with male peers and to discuss topics affecting them [41]. It is possible that male participation could be improved by offering workshops exclusively for men, but respondents in the current study also indicated that attending with spouses or partners could improve male participation. Staff delivering chronic disease and management programs in rural areas in Canada were interviewed in a qualitative study and also reported that spouses were important for encouraging male participation [42].

Other strategies suggested by coordinators and instructors relate to the participation barriers posed by gender roles. Instructors suggested that public support of the programs by male community leaders and advertisements that highlight male participation would help to normalize and increase male participation in the programs. Friedman et al. confirmed that using of mass media, partnering with businesses and churches, enlisting community leaders and role models as spokespeople, and culturally appropriate messages were seen by middle-aged and older African American men as important strategies for promoting physical activity programs [43].

The strategies described in the current study also emphasize addressing content and perceptions of EnhanceFitness to make it more appealing to men. Respondents did not explicitly suggest adapting the other evidence-based programs offered by the HARC, but the barriers they described point to program adaptation as an important strategy for meeting the needs of men.

4.1. Limitations. The main limitation of this study was that the older male participants and nonparticipants were not included in the study. Instructors and coordinator perspectives were examined to understand the barriers to recruiting and engaging older adult men in the region served by the HARC. Future research should examine male gender roles, perceptions of health promotion programs, and preferences among older males who participate and older males who decline the opportunity to participate in EBHP programs.

Another limitation of the study was the low response rate for instructors. Many HARC instructors taught on a volunteer basis and likely did not respond due to the transient nature of their positions as HARC instructors. Also, the majority of the study participants were female which introduces the potential for gender bias. However, analysis did not reveal gender differences in the percentage of instructors reporting agreement with the barriers or the percentage of instructors rating the likelihood of success of strategies. Finally, this study asked instructors and coordinators about EBHP programs in general but it will be important to investigate whether there are similarities across programs or if the factors influencing male participation differ by program.

5. Conclusion

This study provided novel information about barriers to older male participation in evidence-based health promotion programs and strategies to improve participation by older males. The barriers to male participation identified by program coordinators and instructors suggest that men feel outnumbered in health promotion programs, perceive participation as incompatible with the male gender role, and prefer other activities. Overall, the results of this study highlight a number of ways in which the EBHP programs are not well-suited to the needs of older men. The findings indicate that program planners could increase male participation in EBHP programs by tailoring recruiting strategies to men's gender-based perceptions regarding participation in health promotion, adapting health promotion programs to the beliefs and preferences of men, and improving advertising efforts. To advance men's health promotion, research should examine health promotion programs and recruiting strategies to ensure that they are meeting older men's needs and preferences.

Competing Interests

The authors declare that there are no competing interests regarding the publication of this paper.

Acknowledgments

The authors gratefully acknowledge the support of the Health Foundation of South Florida, the HARC community-based agencies, and the program coordinators and instructors.

References

[1] Centers for Disease Control and Prevention, *Healthy Aging: Helping People to Live Long and Productive Lives and Enjoy a Good Quality of Life*, 2011, http://www.aarp.org/content/dam/aarp/livable-communities/learn/health/Healthy-Aging-Helping-People-to-Live-Long-and-Productive-Lives-and-Enjoy-a-Good-Quality-of-Life-2011-AARP.pdf.

[2] Centers for Disease Control and Prevention, *The State of Aging and Health in America 2013*, CDC, US Department of Health and Human Services, Atlanta, Ga, USA, 2013.

[3] W. W. Hung, J. S. Ross, K. S. Boockvar, and A. L. Siu, "Recent trends in chronic disease, impairment and disability among older adults in the United States," *BMC Geriatrics*, vol. 11, article 47, 2011.

[4] A. Batra, M. Melchior, L. Seff, N. Frederick, and R. C. Palmer, "Evaluation of a community-based falls prevention program in South Florida, 2008-2009," *Preventing Chronic Disease*, vol. 9, no. 1, Article ID 110057, 2012.

[5] B. Belza, A. Shumway-Cook, E. A. Phelan, B. Williams, S. J. Snyder, and J. P. LoGerfo, "The effects of a community-based exercise program on function and health in older adults: the enhancefitness program," *Journal of Applied Gerontology*, vol. 25, no. 4, pp. 291–306, 2006.

[6] T. J. Brady, L. Murphy, B. J. O'Colmain et al., "A meta-analysis of health status, health behaviors, and health care utilization outcomes of the Chronic Disease Self-Management Program," *Preventing Chronic Disease*, vol. 10, no. 1, Article ID 120112, 2013.

[7] K. R. Lorig, D. S. Sobel, A. L. Stewart et al., "Evidence suggesting that a chronic disease self-management program can improve health status while reducing hospitalization: a randomized trial," *Medical Care*, vol. 37, no. 1, pp. 5–14, 1999.

[8] M. A. Melchior, L. R. Seff, A. N. Albatineh, H. V. McCoy, T. F. Page, and R. C. Palmer, "Intermediate outcomes of Chronic Disease Self-Management Program offered by members of the Healthy Aging Regional Collaborative in South Florida," *Research on Aging*, vol. 36, no. 4, pp. 431–449, 2014.

[9] M. Tomioka, N. Sugihara, and K. L. Braun, "Replicating the EnhanceFitness Physical Activity Program in Hawai'i's multicultural population, 2007–2010," *Preventing Chronic Disease*, vol. 9, Article ID 110155, 2012.

[10] R. T. Ackermann, B. Williams, H. Q. Nguyen, E. M. Berke, M. L. Maciejewski, and J. P. LoGerfo, "Healthcare cost differences with participation in a community-based group physical activity benefit for medicare managed care health plan members," *Journal of the American Geriatrics Society*, vol. 56, no. 8, pp. 1459–1465, 2008.

[11] Administration for Community Living, "*Administration on Aging: Disease prevention and health promotion services (OAA Title IIID)*," 2014, http://www.aoa.acl.gov/AoA_Programs/HPW/Title_IIID/index.aspx.

[12] National Council on Aging, "Title III-D highest tier evidence-based health promotion/disease prevention programs," 2014, https://www.ncoa.org/wp-content/uploads/Title-IIID-Highest-Tier-Evidence-FINAL.pdf.

[13] H.-R. Han, J. Kang, K. B. Kim, J. P. Ryu, and M. T. Kim, "Barriers to and strategies for recruiting Korean Americans for community-partnered health promotion research," *Journal of Immigrant and Minority Health*, vol. 9, no. 2, pp. 137–146, 2007.

[14] F. Bunn, A. Dickinson, E. Barnett-Page, E. Mcinnes, and K. Horton, "A systematic review of older people's perceptions of facilitators and barriers to participation in falls-prevention interventions," *Ageing & Society*, vol. 28, no. 4, pp. 449–472, 2008.

[15] T. J. Wright and G. C. Hyner, "Principal barriers to health promotion program participation by older adults," *American Journal of Health Studies*, vol. 24, no. 1, pp. 215–222, 2009.

[16] T. J. Wright and G. C. Hyner, "Older adult participation in health promotion programs: perspectives of facility administrators," *Educational Gerontology*, vol. 37, no. 12, pp. 1030–1039, 2011.

[17] A. M. Miller and M. Iris, "Health promotion attitudes and strategies in older adults," *Health Education and Behavior*, vol. 29, no. 2, pp. 249–267, 2002.

[18] K. Biedenweg, H. Meischke, A. Bohl et al., "Understanding older adults' motivators and barriers to participating in organized programs supporting exercise behaviors," *Journal of Primary Prevention*, vol. 35, no. 1, pp. 1–11, 2014.

[19] M. G. Ory, M. L. Smith, E. M. Parker et al., "Fall prevention in community settings: results from implementing Tai Chi: Moving for Better Balance in three states," *Frontiers in Public Health*, vol. 2, pp. 216–221, 2015.

[20] M. L. Smith, M. G. Ory, S. Ahn et al., "National dissemination of chronic disease self-management education programs: an incremental examination of delivery characteristics," *Frontiers in Public Health*, vol. 2, article 227, 2015.

[21] M. L. Smith and M. G. Ory, "Measuring success: evaluation article types for the *Public Health Education and Promotion* Section of *Frontiers in Public Health*," *Frontiers in Public Health*, vol. 2, article 111, pp. 1–6, 2014.

[22] D. H. Yamamoto, "Health care costs—from birth to death," in *Health Care Cost Institute's Independent Report Series*, Report 2013-1, 2013, http://www.healthcostinstitute.org/files/Age-Curve-Study_0.pdf.

[23] W. H. Courtenay, "Behavioral factors associated with disease, injury, and death among men: evidence and implications for prevention," *The Journal of Men's Studies*, vol. 9, no. 1, pp. 81–142, 2000.

[24] M. Robinson and S. Robertson, "Health information needs of men," *Health Education Journal*, vol. 73, no. 2, pp. 150–158, 2014.

[25] R. Coles, F. Watkins, V. Swami, S. Jones, S. Woolf, and D. Stanistreet, "What men really want: a qualitative investigation of men's health needs from the Halton and St Helens primary care trust men's health promotion project," *British Journal of Health Psychology*, vol. 15, no. 4, pp. 921–939, 2010.

[26] U.S. Census Bureau, *Profile of General Population and Housing Characteristics: 2010*, 2010, http://factfinder2.census.gov.

[27] V. Braun and V. Clarke, "Using thematic analysis in psychology," *Qualitative Research in Psychology*, vol. 3, no. 2, pp. 77–101, 2006.

[28] E. S. Ford, M. M. Bergmann, H. Boeing, C. Li, and S. Capewell, "Healthy lifestyle behaviors and all-cause mortality among adults in the United States," *Preventive Medicine*, vol. 55, no. 1, pp. 23–27, 2012.

[29] Centers for Disease Control and Prevention, "*Deaths: Final data for 2011*," 2011, http://www.cdc.gov/nchs/data/sr/nvsr63/nvnvsr63_03.pdf.

[30] W. Bei, R. T. Goins, J. N. Laditka, V. Ignatenko, and E. Goedereis, "Gender differences in views about cognitive health and healthy lifestyle behaviors among rural older adults," *The Gerontologist*, vol. 49, no. 51, pp. 572–578, 2009.

[31] W. H. Courtenay, D. R. McCreary, and J. R. Merighi, "Gender and ethnic differences in health beliefs and behaviors," *Journal of Health Psychology*, vol. 7, no. 3, pp. 219–231, 2002.

[32] W. H. Courtenay, "Constructions of masculinity and their influence on men's well-being: a theory of gender and health," *Social Science & Medicine*, vol. 50, no. 10, pp. 1385–1401, 2000.

[33] C. West and D. H. Zimmerman, "Doing gender," *Gender & Society*, vol. 1, no. 2, pp. 125–151, 1987.

[34] M. E. Addis and J. R. Mahalik, "Men, masculinity, and the contexts of help seeking," *American Psychologist*, vol. 58, no. 1, pp. 5–14, 2003.

[35] T. Peak, J. Gast, and D. Ahlstrom, "A needs assessment of latino men's health concerns," *American Journal of Men's Health*, vol. 4, no. 1, pp. 22–32, 2010.

[36] Z. A. Rivera-Ramos and L. P. Buki, "I will no longer be a man! Manliness and prostate cancer screenings among Latino men," *Psychology of Men and Masculinity*, vol. 12, no. 1, pp. 13–25, 2011.

[37] P. Verdonk, H. Seesing, and A. de Rijk, "Doing masculinity, not doing health? A qualitative study among dutch male employees about health beliefs and workplace physical activity," *BMC Public Health*, vol. 10, article 712, 2010.

[38] J. Gast and T. Peak, "It used to be that if it weren't broken and bleeding profusely, i would never go to the doctor: men, masculinity, and health," *American Journal of Men's Health*, vol. 5, no. 4, pp. 318–331, 2011.

[39] M. L. Ballinger, L. A. Talbot, and G. K. Verrinder, "More than a place to do woodwork: a case study of a community-based Men's Shed," *Journal of Men's Health*, vol. 6, no. 1, pp. 20–27, 2009.

[40] P. Carroll, L. Kirwan, and B. Lambe, "Engaging hard to reach men in community based health promotions," *International Journal of Health Promotion and Education*, vol. 52, no. 3, pp. 120–130, 2014.

[41] D. R. Saunders, C. L. Holt, D. Le et al., "Recruitment and participation of african american men in church-based health promotion workshops," *Journal of Community Health*, vol. 40, no. 6, pp. 1300–1310, 2015.

[42] A. G. Gavarkovs, S. M. Burke, K. C. Reilly, and R. J. Petrella, "Barriers to recruiting men into chronic disease prevention and management programs in rural areas: perspectives of program delivery staff," *American Journal of Men's Health*, 2015.

[43] D. B. Friedman, S. P. Hooker, S. Wilcox, E. L. Burroughs, and C. E. Rheaume, "African american men's perspectives on promoting physical activity: 'we're not that difficult to figure out!'," *Journal of Health Communication*, vol. 17, no. 10, pp. 1151–1170, 2012.

26

Health Indicators of US Older Adults Who Received or did not Receive Meals Funded by the Older Americans Act

Edgar R. Vieira,[1] Joan A. Vaccaro,[2] Gustavo G. Zarini,[3] and Fatma G. Huffman[4]

[1]*Department of Physical Therapy, Florida International University, MMC, 11200 SW 8th St., AHC3-430, Miami, FL 33199, USA*
[2]*Department of Dietetics and Nutrition, Florida International University, MMC, 11200 SW 8th St., AHC5-324, Miami, FL 33199, USA*
[3]*Department of Dietetics and Nutrition, Florida International University, MMC, 11200 SW 8th St., AHC5-300, Miami, FL 33199, USA*
[4]*Department of Dietetics and Nutrition, Florida International University, 11200 SW 8th St., AHC-5, Room 326, Miami, FL 33199, USA*

Correspondence should be addressed to Fatma G. Huffman; huffmanf@fiu.edu

Academic Editor: Antonello Lorenzini

Background. The Older Americans Act (OAA) requires that nutrition programs provide meals and related nutrition services that promote health and help manage chronic diseases. The purpose of this study was to compare health status, food security, functional limitations, and chronic diseases of older adults who received or did not receive OAA meals using data from a representative sample of US adults. *Methods.* Data were from the National Health and Nutrition Surveys 2011–2014 for 2,392 older adults ≥ 65 years of age, including 187 Mexican Americans, 212 other Hispanics, 521 non-Hispanic Blacks, 219 non-Hispanic Asians, and 1253 non-Hispanic Whites. *Results.* Those receiving OAA meals had higher percent of food insecurity and functional disabilities. Adjusting for potential confounders, adults who received OAA meals had higher odds of emphysema (OR = 2.02; 1.05, 3.89) and lower odds of good-to-excellent health (OR = 0.52; 0.36, 0.77). Women and minorities had poorer health status compared to non-Hispanic Whites. *Conclusion.* A higher proportion of older adults who received nutritional services reported poorer health as compared to older adults who do not participate in these services. Future studies should assess nutritional adequacy for older adults who participate in nutritional programs comparing sex and race/ethnicity.

1. Introduction

Nutrition is the cornerstone of healthy aging, yet millions of older adults lack access to sufficient quantities of quality food, placing them at risk for disability, high cholesterol, high blood pressure, obesity, heart disease, cancer, and diabetes [1]. Good nutrition is vital for older adults to maintain health and independence, and it is especially compromised among those in social and economic need [1]. Food insecurity is related to medication nonadherence in low-income, older adults [2]. Medication nonadherence results in chronic disease mismanagement and increased morbidity and mortality [3].

The Older Americans Act (OAA) requires that nutrition programs provide meals and related nutrition services that promote health and help manage chronic diseases [4]. The OAA is now part of the mandate of the Administration for Community Living (ACL) within the Department of Health and Human Services (DHHS). The nutrition program is for adults 60 years of age and older; however, it concentrates assistance on persons with the greatest social or economic need, such as low-income older adults living in rural areas [5]. The ACL provides both home-delivered and congregate meals as part of the agency's fulfillment of the OAA [6]. The states have control for providing the programs and can provide one, two, or three meals 5 to 7 days per week [6]. Each meal must provide one-third of the recommended dietary allowances (RDAs). Congregate meals and government home-delivered meals are critical services provided to help older adults remain independent [6].

According to the Academy of Nutrition and Dietetics, there is limited research on the health outcomes of older adults who participate in the OAA nutrition programs [7]. Older adults receiving congregate or home-delivered meals from the OAA were found to have greater functional decline and more illnesses and to be poorer and at greater risk of institutionalization than the general older adult population [8]. Adults 65 years of age and older are the fastest growing segment of the population, increasing from 36.6 million in 2005 to 47.8 million in 2015 (a 30% increase); their segment is estimated to double by 2060 [9]. Thirty percent of community-dwelling adults receiving Medicare (aged ≥ 65 years) reported difficulty in performing one or more ADLs in 2013 [9]. Limitations in active daily living skills are projected to increase from 2.7 million (2014) to 12.2 million in 2035 among community-dwelling adults 65 years of age and older [10]. Due to the importance of nutrition in healthy aging, the purpose of this study was to compare health status, food security, functional limitations, and chronic diseases of older adults who received or did not receive OAA meals using data from a representative sample of US older adults.

2. Methods

2.1. Description of Sample. We evaluated data from 19,151 people who completed the National Health and Nutrition Examination Survey (NHANES) between 2011 and 2014 that is available for public use [11]. The inclusion criteria were being 65 years of age or older, self-identifying as Mexican American (MA), other Hispanic (OH), non-Hispanic Black (NHB), non-Hispanic Asian (NHA), or non-Hispanic White (NHW), and responding to the question on receiving or not OAA meals (congregate meals or government home-delivered meals). Age ≥ 65 years was a criterion because health insurance is then available through Medicare, even though nutrition programs are already available starting at 60 years old. Those who self-identified as "other" for race/ethnicity which included mixed races were not included due to the small sample size. Based on the inclusion criteria, our final sample size was 2,392 older adults, including 187 MA, 212 OH, 521 NHB, 219 NHA, and 1253 NHW.

2.2. Source of Data and Compliance with Ethical Standards. The NHANES applies a complex, stratified, multistage probability cluster sampling design to obtain a nationally representative sample of the US civilian, noninstitutionalized population. These surveys contain data for approximately 20,000 individuals (5000 per year) of all ages and were generated under the auspices of the National Center for Health Statistics (NCHS), a division of the Centers for Disease Control and Prevention (CDC), a part of the US DHHS. All participants read, understood, and signed informed consent forms. Separate informed consent forms were signed by participants depending on whether they participated in the interview and health examination or just the interview. For this study, the mobile examination center (MEC) sample weight was used to account for unequal probabilities of selection and nonresponse and to conform to the population distribution. Weight and height were measured in a mobile examination center using standardized techniques and equipment. Body mass index (BMI) was calculated as weight in kilograms divided by height in meters squared (kg/m^2). Detailed information concerning the NHANES data collection procedures is available at the NCHS website: https://www.cdc.gov/nchs/ [11].

2.3. Demographic Variables. Body mass index (BMI) categories corresponded to National Institutes of Health (NIH) classification [12]. However, there were not enough individuals in the underweight category (less than 2%), so the underweight category was combined with normal weight category. The BMI categories were as follows: underweight to normal weight (BMI < 25 kg/m^2), overweight (BMI ≥ 25 and <30 kg/m^2), Obesity I (BMI ≥ 30 and <35 kg/m^2), Obesity II (BMI ≥ 35 and <40 kg/m^2), and Obesity III (BMI ≥ 40 kg/m^2).

Food security level was classified based on household interview data using a validated questionnaire, US Food Security Survey Module, developed by the United States Department of Agriculture (USDA) [13]. People were classified as having full food security level, marginal food security level, low food security level, or very low food security level. In addition, food security was assessed based on being afraid of running out of food over the past 12 months (yes/no). *Poverty level* was measured as the ratio of monthly income to poverty, based on the 2011–2014 Department of Health and Human Services (HHS) poverty guidelines, and used by NHANES to calculate the index. *Poverty level* was constructed as a binary variable with a ratio < 1 considered as poverty (as per the US government).

Marital status was classified as "currently married/partnered or not" (single, widowed, or divorced). Finally, *smoking status* was classified as "current smoking or not" (including former smokers and never smokers).

2.4. Health Status. Physical function was classified as impaired when people said they had limitations for the amount of work they could do, or that they needed to use walking equipment (assistive devices). The *presence of a disease* was assessed based on an affirmative response to the question, "Have you ever been told by a doctor or other medical professional that you had ____________ (the disease)?" *Cognitive status* was classified as impaired when people said they had problems with memory. *The actual question asked to the individuals was as follows*: "Are you limited in any way because of difficulty remembering or because you experience periodic confusion?" And the response was dichotomous (yes/no). *Self-rated health* was assessed using the question, "In the past 12 months, how would you rate your health?" The original five categories (excellent, very good, good, fair, and poor) were collapsed to a binary variable: poor-to-fair or good-to-excellent health. Self-rated health has been validated against actual health in older adults, and it is an independent predictor of mortality [14–16].

2.5. Data Analysis. Descriptive statistics of the sample characteristics were presented as cross-tabulations (frequencies in percent and 95 percent confidence intervals) comparing those who received and did not receive OAA funded meals (congregate meals and/or home-delivered meals). Significance was based on the adjusted F, a variant of the second-order Rao-Scott adjusted chi-square statistic and its degrees of freedom. A logistic regression model was constructed

TABLE 1: Demographics and health issues of the combined sample receiving/not receiving OAA meals.

Variable	Parameter	Percent (95% CI)
Received funded meals	Yes	10.1 (8.0, 12.7)
	No	89.9 (87.3, 92.0)
Sex	Male	44.0 (42.2, 45.9)
	Female	56.0 (54.1, 57.8)
Race/ethnicity	Mexican American	3.4 (2.1, 5.6)
	Other Hispanics	3.8 (2.6, 5.6)
	Non-Hispanic Blacks	8.6 (6.6, 11.3)
	Non-Hispanic Asians	4.1 (3.1, 5.5)
	Non-Hispanic Whites	80.0 (75.3, 83.6)
Marital status	Married/partnered	60.7 (57.6, 63.7)
	Single, widowed, or divorced	39.3 (36.3, 42.4)
Smoking status	Current smoker	8.3 (7.1, 9.7)
	Not smoking	91.7 (90.3, 93.9)
Body mass index category	Underweight/normal weight	29.0 (26.4, 31.7)
	Overweight	36.5 (34.4, 39.7)
	Mild obesity	21.2 (18.7, 23.9)
	Moderate obesity	9.1 (7.8, 10.5)
	High obesity	4.3 (3.2, 5.5)
Fear of running out of food	Yes	10.2 (8.9, 11.8)
	No	89.8 (88.2, 91.1)
Poverty	Yes	11.1 (9.4, 13.2)
	No	88.9 (86.8, 90.6)
Self-rated health	Poor to fair	23.2 (20.8, 25.9)
	Good to excellent	76.8 (74.1, 79.2)
Stroke	Yes	9.0 (8.1, 10.0)
	No	91.0 (90.0, 91.9)
Emphysema	Yes	5.3 (4.3, 6.6)
	No	94.7 (93.4, 95.7)
Memory problems	Yes	13.0 (11.5, 14.5)
	No	87.0 (85.5, 88.5)
Need equipment for walking	Yes	19.6 (17.4, 22.1)
	No	80.4 (77.9, 82.6)
Limited in amount of work can do	Yes	31.2 (27.9, 34.8)
	No	68.8 (65.2, 72.1)

Notes. Data presented as percent (95% confidence intervals). Parameters were $p < .001$ from each other for all variables, based on the adjusted F, a variant of the second-order Rao-Scott adjusted chi-square statistic and its degrees of freedom. Poverty was considered at <1.00 poverty index. Complex analysis for the population frequencies was based on the unweighted sample, $n = 2{,}392$. Significance was considered at $p < .05$. OAA: Older Americans Act.

using major demographics (gender, race/ethnicity, and marital status) and health indicators that were significant in the cross-tabulation analysis. All data were analyzed with the module for complex sample design analysis and sample weights, considering the differential probabilities of selection, with the Statistical Package for the Social Sciences (IBM SPSS, version 24) using the Taylor series linearization. For logistic regression, the Wald F test statistic was used for model fit with a model effect of $p < .01$ and a correct classification of cases ≥ 75%. To achieve model fit, all potential adjustment variables were added, retained only with a partial p value of .2 or less. A p value of less than .05 (two-sided) was considered statistically significant for variables.

3. Results

Table 1 presents the demographics and health indicators of the sample. Approximately 10% of older adults reported having received congregate meals and/or government home-delivered meals. There was a slightly larger proportion of females in the sample; most participants were non-Hispanic Whites and married. Less than 10% were smokers, but more than two-thirds were overweight or obese. About 10% reported fear of running out of food. More than three-fourths of the sample considered their health to be good to excellent, and the percentage of stroke, emphysema, and memory problems varied between 5 and 15%. About one-fifth

TABLE 2: Comparison between participants who received and did not receive meals funded by the Older Americans Act (OAA).

Variable	Received meals funded by the OAA Yes	No	p
Sex			
Male	33.4 (27.0, 40.5)	45.2 (43.6, 46.9)	.001
Female	66.6 (59.5, 73.0)	54.8 (53.2, 56.4)	
Race/ethnicity			
Mexican Americans	4.0 (1.8, 8.7)	3.4 (2.0, 5.0)	
Other Hispanics	2.9 (1.6, 5.1)	4.0 (2.6, 5.9)	
Non-Hispanic Blacks	12.7 (7.7, 10.2)	8.2 (6.2, 10.7)	.105
Non-Hispanic Asians	2.6 (1.4, 4.8)	4.3 (3.2, 5.7)	
Non-Hispanic Whites	77.7 (67.6, 85.4)	80.2 (75.2, 83.7)	
Marital status			
Married/partnered	38.8 (31.4, 46.8)	63.2 (60.2, 66.1)	<.001
Single, widowed, or divorced	61.3 (53.2, 68.6)	36.8 (33.9, 39.8)	
Smoking status			
Current smoker	7.6 (5.5, 10.5)	8.4 (7.0, 9.9)	.611
Not smoking	92.4 (89.5, 93.5)	91.6 (90.1, 93.0)	
BMI category			
Underweight/normal weight	32.0 (26.4, 38.3)	28.7 (26.1, 31.4)	
Overweight	36.6 (34.0, 43.4)	36.3 (33.9, 38.8)	.281
Obesity I	19.8 (15.2, 25.5)	21.4 (18.8, 24.2)	
Obesity II	6.5 (4.2, 9.9)	9.3 (8.0, 10.9)	
Obesity	3.1 (1.6, 6.0)	4.3 (3.3, 5.6)	
Fear of running out of food			
Yes	14.9 (11.8, 18.5)	9.7 (8.3, 11.4)	.002
No	85.1 (81.5, 88.2)	90.3 (88.6, 91.7)	
Poverty			
Yes	23.4 (17.7, 30.4)	9.7 (8.0, 11.9)	<.001
No	76.6 (69.6, 82.3)	90.3 (88.1, 92.0)	
Self-rated health			
Good to excellent	44.0 (38.6, 49.6)	29.8 (26.1, 33.7)	<.001
Fair to poor	56.0 (50.4, 61.4)	70.2 (66.3, 73.9)	
Stroke			
Yes	15.8 (11.1, 22.2)	8.3 (7.4, 9.2)	.001
No	84.2 (77.9, 88.9)	91.7 (90.8, 92.6)	
Emphysema			
Yes	9.4 (6.4, 13.6)	4.9 (3.9, 6.2)	.005
No	90.6 (86.4, 93.6)	95.1 (93.8, 96.1)	
Memory problems			
Yes	24.8 (20.4, 30.0)	11.6 (10.3, 13.2)	<.001
No	75.1 (17.0, 79.6)	88.4 (86.8 89.8)	
Need equipment for walking			
Yes	32.7 (27.7, 38.0)	18.1 (15.9, 20.6)	<.001
No	67.3 (62.0, 72.3)	81.9 (79.4, 84.1)	
Limited in amount of work can do			
Yes	44.0 (38.6, 49.6)	29.8 (26.1, 33.7)	<.001
No	56.0 (50.4, 61.4)	70.2 (66.3, 73.9)	

Data are presented as percent (95% confidence intervals). The percentages are weighted (sample weights, applied). Variables are totaled to 100% for "yes" and 100% for "no" responses. BMI: body mass index (kg/m^2). Categories are defined as underweight (<18.5) to normal weight (18.5–24.9), overweight (25–29.9), Obesity I (30–34.9), Obesity II (35–39.9), and Obesity III (≥40). Poverty was considered at <1.00 poverty index. Significance was based on the adjusted F, a variant of the second-order Rao-Scott adjusted chi-square statistic and its degrees of freedom. Significance was considered at $p < .05$.

of the population required an assistive device for walking and about 30% reported limitations in the amount of work they could do.

The frequency of those receiving OAA meals (congregate or home-delivered) was 287 (unweighted count, weighted frequency: 10.1% (8.0, 12.7)) as compared to those not receiving these services (2105, unweighted count, weighted frequency: 89.9% (87.3, 92.0)). Differences between participants who received and did not receive meals funded by the OAA are shown in Table 2. Twice the number of females, as compared to males, participate in the nutrition programs

TABLE 3: Logistic regression analysis of demographics and health indicators for participation in OAA nutrition program compared to nonparticipation.

Variable	Parameter	OR (95% CI)	p
Gender	Male	0.83 (0.62, 1.11)	.203
	Female (reference)	1.00	—
Age (years)		2.23 (2.08, 1.17)	<.001
Poverty level	Index < 1.0	2.09 (1.18, 3.72)	.013
	(reference)	1.00	
Race/ethnicity	—	—	.245
	Mexican American	0.96 (0.44, 2.10)	.911
	Other Hispanics	0.52 (0.22, 1.23)	.131
	Non-Hispanic Blacks	1.34 (0.71, 2.54)	.359
	Non-Hispanic Asians	0.61 (0.26, 1.43)	.247
	Non-Hispanic Whites (reference)	1.00	—
Marital status	Married/partnered	0.52 (0.32, 0.86)	.013
	Other (single, widowed, or divorced; reference)	1.00	—
Current smoker	Yes	0.93 (0.59, 1.45)	.733
	No (reference)	1.00	—
BMI category	—	—	.506
	<25 (under/normal wt.)	1.50 (0.70, 3.20)	.286
	25–29.9 (overweight)	1.55 (0.72, 3.34)	.249
	30–34.5 (Obesity I)	1.39 (0.64, 2.98)	.391
	35–39.9 (Obesity II)	1.02 (0.43, 2.46)	.957
	≥40 (Obesity III, reference)	1.00	—
Food insecurity (fear of running out of food)	Yes	1.12 (0.75, 1.69)	.559
	No (reference)	1.00	
Self-rated health	Good to excellent	0.52 (0.36, 0.77)	.002
	Fair to poor (reference)	1.00	—
Stroke	Yes	1.33 (0.84, 2.10)	.213
	No (reference)	1.00	—
Emphysema	Yes	2.02 (1.05, 3.89)	.035
	No (reference)	1.00	—
Memory problems	Yes	1.25 (0.96, 1.64)	.095
	No (reference)	1.00	
Need equipment walking	Yes	0.97 (0.71, 1.32)	.830
	No (reference)	1.00	—
Limited in amount of work can do	Yes	0.92 (0.65, 1.30)	.634
	No (reference)	1.00	—

Note. Dependent variable: participation in congregate meals and/or government delivered meals. Nutrition program = home-delivered meals, congregate meals, or both. BMI: body mass index; wt.: body weight; OAA: Older Americans Act. Model fit was considered at $p < .01$ with correct classification of cases ≥ 75%.

(home-delivered meals, congregate meals, or both). Those who reported using nutritional services had a higher percent of reporting being single as compared to married/partnered individuals, having had a stroke, having memory problems, being food insecure, having emphysema, needing equipment for walking, being limited in the work they could do, and having poorer health.

Reports of chronic diseases were compared for program participants versus nonparticipants using complex cross-tabulation. Having any cardiovascular disease, stroke, coronary heart disease, and emphysema was significantly more prevalent (higher percent) for individuals receiving meals as compared to their counterparts. Diabetes, high cholesterol, high blood pressure, arthritis, bronchitis, and cancer were not significantly different. A higher percentage of persons receiving OAA meals (congregate or meals on wheels) were living at or below the poverty level compared to those not receiving meals. A final logistic regression model is presented by Table 3. Participants did not differ by gender or race/ethnicity, but married or partnered ones had lower odds of participation as compared to single, widowed, or divorced individuals. Individuals reporting going to congregate meals or receiving government meals had poorer self-rated health (SRH) and greater odds of emphysema. Food insecurity and physical function (needing equipment to walk and limited in the amount of work one can perform) were no longer significant, adjusting for demographics. The model was fit with $p < .001$ and 90.1% correct classification (Table 3).

Cross-tabulations of health factors were performed for the combined population (participants and nonparticipants of OAA) by gender and race/ethnicity. Females had a higher percent reporting memory problems [14.8 (23.8, 17.0) versus 10.6 (9.1, 12.3)], $p = .001$, food insecurity (fear of running out of food) [11.6 (9.9, 13.6) versus 8.5 (6.9, 10.4)], $p = .005$, and needing walking equipment [21.7 (19.0, 24.7) versus 17.0 (13.9, 20.5)] as compared to men, $p = .027$. Mexican Americans and other Hispanics had a higher percent of reporting memory problems [23.5 (17.2, 31.2) and 24.7 (18.7, 31.9)], respectively, as compared to NHW [11.7 (9.9, 13.8)], $p < .001$. Other Hispanics [27.5 (22.5, 33.2)] and NHB [28.3 (23.4, 32.5)] had a higher percent of reported needing walking equipment as compared to NHW [18.2 (15.6, 21.3)], $p < .001$. Other Hispanics had a higher percent of reporting having to limit the amount of work they can do as compared to NHW [40.4 (34.2, 46.9) versus 30.5 (26.5, 34.8)], $p = .010$. Higher percent of food insecurity (fear of running out of food) was reported for MA [28.5 (22.3, 35.6)], OH [30.7 (22.9, 39.7)], and NHB [22.0 (16.4, 28.9)] as compared to NHW [7.2 (6.0, 8.6)], $p < .001$.

4. Discussion

We found a higher proportion of older adults (unadjusted) who receive nutritional services (home-delivered meals, congregate meals, or both) to have physical disabilities, report poorer health, and suffer from debilitating chronic diseases as compared to older adults who do not participate in these services. Even after adjusting for potential confounders, poorer self-rated health and emphysema were more likely for those receiving nutrition services. Our results parallel data from a national survey of OAA participants where 71% of home-delivered meal participants and 57% of congregate meal participants had five or more chronic diseases [8]; however, this survey did not compare OAA participants with nonparticipants. The Administration for Community Living [6] recommends that congregate meal sites have fitness classes to improve the health and function of participants. Our study did not have data on exercise class attendance; however, there is some evidence to support fitness classes; physical activity classes at congregate meal sites improved physical activity effort and physical function for older adults, even those with a history of depression [17, 18].

Food insecurity was a contributing factor of poor physical function for congregate meal attendees [19]. Older adults attending congregate meals have a higher percent of food insecurity (18.1%) [20] compared to the national average in older adults (6.5%) [21]. The goal of OAA is to reach older adults with food insecurity, yet there are instances of inequity among some communities. Weddle and colleagues [22] reported that, for community-dwelling, older African Americans, nutrition risk was higher among nonparticipants compared to participants of congregate meal services. Home-delivered meals improved dietary status and reduced food insecurity of recipients in 6 out of 8 studies, according to a systematic review [23]. Meal enhancements such as delivered snacks and local fruits and vegetables and nutritional supplements for those that need them have demonstrated reductions in food insecurity and improvements in functional status [24]. Nutritional adequacy may not be equal across demographics. Women and Blacks who received home-delivered meals had lower nutritional intake compared to their counterparts, regardless of health condition [25]. Food adequacy may be a confounder for health status (chronic disease and physical function) and program participation. Participants receiving OAA meals had a higher percent of food insecurity as defined by "fear of running out of food" as compared to those not receiving OAA meals. Although participation in nutritional services (home-delivered meals, congregate meals, or both) did not differ by race/ethnicity in the present study, there were a greater proportion of minorities with food insecurity as compared to NHW [26]. Older Blacks and Hispanics have more than twice the rate of food insecurity as compared to NHW [26]. A greater proportion of restricted eating was reported for Blacks who had food insecurity and who were obese as compared to their White counterparts [27]. In an earlier study, investigators reported that a higher percentage of older adults with food insecurity were obese (37%) as compared to older adults, nationally (23%) [28].

There was a significant percent of older adults with obesity in our study. Malnutrition is possible for older adults with obesity when diet quality is inadequate [29]. We found no significant difference in obesity for participants versus nonparticipants. This may be due to the alarmingly high rates of obesity among older adults, particularly women. Obesity was associated with abnormal eating behaviors, certain food group intake, and mental health symptoms in a predominately African American and female, urban congregate meal site [30]. Obesity rates from 2011–2014 were reported as 41% (those aged 65–74 years) and 31% (those aged 75 years and older) for women and 24% (those aged 65–74 years) and 13% (those aged 75 years and older) for men [31]. There are controversial reports for weight-loss interventions with physical activity as a treatment for physical disability in older adults [32]. Obesity was associated with disabilities for older adults (17.4%) [19]. Furthermore, there may be differences by sex and race/ethnicity for overweight and mild obesity protective effects with exercise [32]. Prior to developing nutrition interventions at community sites for older adults with obesity, more evidence is needed on how to treat this population [24].

Emphysema and poorer self-rated health were more prevalent for those receiving OAA meals as compared to their counterparts. The current study supports previous findings that older adults participating in nutrition programs have poorer health and lower socioeconomic status, compared to the general population of older adults [8]; however, functional decline did not differ by participation level, adjusting for sociodemographics. The current study indicated that participation/nonparticipation in nutrition programs did not differ by race/ethnicity and that women and minorities had poorer health status than non-Hispanic Whites, regardless of their participation level in nutrition programs. These findings suggest that greater outreach is needed for OAA meals and that interventions to improve health status should be addressed within these programs to help reduce health disparities.

This study has several limitations. Although data was from a nationally representative sample of US older adults, the study was cross-sectional and cause and effect cannot be assumed. The percent of home-delivered meal participants in our study was less than 10%, so they were combined with congregate meal participants for all analyses. Although the interviewers were trained to administer questions, some responses by participants might have been what they perceived as socially acceptable. Memory loss was assessed by interview and not with an objective assessment tool. Another limitation was that race/ethnicity interaction with nutrition program participation could not be assessed due to limited power. Despite these limitations, this study has several strengths: (1) the use of data from a national representative sample of US adults, (2) filling a gap in the literature by comparison of chronic diseases and functional limitations by participating versus not participating in nutrition programs, and (3) comparison of sociodemographics of participants and nonparticipants in a relatively large sample of older adults.

5. Conclusion

Older adults receiving congregate meals and/or government home-delivered meals had overall poorer physical function and health as compared to their counterparts who did not participate in nutritional services. Future studies should assess nutritional adequacy for older adults who participate in nutritional programs comparing sex and race/ethnicity. Clinical studies are needed to determine nutritional needs of older adults with obesity [24]. It is recommended that OAA meal programs provide adequate nutrition education and counseling that address and help to reduce food insecurity [24]. OAA meal programs should provide nutritionally dense meals and meal enhancements for older adults with undernutrition and possibly for obese, older adults with malnutrition [24, 29].

Conflicts of Interest

The authors declare that they have no conflicts of interest.

Authors' Contributions

All authors have contributed significantly to the research concept, literature review, and objectives. They all are in agreement with the content of the manuscript. All authors approved the manuscript and this submission.

References

[1] N. Kowlessar, K. Robinson, C. Schur, and Social & Scientific Systems Inc., "Older Americans Benefit from Older Americans Act Nutrition Programs," Research Brief No. 8. Administration for Community Living, Agency for Older Adults, 2015, https://www.acl.gov/sites/default/files/programs/2016-11/AoA-Research-Brief-8-2015.pdf.

[2] E. L. P. Sattler and J. S. Lee, "Persistent Food Insecurity Is Associated With Higher Levels of Cost-Related Medication Nonadherence in Low-Income Older Adults," *Journal of Nutrition in Gerontology and Geriatrics*, vol. 32, no. 1, pp. 41–58, 2013.

[3] J. G. Hugtenburg, L. Timmers, P. J. M. Elders, M. Vervloet, and L. van Dijk, "Definitions, variants, and causes of nonadherence with medication: a challenge for tailored interventions," *Patient Preference and Adherence*, vol. 7, pp. 675–682, 2013.

[4] N. S. Wellman, D. O. Weddle, B. Kamp et al., "Older Americans nutrition program toolkit," in *National Policy and Resource Center on Nutrition and Aging*, Florida International University, Miami, FL, USA, 2005, http://nutrition.fiu.edu/OANP_Toolkit/toolkit%20update%202.7.06.pdf.

[5] National Committee to Preserve Social Security and Medicare (NCPSSM), "Government Relations and Policy," 2016, http://www.ncpssm.org/PublicPolicy/OlderAmericans/Documents/ArticleID/1171/Older-Americans-Act.

[6] Administration for Community Living (ACL), "Nutrition Services," 2017, https://www.acl.gov/programs/health-wellness/nutrition-services.

[7] M. Bernstein, N. Munoz, and Academy of Nutrition and Dietetics, "Position of the Academy of Nutrition and Dietetics: food and nutrition for older adults: promoting health and wellness," *Journal of the Academy of Nutrition and Dietetics*, vol. 112, no. 8, pp. 1255–1277, 2012.

[8] J. L. Lloyd and N. S. Wellman, "Older Americans Act Nutrition Programs: A Community-Based Nutrition Program Helping Older Adults Remain at Home," *Journal of Nutrition in Gerontology and Geriatrics*, vol. 34, no. 2, pp. 90–109, 2015.

[9] Administration on Aging, "A Profile of Older Americans: 2016," Administration on Aging (AoA), Administration for Community Living, U.S. Department of Health and Human Services, 2016, https://www.acl.gov/sites/default/files/Aging%20and%20Disability%20in%20America/2016-Profile.pdf.

[10] Joint Center for Housing Studies (JCHS) "Disabilities among older adults," 2014, http://www.jchs.harvard.edu/sites/jchs.harvard.edu/files/harvard_jchs_housing_growing_population_2016_chapter_3.pdf.

[11] National Center for Health Statistics (NCHS), "Questionnaires, Datasets, and Related Documentation," 1600 Clifton Road Atlanta, GA 30329-4027 USA: author, 2015, http://www.cdc.gov/nchs/nhanes/nhanes_questionnaires.htm.

[12] National Heart, Lung, and Blood Institute (NHLBI), "National Institutes of Health. Classification according to waist circumference and body mass index," http://www.nhlbi.nih.gov/health-pro/guidelines/current/obesity-guidelines/e_textbook/txgd/4142.htm.

[13] G. Bickel, M. Nord, C. Price, W. Hamilton, and J. Cook, "Guide to Measuring Household Food Security, Revised 2000," Alexandria, VA; U.S. Department of Agriculture, Food and Nutrition Service, 2000, https://www.fns.usda.gov/guide-measuring-household-food-security-revised-2000.

[14] E. L. Idler and Y. Benyamini, "Self-rated health and mortality: a review of twenty-seven community studies," *Journal of Health and Social Behavior*, vol. 38, no. 1, pp. 21–37, 1997.

[15] K. B. DeSalvo, N. Bloser, K. Reynolds, J. He, and P. Muntner, "Mortality prediction with a single general self-rated health question: a meta-analysis," *Journal of General Internal Medicine*, vol. 21, no. 3, pp. 267–275, 2006.

[16] J. M. Ocampa, "Self-rated health: Importance of use in elderly adults," *Colombia Medical*, vol. 41, no. 3, 2010.

[17] T. L. Moore-Harrison, M. A. Johnson, M. E. Quinn, and M. E. Cress, "An evidence-based exercise program implemented in congregate-meal sites," *Journal of Physical Activity & Health*, vol. 6, no. 2, pp. 247–251, 2009.

[18] K. N. Porter, J. G. Fischer, and M. A. Johnson, "Improved physical function and physical activity in older adults following a community-based intervention: Relationships with a history of depression," *Maturitas*, vol. 70, no. 3, pp. 290–294, 2011.

[19] D. P. Brewer, C. S. Catlett, K. N. Porter et al., "Physical limitations contribute to food insecurity and the food insecurity-obesity paradox in older adults at senior centers in Georgia," *Journal of Nutrition for the Elderly*, vol. 29, no. 2, pp. 150–169, 2010.

[20] F. Huffman, J. Vaccaro, E. Vieira, and G. Zarini, "Health-Related Characteristics of Older Adults Who Attend Congregate Meal Sites in the United States," *Geriatrics*, vol. 2, no. 3, p. 22, 2017.

[21] S. Strickhouser, J. D. Wright, and A. M. Donley, "Food insecurity among older adults: full report, 2015 update," AARP, http://www.aarp.org/content/dam/aarp/aarp_foundation/2015-PDFs/AF-Food-Insecurity-2015Update-Final-Report.pdf.

[22] D. Weddle, F. L. Wilson, S. D. Berkshire, and R. Heuberger, "Evaluating Nutrition Risk Factors and Other Determinants of Use of an Urban Congregate Meal Program by Older African Americans," *Journal of Nutrition in Gerontology and Geriatrics*, vol. 31, no. 1, pp. 38–58, 2012.

[23] H. Zhu and R. An, "Impact of home-delivered meal programs on diet and nutrition among older adults: A review," *Nutrition and Health*, vol. 22, no. 2, pp. 89–103, 2013.

[24] J. Tilly, "Opportunities to improve nutrition for older adults and reduce poor health outcomes," Administration for Community Living, Center for Policy and Evaluation, 2017, http://nutritionandaging.org/wp-content/uploads/2017/03/Malnutrition-Issue-Brief-final-3-2017.pdf.

[25] J. R. Sharkey, L. G. Branch, N. Zohoori, C. Giuliani, J. Busby-Whitehead, and P. S. Haines, "Inadequate nutrient intakes among homebound elderly and their correlation with individual characteristics and health-related factors," *American Journal of Clinical Nutrition*, vol. 76, no. 6, Article ID 12450914, pp. 1435–1445, 2002.

[26] Office of Minority Health (OMH), "Department of Health and Human Services, Policy and data, Minority health," 2017, https://www.minorityhealth.hhs.gov/omh/browse.aspx?lvl=2&lvlid=26.

[27] T. Myles, K. N. Porter Starr, K. B. Johnson, J. Sun Lee, J. G. Fischer, and M. Ann Johnson, "Food Insecurity and Eating Behavior Relationships Among Congregate Meal Participants in Georgia," *Journal of Nutrition in Gerontology and Geriatrics*, vol. 35, no. 1, pp. 32–42, 2016.

[28] C. L. Ogden, M. D. Carroll, M. A. McDowell, and K. M. Flegal, "Obesity among adults in the United States—no change since 2003-2004," *NCHS Data Brief*, vol. 1, Article ID 19389313, pp. 1–8, 2007.

[29] K. N. Porter Starr, S. R. McDonald, J. A. Weidner, and C. W. Bales, "Challenges in the management of geriatric obesity in high risk populations," *Nutrients*, vol. 8, no. 5, article no. 262, 2016.

[30] K. Porter Starr, J. G. Fischer, and M. A. Johnson, "Eating Behaviors, Mental Health, and Food Intake Are Associated With Obesity in Older Congregate Meal Participants," *Journal of Nutrition in Gerontology and Geriatrics*, vol. 33, no. 4, pp. 340–356, 2014.

[31] Federal Interagency Forum on Aging-Related Statistics, "Older Americans 2016: Key Indicators of Well-Being, Federal Interagency Forum on Aging-Related Statistics, Washington, DC," 2016, http://volumes/MAIN_JOB/WORKING/aaaaaaa-CHILD%20after%20school%20GRANTS/Older-Americans-2016-Key-Indicators-of-WellBeing.pdf.

[32] W. J. Rejeski, A. P. Marsh, E. Chmelo, and J. J. Rejeski, "Obesity, intentional weight loss and physical disability in older adults," *Obesity Reviews*, vol. 11, no. 9, pp. 671–685, 2010.

27

Sustainability Literacy of Older People in Retirement Villages

Bo Xia,[1] Jian Zuo,[2] Martin Skitmore,[1] Laurie Buys,[3] and Xin Hu[1]

[1]*School of Civil Engineering and Built Environment, Queensland University of Technology, Garden Point Campus, 2 George Street, Brisbane, QLD 4001, Australia*
[2]*School of Natural and Built Environments, University of South Australia, City East Campus, North Terrace, Adelaide, SA 5001, Australia*
[3]*School of Design, Queensland University of Technology, Garden Point Campus, 2 George Street, Brisbane, QLD 4001, Australia*

Correspondence should be addressed to Bo Xia; paul.xia@qut.edu.au

Academic Editor: Elke Bromberg

With many developed countries experiencing the aging of the population, older people play a large role in contributing to environmental problems but also to environmental solutions. The purpose of this research is to understand the awareness and behavior of current older people living in retirement villages towards sustainability development. To achieve this, a sustainability literacy survey was conducted with 65 older residents of a private retirement village located 10 Km outside the Brisbane, Australia's central business district (CBD). Most of residents recognized the importance of environment protection and would like to lead a more environmentally friendly lifestyle. In addition, the majority were willing to pay higher prices for a living environment with sustainable features. The importance of positive social communications was emphasized with most residents having established good relationships with others in the village. The findings provide an important insight into consumer perspectives regarding the sustainable features that should and can be incorporated into the village planning and development.

1. Introduction

Sustainable development, defined as "development that meets the needs of the present without compromising the ability of future generations to meet their own needs" [1], has gained momentum in the current era and visualizes a cleaner environment, the efficient use of natural resources, and a more inclusive society with widely shared benefits of increased economic prosperity [2]. In terms of the built environment, this implies the conservation of a wide variety of resources, such as energy and water [3].

With the increasing proportion of aging population around the world, the actions of older people are likely to have a corresponding increasingly important role in the sustainable development of the community. Older people are expected to consume more energy due to both their increased numbers and their lifestyles, such as spending more time at home (requiring more electricity and water) and using their cars frequently [4, 5].

However, older people can also make major contributions to solving environmental problems [6, 7]. Older people are generally aware of resource consumption and would like their habitat and community to be more sustainable [8]. They can therefore play a positive role in engaging in sustainable activities, such as recycling, food production, renewable energy use, and using alternative transport options. Additionally, environmental volunteerism creates opportunities for social integration in later life, offering meaningful civic engagement in productive activities while providing volunteer resources to promote environmental stewardship [9].

Due to the increasingly significant potential impact of older people on both environmental problems and solutions, it is important to understand their current attitudes and behaviors concerning sustainable development, considered as one of the highest priority topics for research on aging and environmental sustainability [9]. Older people may experience reduced physical capabilities and particular ergonomic requirements (easy access, companionship, security, etc.) and generally value a combination of independence, security, friendships, and community support [10]. The realization of the sustainable agenda (e.g., sustainable buildings and environmental friendly lifecycle) needs to take into consideration these requirements. Furthermore, due to changes in financial circumstances during retirement, additional costs involved in sustainable development inevitably become a major concern [11]. A clear understanding of older peoples' perceptions of sustainable development is, therefore, necessary for devising sustainability policies and programs.

However, few studies have documented older people's attitudes and knowledge relating to sustainable development. Understanding and knowledge of sustainability issues have been termed sustainability literacy, which is "... the understanding, skills, attitudes, and attributes to take informed action for the benefit of oneself and others, now and into a long term future" [12]. Older people living in different accommodation forms, ranging from independent-living alternatives to high-level care, may have different perceptions and knowledge of sustainability and sustainable development. According to Murray and Cotgrave [13], a sustainability literate person understands the need for change to a sustainable way of doing things individually and collectively, has sufficient knowledge and skills to decide to act in a way that favors sustainable development, and is able to recognize and reward other people's decisions and actions that favor sustainable development [14]. The first sustainability literacy surveys were originally developed to assess student sustainability knowledge, sustainable practices, attitudes concerning sustainability topics, and awareness of sustainability initiatives at the Arizona State University, Meredith College, and Maryland University in the USA.

Retirement villages are becoming accepted as a viable accommodation option and house over five percent of Australians aged 65 years and over. A survey of 76 older people living in not-for-profit retirement villages in South Australia found that they are both very conscious of resource consumption and concerned about energy costs [8]. To date, however, nothing is known of the detailed views of residents or of those living in for-profit retirement villages outside South Australia. Further north in Queensland, for example, the warmer climate and reputation for a more relaxed lifestyle are popular for retirees who want to relocate. Queensland has a reputation for having an entrepreneurial approach to business which provides an opportunity to incorporate attitudes of residents within the planning and development processes.

This research explores the perceptions of older people, living in a comparatively large and luxurious Queensland for-profit retirement village, regarding sustainable issues relating to environmental, economic, and social aspects of sustainability. This paper focuses on resident's sustainability concerns, impacts on activities of daily life, and sustainability literacy.

2. Methods

The study sought to investigate the sustainability literacy of residents living in a Queensland for-profit retirement village. Data were collected from October to December 2012. Ethical approval was granted by the Queensland University of Technology Human Research Ethics Committee. Approval from the target regiment village was also obtained to provide necessary assistance for data collection.

The survey was conducted in a private retirement village in a suburb of Brisbane, Queensland, Australia, located approximately 10 kilometers northwest of the Brisbane central business district (CBD) close to amenities such as transport, health services, stores, and libraries. The retirement village developer aspires to be a leader in sustainable property and infrastructure, focusing on transitioning to a low-carbon, energy-efficient, and resource-conservation model that reflects and advances social and environmental best practice. The village contains 254 one-, two-, or three-bedroom homes.

Based on sustainability literacy surveys for university students, a survey was developed focusing on attitudes and behaviors concerning sustainable development. The questionnaire included questions on environmental, economic, and social issues and comprised two main parts (see Table 1). The first part addressed older people's awareness of sustainability issues (using 1: strongly disagree, 2: disagree, 3: agree, and 4: strongly agree); and the second part explored the frequency of daily sustainability-related activities (using 1: never, 2: rarely, 3: usually, and 4: always). The unique aspects of older people living in retirement village were also taken into consideration in the questionnaire design.

Survey forms were placed in the village's community center's reception room from October 26, 2012, until December 4, 2012, with a covering letter explaining the purpose of the research.

3. Results

Sixty-five residents returned the completed questionnaire, providing an overall response rate of approximately 25%.

Figure 1 summarizes the respondents' demographics with the majority of the residents being female and older than 70 years.

The frequencies of degree of agreement of the importance of sustainability activities as well as the median score and interquartile ranges (IQR) are shown in Table 2. Most respondents agree or strongly agree on the importance of these activities to sustainable development. Most of the median scores of importance perceptions are 3 or higher, particularly for "recycling items when possible," "buying local products," and "cutting down on the use of products that are harmful to the environment," where all the respondents agree on their importance. Interestingly, the majority (67%) of residents agree on the necessity of paying a higher price for a home that has environmentally friendly features.

Table 3 describes the frequencies of residents carrying out activities that relate to sustainability as well as the median score and interquartile ranges (IQR). More than 50% of respondents "always" separate landfill waste and recycled waste (63%) and turn off lights and electronic devices when not in use (52%). In contrast, 43% of respondents "rarely"

TABLE 1: Cluster of the questionnaire.

(a)

Category	Sustainability awareness
Environment	Saving electricity and water Using recycled water for gardening or laundering Choosing more durable items to maximize their lifespan Cutting down on the use of products that are harmful to the environment Selling or giving away items that are no longer being used Creating new items from old and unused materials Recycling items when possible Reporting any housing issues to facility manager to repair
Economic	Paying a higher price for a home that has environmentally friendly features Buying local products Gardening Planting fruits or vegetables in own garden or community garden
Social	Attending social group activities Actively involved in community projects Having a good engagement with other village residents

(b)

Category	Daily activities on sustainability awareness
Environment	Turning off lights and electronic devices when not in use Using as little water as necessary in the kitchen and bathroom Using a rainwater tank for gardening or laundering Using reusable bags when shopping Creating crafts from recycled material or old stuff Making compost from leaves, litter, or food waste Separating landfill waste and recycled waste
Economic	Donating or selling items that are no longer used Buying local products
Social	Attending social group activities, such as community meetings or community events, with other village residents Having activities such as community gardening, barbeque, sports, dancing, or making crafts with other village residents

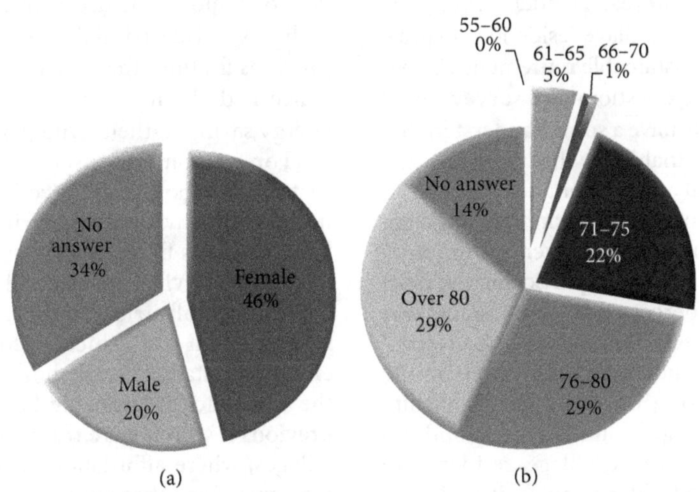

FIGURE 1: (a) Respondents' gender distribution. (b) Respondents' age distribution.

TABLE 2: Percentage of respondents agreeing on the importance of sustainability activities.

Sustainability awareness	Degree of importance				Number	Median	IQR
	1	2	3	4			
Reporting housing issues to the facility manager for repair	0	2	32	**66**	65	4	1
Saving electricity and water	2	0	40	**58**	65	4	1
Recycling items when possible	0	0	46	**54**	65	4	1
Buying local products	0	0	50	**50**	64	3.5	1
Having a good engagement with other village residents	0	3	48	**49**	65	3	1
Attending social group activities	0	8	45	**47**	62	3	1
Paying a higher price for a home that has environmentally friendly features	3	17	**67**	13	60	3	0
Using recycled water for gardening or laundering	0	7	**64**	29	55	3	1
Being actively involved in community projects	0	13	**55**	32	62	3	1
Cutting down on the use of products that are harmful to the environment	0	0	**55**	45	64	3	1
Creating new items from old and unused items	2	29	**54**	15	61	3	1
Choosing more durable items to maximise their lifespan	0	2	**53**	45	64	3	1
Selling or giving away items that are no longer used	0	5	**50**	45	64	3	1
Gardening	8	18	**40**	34	62	3	1.75
Planting fruit or vegetables in own or community garden	3	31	33	**33**	58	3	2

Note: 1: strongly disagree, 2: disagree, 3: agree, and 4: strongly agree.

create crafts from recycled materials or old stuff and 74% "never" use rainwater tanks for gardening or laundering.

Based on survey results, the relationship between sustainable awareness of respondents and their daily activities is drawn (see Figure 2). In general, high levels of sustainability awareness of respondents lead to high frequencies of sustainability activities in their daily life.

4. Discussion

Given their increasing number in our society, older people play an important role in fulfilling the sustainability agenda. It is predicted that a growing proportion of older people will live in retirement villages in the next 10 years. Understanding the attitude and behavior of retirement village residents is of great importance for the delivery of sustainable retirement villages in the future. The results of the questionnaire survey reveal that the majority of respondents have a sound understanding on the holistic aspects of sustainability, which requires the reconciliation of environmental and economic demands and the need for social equity. In other words, there was sufficient sustainable literacy within the senior citizen community living in the studied retirement village. In particular, the most important sustainability issue perceived by respondents was "reporting housing issues to the facility manager for repair." This clearly indicated that respondents are fully aware of the effectiveness of resolving housing issues by having facility management professionals engaged. Similarly, respondents perceived the interaction with other village residents to be very important. This showed older people's attention to social sustainability-related issues. Environmental sustainability issues, such as energy, resource, and water efficiency, were also assigned high priority by respondents for achieving sustainability.

This sustainability literacy of retirement village residents is correlated with their behavior in terms of daily activities. A sustainable development not only protects the natural environment (environmentally sustainable) and increases economic growth (economically sustainable) but also promotes social progress that takes into account the needs of everyone (socially sustainable). For environmental sustainability, most respondents agree on the importance of energy and water saving, recycling, and using fewer products that are harmful to the environment. Furthermore, most respondents manage to save energy in their daily activities. For example, more than 90% of respondents use as little water as necessary and turn off lights and electrical devices when not in use. This confirms previous findings that older people in retirement villages are concerned about environmental issues and welcome more energy saving in their living environment [8, 15].

For economical sustainability, it is interesting to find that most respondents agreed with paying a higher price for homes with environmental friendly features. This is different from previous findings that although nearly all the residents in retirement villages would like to have their facilities more environmentally friendly, most are concerned about the costs involved and are reluctant to pay a higher price for an environmentally friendly home [8, 15]. The major reason for the difference is probably because the respondents in this previous research were residents in not-for-profit retirement villages, where affordability is of the highest importance to residents. The retirement village investigated in this research is a private one that has a very low ongoing vacancy rate (6–8%). This difference provides interesting implications for

TABLE 3: Percentage of respondent carrying out sustainability activities.

Daily activities	Frequency 1	2	3	4	Number	Median	IQR
Separate landfill waste and recycled waste	13	6	17	**63**	63	4	1
Turn off lights and electronic devices when not in use	0	6	42	**52**	65	4	1
Use as little water as necessary in the kitchen and bathroom	0	3	48	**49**	65	3	1
Attend social group activities such as community meeting or community events with other village residents	3	9	42	**46**	65	3	1
Use reusable bags when shopping	5	19	33	**44**	64	3	1
Buy local products	2	3	**66**	30	64	3	1
Donate or sell items that are no longer used	0	6	**48**	45	64	3	1
Have activities such as community gardening, barbeque, sports, dancing, or making crafts with other village residents	6	17	**41**	36	64	3	1
Create crafts from recycled material or old stuff	37	**43**	16	5	63	2	1
Use rainwater tanks for gardening or laundering	**74**	16	5	5	62	1	1
Make compost from leaves, litter, or food waste	**39**	26	19	16	62	2	2

Note: 1: never, 2: rarely, 3: usually, and 4: always.

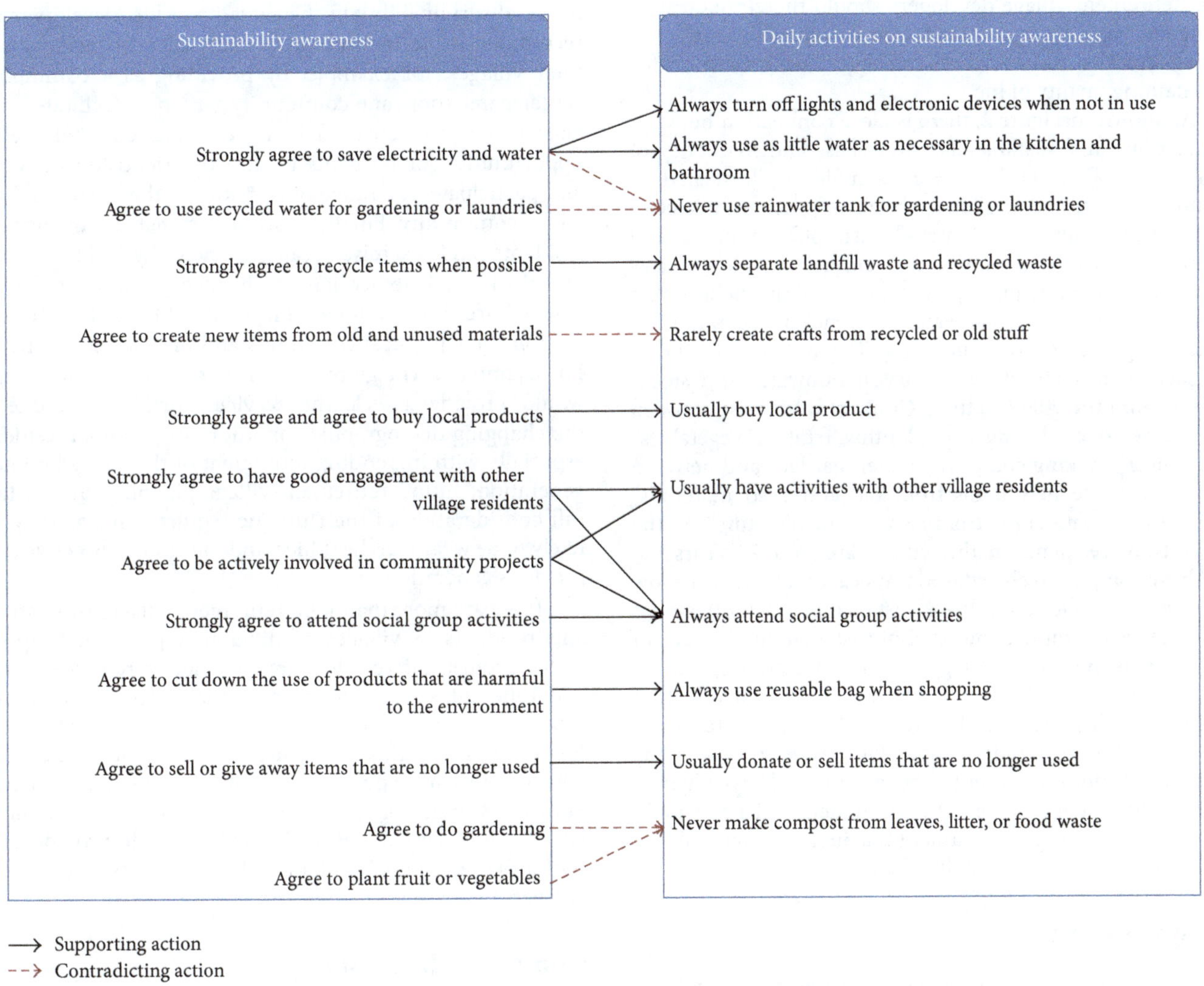

FIGURE 2: Relationship of sustainability awareness and daily activities.

future retirement village planning. For example, the "baby boomer" generation represents the potential residents of retirement villages of the future. Considering that baby boomers normally have better financial circumstances than previous generations, they are likely to be more inclined to pay additional cost associated with sustainability features of living environment. The retirement village industry may want to take full consideration of this emerging demographical change and endeavor to satisfy the changing requirements involved.

For social sustainability, it is within expectations that most of the respondents agree with the importance of attending social group activities and having sufficient engagement with other village residents. In fact, almost all the residents have very good relationships with their neighbors and village managers and attend social group activities quite often (with 42% "usually" and 46% "always"). As confirmed by the findings of previous research, social activities, friendships, and social networks are important for the residents' quality of life [8, 16–18]. Older people need to remain socially active and it is crucial in personal functioning of later life [19, 20]. Retirement village developers should therefore create a living environment/community that facilitates the residents' social activities and social relationships that are critical for maintaining quality of life.

As shown in Figure 2, there is close connection between the respondents' sustainability awareness and frequency of daily sustainable activities. For example, as illustrated in Figure 2, if respondents "strongly agree" with saving electricity and water, they "always" turn off the lights and electrical devices when not in use and use as little water as necessary. However, although most respondents believe that it is important to recycle water, they never use rainwater tanks for gardening or laundering. This outcome is due to the lack of infrastructure to harvest rainwater and storm water within the village setting. Contrasts also exist between the "agree to gardening and planting fruit or vegetables" and "never" making compost for their gardens and between "agree to create new items from old and used materials" and "rarely create crafts from recycled or old stuff." As the majority of residents in this village are over 75 years old and have comparatively reduced physical capabilities, the low frequency of conducting these sustainability activities does not necessarily imply a low level of sustainability literacy of respondents. Instead, this suggests an important implication for the retirement village industry in which the introduction of sustainability features should take full consideration of the physical limit of older people. Otherwise, as with many current communities, some public facilities will have physical barriers for older people [21]. Retirement villages should provide a supportive environment that increases accessibility to and usability of sustainability features.

5. Conclusions

The study described in the paper conducted a sustainability literacy survey of residents of a private retirement village in Queensland in order to explore their attitudes and activities relating to sustainability issues. The survey results show that most residents have sufficient literacy as they recognize the importance of environment protection and would like to lead a more environmentally friendly lifestyle. In addition, the majority of respondents are willing to pay a higher price for a living environment with sustainable features. Furthermore, almost all the respondents agree with the importance of social communications and good relationships with other residents in the village. Results also showed a close connection between village residents' sustainability literacy and their behavior in terms of daily activities.

These findings provide useful inputs into the type of sustainable features to incorporate into retirement villages. As residents are very aware of energy and water saving, energy-efficient designs (e.g., north-facing windows, open floor plan, and the location of internal walls) and materials (e.g., double-brick walls, double glazed windows, and thermally insulated roof) and water saving fixtures (e.g., in tap ware, toilets, and showerheads) can be adopted. In addition, given that retirement village residents regularly attend social group activities and recognize the importance of social sustainability in their quality of life, developers are recommended to incorporate socially friendly facilities into their villages, for example, by providing as a community center, game room and community garden, to facilitate social engagement and create a living environment that creates opportunities for residents to develop friendship networks and participate in a range of activities in the village and the wider community. Finally, considering that the majority of residents rarely exercise because of their physical limitations or lack of sustainability literacy, the incorporation of sustainable features in retirement villages should take into consideration their physical conditions and unique requirements. For example, a village bus (within and outside the village) would provide a welcome service. Furthermore, due to the changing demographic conditions of potential residents especially with impending retirement of the "baby boomer" generation, future retirement village planning should take full consideration of their unique requirements as they are likely to be wealthier, healthier, and more socially active than previous generations.

There are more than 1800 retirement villages in Australia and residents in villages of different types (not-for-profit or for-profit), different locations (urban or remote suburb) and different sizes, and so forth may have different perceptions and behaviors relating to sustainable development. For example, as this study has shown, issues concerning affordability can be quite different in different circumstances. Future research opportunities therefore exist to conduct a larger scale survey at national level in order to provide a full profile of the sustainable literacy of the residents of retirement villages.

Conflict of Interests

The authors declare that there is no conflict of interests regarding the publication of this paper.

Acknowledgment

The work described in the paper was supported by the Research Trust of the Royal Institute of Chartered Surveyors (RICS).

References

[1] Brutland Report, "Our Common Future, Chapter 2: Towards Sustainable Development. World Commission on Environment and Development," 1987, http://www.un-documents.net/ocf-02.htm.

[2] Department of the Environment, Transport, and the Regions, *Building a Better Quality of Life: A Strategy for More Sustainable Construction*, Department of the Environment, Transport and the Regions, London, UK, 2000.

[3] P. Brandon and P. Lombardi, *Evaluating Sustainable Development in the Built Environment*, John Wiley & Sons, Chichester, UK, 2010.

[4] O. Guerra Santin, L. Itard, and H. Visscher, "The effect of occupancy and building characteristics on energy use for space and water heating in Dutch residential stock," *Energy and Buildings*, vol. 41, no. 11, pp. 1223–1232, 2009.

[5] S. Farag and G. Lyons, "To use or not to use? An empirical study of pre-trip public transport information for business and leisure trips and comparison with car travel," *Transport Policy*, vol. 20, pp. 82–92, 2012.

[6] K. Pillemer and L. P. Wagenet, "Taking action: Environmental volunteerism and civic engagement by older people," *Public Policy and Aging Report*, vol. 18, no. 2, pp. 1–27, 2008.

[7] C. Bridge, "Cities, environmental stressors, ageing and chronic disease," *Australasian Journal on Ageing*, vol. 31, no. 3, pp. 140–140, 2012.

[8] J. Barker, J. Zuo, B. Xia, and G. Zillante, "Sustainable retirement living: what matters," in *Proceedings of 37th Annual Conference of Australasian University Building Educators Association (AUBEA '12)*, New South Wales, Australia, 2012.

[9] K. Pillemer, N. M. Wells, L. P. Wagenet, R. H. Meador, and J. T. Parise, "Environmental sustainability in an aging society: a research agenda," *Journal of Aging and Health*, vol. 23, no. 3, pp. 433–453, 2011.

[10] N. Gracia, W. Moyle, D. Oxlade, and K. Radford, "Addressing loneliness in a retirement village community: a pilot test of a print-delivered intervention," *Australasian Journal on Ageing*, vol. 29, no. 4, pp. 179–182, 2010.

[11] K. Willis, R. Scarpa, R. Gilroy, and N. Hamza, "Renewable energy adoption in an ageing population: heterogeneity in preferences for micro-generation technology adoption," *Energy Policy*, vol. 39, no. 10, pp. 6021–6029, 2011.

[12] S. Diamond and B. Irwin, "Using e-learning for student sustainability literacy: framework and review," *International Journal of Sustainability in Higher Education*, vol. 14, no. 4, pp. 338–348, 2013.

[13] P. E. Murray and A. J. Cotgrave, "Sustainability literacy: the future paradigm for construction education?" *Structural Survey*, vol. 25, no. 1, pp. 7–23, 2007.

[14] S. Parkin, A. Johnson, H. Buckland, and E. White, *Learning and Skills for Sustainable Development: Developing a Sustainability Literate Society*, HEPS, London, UK, 2004.

[15] J. Zuo, B. Xia, J. Barker, and M. Skitmore, "Green buildings for greying people: a case study of a retirement village in Australia," *Facilities*, vol. 32, no. 7-8, pp. 365–381, 2014.

[16] L. R. Buys, "Care and support assistance provided in retirement villages: expectations vs reality," *Australasian Journal on Ageing*, vol. 19, no. 3, pp. 149–151, 2000.

[17] K. Croucher, *Making the Case for Retirement Villages*, York Publishing Services, York, UK, 2006.

[18] B. Xia, M. Skitmore, J. Zuo, and L. Buys, "Review of community facilities in Australian retirement villages: a content analysis," *Australasian Journal on Ageing*, 2014.

[19] J. Golden, R. M. Conroy, and B. A. Lawlor, "Social support network structure in older people: underlying dimensions and association with psychological and physical health," *Psychology, Health and Medicine*, vol. 14, no. 3, pp. 280–290, 2009.

[20] E. Grundy and S. Read, "Social contacts and receipt of help among older people in england: are there benefits of having more children?" *The Journals of Gerontology B: Psychological Sciences and Social Sciences*, vol. 67, no. 6, pp. 742–754, 2012.

[21] A. Fänge, S. Iwarrson, and Å. Persson, "Accessibility to the public environment as perceived by teenagers with functional limitations in a south Swedish town centre," *Disability and Rehabilitation*, vol. 24, no. 6, pp. 318–326, 2002.

Permissions

All chapters in this book were first published in JAR, by Hindawi Publishing Corporation; hereby published with permission under the Creative Commons Attribution License or equivalent. Every chapter published in this book has been scrutinized by our experts. Their significance has been extensively debated. The topics covered herein carry significant findings which will fuel the growth of the discipline. They may even be implemented as practical applications or may be referred to as a beginning point for another development.

The contributors of this book come from diverse backgrounds, making this book a truly international effort. This book will bring forth new frontiers with its revolutionizing research information and detailed analysis of the nascent developments around the world.

We would like to thank all the contributing authors for lending their expertise to make the book truly unique. They have played a crucial role in the development of this book. Without their invaluable contributions this book wouldn't have been possible. They have made vital efforts to compile up to date information on the varied aspects of this subject to make this book a valuable addition to the collection of many professionals and students.

This book was conceptualized with the vision of imparting up-to-date information and advanced data in this field. To ensure the same, a matchless editorial board was set up. Every individual on the board went through rigorous rounds of assessment to prove their worth. After which they invested a large part of their time researching and compiling the most relevant data for our readers.

The editorial board has been involved in producing this book since its inception. They have spent rigorous hours researching and exploring the diverse topics which have resulted in the successful publishing of this book. They have passed on their knowledge of decades through this book. To expedite this challenging task, the publisher supported the team at every step. A small team of assistant editors was also appointed to further simplify the editing procedure and attain best results for the readers.

Apart from the editorial board, the designing team has also invested a significant amount of their time in understanding the subject and creating the most relevant covers. They scrutinized every image to scout for the most suitable representation of the subject and create an appropriate cover for the book.

The publishing team has been an ardent support to the editorial, designing and production team. Their endless efforts to recruit the best for this project, has resulted in the accomplishment of this book. They are a veteran in the field of academics and their pool of knowledge is as vast as their experience in printing. Their expertise and guidance has proved useful at every step. Their uncompromising quality standards have made this book an exceptional effort. Their encouragement from time to time has been an inspiration for everyone.

The publisher and the editorial board hope that this book will prove to be a valuable piece of knowledge for researchers, students, practitioners and scholars across the globe.

List of Contributors

Pia Rotshtein
School of Psychology, University of Birmingham, Birmingham B15 2TT, UK

Alla Yankouskaya
School of Psychology, University of Birmingham, Birmingham B15 2TT, UK
Department of Experimental Psychology, University of Oxford, Oxford OX1 3UD, UK

Glyn W. Humphreys
Department of Experimental Psychology, University of Oxford, Oxford OX1 3UD, UK

Albert Westergren
The PRO-CARE Group, School of Health and Society, Kristianstad University, 291 88 Kristianstad, Sweden

Carol Fitz Gerald, Una Cronin, Yang Gao and Eileen O'Herlihy
Centre for Gerontology and Rehabilitation, University College Cork, St. Finbarr's Hospital, Douglas Road, Cork, Ireland

D. William Molloy and Rónán O'Caoimh
Centre for Gerontology and Rehabilitation, University College Cork, St. Finbarr's Hospital, Douglas Road, Cork, Ireland
COLLAGE (Collaboration on Ageing), University College Cork, Cork City and Louth Age Friendly County Initiative, County Louth, Ireland

Anton Svendrovski
UZIK Consulting Inc, 86 Gerrard Street E, Unit 12D, Toronto, ON, Canada M5B 2J1

Elizabeth Healy
Centre for Public Health Nursing, Ballincollig and Bishopstown, County Cork, Ireland

Elizabeth O'Connell
Centre for Public Health Nursing, Mahon and Ballin temple, Cork, Ireland

Gabrielle O'Keeffe
Health Service Executive, South Lee, St. Finbarr's Hospital, Cork, Ireland

Patricia Leahy-Warren, Elizabeth Weathers and Nicola Cornally
School of Nursing and Midwifery, University College Cork, Brookfield Health Sciences Complex, College Road, Cork, Ireland

Francesc Orfila
Primary Healthcare University Research Institute, IDIAP Jordi Gol, Barcelona, Spain

Constança Paúl
UNIFAI/ICBAS, Institute of Biomedical Sciences Abel Salazar, University of Porto, 4050-313 Porto, Portugal

Roger Clarnette
School of Medicine and Pharmacology, University of Western Australia, 35 Stirling Hwy, Crawley, WA 6009, Australia

John G. Gaspar and Arthur F. Kramer
Department of Psychology and Beckman Institute for Advanced Science and Technology, University of Illinois at Urbana-Champaign, Urbana, IL 61801, USA

Mark B. Neider
Department of Psychology, University of Central Florida, Orlando, FL 32816, USA

Catriona M. Steele
Toronto Rehabilitation Institute, University Health Network, 550 University Avenue, Toronto, ON, Canada M5G 2A2

Raymond L. Ownby and Robin J. Jacobs
Department of Psychiatry and Behavioral Medicine, Nova Southeastern University, Fort Lauderdale, FL 33314, USA

Amarilis Acevedo
Center for Psychological Studies, Nova Southeastern University, Fort Lauderdale, FL 33314, USA

Drenna Waldrop-Valverde
Nell Hodgson Woodruff School of Nursing, Emory University, Atlanta, GA 30322, USA

Jian Chen
School of Human Kinetics, Laurentian University, 935 Ramsey Lake Road, Sudbury, ON, Canada P3E 2C6

Kara King and Jian X. Zhang
Biology Department, University of North Carolina, 9201 University City Bulevard, Charlotte, NC 28223, USA

Rosemary L. Aird and Laurie Buys
School of Design, Queensland University of Technology, Brisbane, QLD4001, Australia

Lily Nosraty, Antti Hervonen and Marja Jylhä
Gerontology Research Center and School of Health Sciences, 33014 University of Tampere, Tampere, Finland

Tytti Sarkeala
Finnish Cancer Registry, Institute of Statical and Epidemiological Cancer Research, Pieni Roobertinkatu 9, 00130 Helsinki, Finland

David Predovan, Sarah A. Fraser and Mélanie Renaud
Centre de Recherche, Institut universitaire de gériatrie de Montréal, Montréal, QC, Canada H3W 1W5
Département de Psychologie, Universitédu Québeca Montréal, Montréal, QC, Canada H3C 3P8

Louis Bherer
Centre de Recherche, Institut universitaire de gériatrie de Montréal, Montréal, QC, Canada H3W 1W5
PERFORM Centre and Department of Psychology, Concordia University, Montréal, QC, Canada H4B 1R6

Lucas Whitcher
Department of Applied Arts and Sciences, University of Montana-Missoula College, Missoula, MT 95812, USA

Charilaos Papadopoulos
Department of Kinesiology, Pacific Lutheran University, Tacoma, WA 98447, USA

Lisa B. Caruso and Gary H. Brandei
Boston University Geriatric Services, Boston University School of Medicine, Boston Medical Center, 88 East Newton Street, Robinson 2, Boston, MA 02118, USA

Soe Thwin
Boston University Geriatric Services, Boston University School of Medicine, Boston Medical Center, 88 East Newton Street, Robinson 2, Boston, MA 02118, USA
Massachusetts Veterans Epidemiology Research and Information Center (MAVERIC), New England VA Healthcare System, 150 South Huntington Avenue, Boston, MA 02130, USA

J. van Hoof, M. M. Verhagen and E. J. M. Wouters
Centre for Healthcare and Technology (Fontys EGT), Fontys University of Applied Sciences, Dominee Theodor Fliednerstraat 2, 5631 BN Eindhoven, Netherlands
Institute of Allied Health Professions, Fontys University of Applied Sciences, Dominee Theodor Fliednerstraat 2, 5631 BN Eindhoven, Netherlands

M. D. Rijnaard
Institute of Allied Health Professions, Fontys University of Applied Sciences, Dominee Theodor Fliednerstraat 2, 5631 BN Eindhoven, Netherlands

B. M. Janssen
Section of Applied Gerontology, Institute of Nursing, Fontys University of Applied Sciences, Dominee Theodor Fliednerstraat 2, 5631 BN Eindhoven, Netherlands

H. R. Marston
Centre for Research Computing, Faculty of Mathematics, Computing and Technology, Open University, Milton Keynes, Buckinghamshire, MK6 7AA, UK

Kyle Y. Whitfield and Jason S. Daniels
Faculty of Extension, University of Alberta, Enterprise Square, Room 2-215, 10230 Jasper Avenue, Edmonton, Alberta, Canada T5J 4P6

Keri Flesaker
Department of Educational Psychology, University of Alberta, 6-102 Education North, Edmonton, Alberta, Canada T6G 2G5

Doneka Simmons
Senior Association of Greater Edmonton, 15 Sir Winston Churchill Square, Edmonton, Alberta, Canada T5J 2E5

Prudence Plummer-D'Amato, Briana Brancato, Mallory Dantowitz, Stephanie Birken, Christina Bonke and Erin Furey
Department of Physical Therapy, Northeastern University, 360 Huntington Avenue, 6 Robinson Hall, Boston, MA 02115-5000, USA

Deborah L. Huang
Veterans Affairs Puget Sound Health Care System, Geriatric Research, Education and Clinical Center (S-182), 1660 South Columbian Way, Seattle, WA 98108, USA

Dori E. Rosenberg
Group Health Research Institute, 1730 Minor Avenue, Suite 1600, Seattle, WA 98101, USA

Shannon D. Simonovich
Department of Biobehavioral Nursing and Health Systems, School of Nursing, University of Washington, Seattle, WA 98195, USA

Basia Belza
Health Promotion Research Center, University of Washington, Seattle, WA 98195, USA

Flávia Cristina Drumond Andrad
Department of Kinesiology and Community Health, University of Illinois at Urbana-Champaign, 1206 South 4th Street, Champaign, IL 61820, USA

Ahmad Iqmer Nashriq Mohd Nazan
Zilber School of Public Health, University of Wisconsin-Milwaukee, 1240 N. 10th Street, Milwaukee, WI 53205, USA

Maria Lúcia Lebrão
School of Public Health, Departament of Epidemiology, University of São Paulo, Avenida Dr. Arnaldo, 715 Pinheiros, 01246-904 São Paulo, SP, Brazil

Yeda Aparecida de Oliveira Duarte
School of Nursing, Department of Medical-Surgical Nursing, University of São Paulo, Avenida Dr. Enéas de Carvalho Aguiar, 419 3o andar, Sala 318, Cerqueira Cesar, 05403-000 São Paulo, SP, Brazil

Jonathan Desaulniers, Sophie Desjardins and Sylvie Lapierre
Department of Psychology, Université du Québecà Trois-Riviéres, C.P. 500, Trois-Riviéres, Québec, Canada G9A 5H7

Alain Desgagné
Department of Mathematics, Université du Québecà Montréal, C.P. 8888, Succursale Centre-ville, Montréal, Québec, Canada

Terceira A. Berdahl
Division of Research and Modeling, Center for Financing, Access and Cost Trends, Agency for Healthcare Research and Quality, 5600 Fishers Lane, Rockville, MD 20852, USA

Julia McQuillan
University of Nebraska-Lincoln, 709 Old father Hall, Lincoln, NE 68588-0324, USA

Yaena Min, Pramit A. Nadpara and Patricia W. Slattum
Department of Pharmacotherapy and Outcomes Science, School of Pharmacy, Virginia Commonwealth University, Richmond, VA 23298-0533, USA

Chantrell Antoine Parker and Rebecca Ellis
Georgia State University, Atlanta, GA 30302, USA

G. Kevin Randall
CC Wheeler Institute, Bradley University, 05 Bradley Hall, 1501 W. Bradley Avenue, Peoria, IL 61625, USA

Peter Martin
Gerontology Program, Iowa State University, 1096 Le Baron Hall, Ames, IA 50011 1120, USA

Mary Ann Johnson
Department of Foods and Nutrition, The University of Georgia, 143 Barrow Hall, 115 DW Brooks Dr, Athens, GA 30602, USA

Leonard W. Poon
Institute of Gerontology, College of Public Health, The University of Georgia, 255 E. Hancock Avenue, Athens, GA 30602-5775, USA

Melanie Birks
Nursing, Midwifery, and Nutrition, Centre for Nursing and Midwifery Research, College of Healthcare Sciences, James Cook University, Townsville, QLD, Australia

Marie Bodak
Nursing, Midwifery, and Nutrition, College of Healthcare Sciences, James Cook University, Townsville, QLD, Australia

Joanna Barlas
Clinical Psychology, College of Healthcare Sciences, James Cook University, Singapore Campus, Singapore

June Harwood
Aged Care Services Australia Group, Launceston, TAS, Australia

Mary Pether
Regis Aged Care, Townsville, QLD, Australia

Michael J. Turner
Laboratory of Systems Physiology, University of North Carolina at Charlotte, Charlotte, NC 28223, USA

Emily E. Schmitt
Biology of Physical Activity Laboratory, Texas A&M University, College Station, TX 77843, USA

Tricia Hubbard-Turner
Biodynamics Research Laboratory, Department of Kinesiology, University of North Carolina at Charlotte, Charlotte, NC 28223, USA
Center for Biomedical Engineering and Science, University of North Carolina at Charlotte, Charlotte, NC 28223, USA

Chelsie Anderson, Laura R. Seff, Anamika Batra, Chintan Bhatt and Richard C. Palmer
Florida International University, Miami, FL 33199, USA

Edgar R. Vieira
Department of Physical Therapy, Florida International University, MMC, 11200 SW 8th St., AHC3-430, Miami, FL 33199, USA

Joan A. Vaccaro
Department of Dietetics and Nutrition, Florida International University, MMC, 11200 SW 8th St., AHC5-324, Miami, FL 33199, USA

Gustavo G. Zarini
Department of Dietetics and Nutrition, Florida International University, MMC, 11200 SW 8th St., AHC5-300, Miami, FL 33199, USA

Fatma G. Huffman
Department of Dietetics and Nutrition, Florida International University, 11200 SW 8th St., AHC-5, Room 326, Miami, FL 33199, USA

Bo Xia, Martin Skitmore and Xin Hu
School of Civil Engineering and Built Environment, Queensland University of Technology, Garden Point Campus, 2 George Street, Brisbane, QLD 4001, Australia

Jian Zuo
School of Natural and Built Environments, University of South Australia, City East Campus, North Terrace, Adelaide, SA 5001, Australia

Laurie Buys
School of Design, Queensland University of Technology, Garden Point Campus, 2 George Street, Brisbane, QLD4001, Australia

Index

R

S

T

U

V

W

www.ingramcontent.com/pod-product-compliance
Lightning Source LLC
LaVergne TN
LVHW060519210926
848485LV00005B/1110
9781639270064